ARGON LASER PHOTOCOAGULATION

ARGON LASER PHOTOCOAGULATION

H. Christian Zweng, M.D.

Palo Alto Retinal Medical Group, Inc.;
Clinical Professor of Surgery (Ophthalmology),
Stanford University School of Medicine,
Stanford, California

Hunter L. Little, M.D.

Palo Alto Retinal Medical Group, Inc.;
Associate Clinical Professor of Surgery (Ophthalmology),
Stanford University School of Medicine,
Stanford, California

In collaboration with

Arthur Vassiliadis, Ph.D.

Staff Scientist
Palo Alto Retinal Research Foundation,
Menlo Park, California

401 illustrations; graphs and drawings by Carol Mead

The C. V. Mosby Company

Saint Louis   1977

Printed in the United States of America

Distributed in Great Britain by Henry Kimpton, London

The C. V. Mosby Company
11830 Westline Industrial Drive, St. Louis, Missouri 63141

Library of Congress Cataloging in Publication Data

Zweng, H   Christian.
    Argon laser photocoagulation.

    Bibliography: p.
    Includes index.
    1. Laser coagulation.   2. Retina—Diseases.
3. Argon lasers.   I. Little, Hunter L., joint author.   II. Title.
RE992.P5Z78   617.7′3′05   76-58392
ISBN 0-8016-5706-7

TS/CB/B   9   8   7   6   5   4   3   2   1

To our families

PREFACE

This book is a distillate of our experiences from May 1969 to February 1976 in applying argon laser light to eye tissues through a slit-lamp delivery system. As such, this is a professionally personal volume, although we include many references to the work of others in the fields of photocoagulation and retinal diseases generally. As of this writing, we have treated approximately 2,500 eyes in about 9,500 treatment sessions. Obviously we have learned a great deal from such a large experience; what we have learned is the subject matter of this book.

We introduced argon laser slit-lamp photocoagulation by developing a prototype instrument at the Stanford Research Institute, with Norman Peppers, Lloyd Alterton, and Robert Myers, between 1966 and 1969. Now about 1,000 instruments based on our prototype are being used throughout the world by several thousand ophthalmologists. We feel, therefore, a great responsibility to disseminate to those ophthalmologists and their patients the knowledge gained by our experiences. To be more specific, in setting forth this work we are moved by a desire to help other ophthalmologists who perform argon laser photocoagulation to avoid our mistakes; to inform general ophthalmologists of indications, contraindications, and complications of argon laser photocoagulation; and to deepen the often shallow knowledge possessed by the general physician and internist of retinal diseases, most of which have implications for the patient's general health.

Since January 1971 we have given fourteen courses in argon laser photocoagulation in Menlo Park; six additional courses have been given in New York and Baltimore. Other Laser Course faculty members include Drs. Robert L. Jack of Palo Alto, Francis A. L'Esperance, Jr., of New York, Arnall Patz and Stuart Fine of Baltimore, Lloyd Aiello of Boston, Robert Peabody of Sacramento, and Howard Schatz of San Francisco. Approximately 900 ophthalmologists have taken these twenty courses. The course faculty members have had an opportunity to share their experiences and thoughts every 3 months. This frequent and free communication among the faculty has clarified the place of argon laser photocoagulation therapy much more rapidly than communications through the literature and meetings normally allow. We wholeheartedly acknowledge the immense additions to our own experience made by the other Laser Course faculty members. While we do not hold them responsible for the contents of this volume, we are very grateful to them for their curiosity and acumen in observation and their candor and clarity in discussion.

This volume is the latest word on argon laser photocoagulation but not the last. Indications and contraindications must be sharpened further, techniques still improved, and complications more completely avoided. Many ophthalmologists will make invaluable contributions, and our own research continues. Beyond doubt, however, a patient now being considered by us for argon laser photocoagulation receives a more informed examination and, if treated, a wiser treatment than was possible several years ago. We hope that as a result of this book all patients will benefit whenever such examinations and treatments are given. Mistakes are often tragic.

We wish to thank everyone already cited in this preface for their input into our work and therefore into this book. In addition, we also thank Miss Ann Hammond, Mrs. Pat Hill, Mrs. Louise Porteous, and Miss Janette Boehm for their help in treating patients, gathering data, and preparing this manuscript.

We wish to acknowledge and thank the ophthalmic photographers who have assisted us between 1969 and the present: Andy Bell, Dr. Philip Sloan, Richard Thompson, Bruce Kunde, and Arthur Smialowski.

We especially thank the National Eye Institute for its support through many years of photocoagulation research, from 1959 to 1976. Without the Institute's help, our work would not have been done and this book not written.

H. Christian Zweng
Hunter L. Little
Arthur Vassiliadis

CONTENTS

ARGON LASER PHOTOCOAGULATION

1
LIGHT, LASERS, AND THE RETINA

The use of optical radiation to treat eye problems by photocoagulation was pioneered by G. Meyer-Schwickerath[10] in 1946. He first used solar radiation, but his great success was achieved when the xenon arc bulb was applied to photocoagulation. Although, as will be seen, natural sources of light suffer from limitations that make it difficult to concentrate the radiation sufficiently to obtain intense small spots of radiation, their application in ophthalmology was accepted and used with success.

It is not surprising, therefore, that when the laser was first announced in 1960[9] it immediately became apparent to a number of experimenters that this radiation could be applied to ophthalmology with even greater success than could conventional light sources. As early as 1962-1963 several groups[4,5,14,15] had used and reported results with ruby laser in photocoagulation, thus initiating not only laser photocoagulation but development of quantitative photocoagulation.

A review of a number of basic concepts related to optical radiation and its application to photocoagulation is presented in this chapter. Specifically, the fundamentals of optical radiation and the nature of atoms and molecules and how they interact with radiation are summarized. This is followed by a discussion of natural and conventional light sources and lasers—how they operate and what their characteristics are.

Interaction of radiation and living cells depends on the wavelength of the radiation. The various interactions possible are discussed, and it is shown that thermal damage is the effective mechanism in photocoagulation. Interaction of radiation and the fundus is discussed in terms of a simple thermal model, providing insight into a number of important considerations that must be used for effective quantitative photocoagulation.

CHARACTERISTICS OF LIGHT
Background

Light is radiation that comprises a small part of the electromagnetic spectrum. The optical part of the spectrum is usually considered as including the visible

1

region (400 to 700 nm) and the flanking regions. Ultraviolet radiation is on the short wavelength side and infrared radiation is on the long wavelength side. At more remote parts of the electromagnetic spectrum, radio and microwave radiation are found on the very long wavelength side, and on the very short wavelength side are found the familiar X rays and gamma rays.

It is surprising that these widely differing types of radiation are identical in form, the only difference being the wavelength of the radiation. Therefore, wavelength is a very important characteristic of radiation.

In 1900 Planck made his revolutionary hypothesis that material oscillators could only give up or absorb energy in discrete or quantized amounts of energy, rather than in a continuous manner.[1] Shortly thereafter, in 1905, Einstein proposed that light radiation consists of quanta, which he called photons, whose energy, E, is given by

$$E = h\nu = hc/\lambda$$

where h is Planck's constant, ν is the frequency of the radiation, c is the velocity of light, and λ is the wavelength. With this hypothesis, Einstein showed that it was possible to explain a number of phenomena, including the photoelectric effect, that could not be explained by the classic theory of the time, which assumed that radiation was continuous.

Because radiation is quantized, the minimum energy that can enter an interaction must be a single photon. The energy of the individual photon depends on the wavelength, as previously shown. As the wavelength becomes shorter, the energy of the photon becomes larger. Thus, at shorter wavelengths the photons have more energy than do photons of longer wavelength; consequently, interactions at short wavelengths will be more violent or disruptive than interactions at long wavelengths.

Radiation sources

All matter in nature radiates electromagnetic radiation. The radiation of a typical source depends on the temperature of the material, and it has some inherent characteristics:

1. Radiation is spectrally broad (i.e., it consists of components of many different wavelengths).
2. Radiation is emitted in all directions (i.e., various parts of the source emit independently and in random directions).

The emission of natural and artificial sources of light (other than lasers) is, in terms of wavelength, wide in spectral extent. The radiation is usually a superposition of a continuum, approaching the characteristics of a blackbody radiation curve (Fig. 1-1) and the characteristic emission or absorption lines of the atoms in the material. Blackbody radiation characteristics can be fully explained by the quantization of material sources proposed by Planck, but not by classical theory.

As the temperature of a source is increased, the source becomes brighter

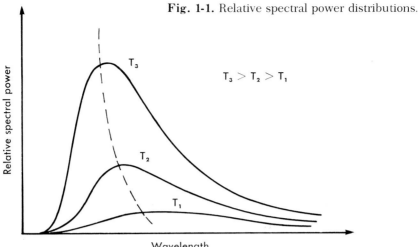

Fig. 1-1. Relative spectral power distributions.

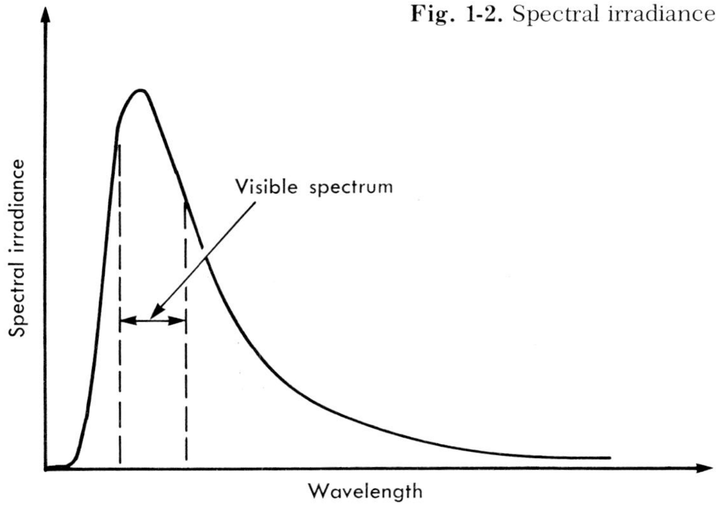

$T_3 > T_2 > T_1$

Fig. 1-2. Spectral irradiance of the sun.

(more power is emitted at all wavelengths), and the peak of the radiation shifts to shorter wavelengths (Fig. 1-1). For example, solar temperature is approximately 5,900 K. At this temperature, the dominant part of the radiation extends from the ultraviolet, through the visible, and well into the infrared part of the spectrum; indeed, only about 40% of the radiation is in the visible part of the spectrum (Fig. 1-2). It is apparent that the radiation is extensive insofar as wavelength is concerned and that there are photons of widely varying energies in the radiation.

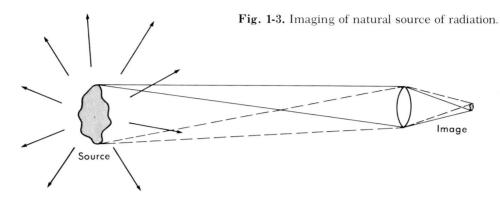

Fig. 1-3. Imaging of natural source of radiation.

The spectral range of radiation can be limited for a specific application by using filters, prisms, or gratings, depending on the spectral width desired. However, because natural sources contain power in a wide range of wavelengths, only a small portion of the total power would be available in a limited wavelength range. Thus, starting with natural sources, there are severe limitations on the power that can be obtained in a narrow wavelength range.

The other important characteristic of naturally occurring sources is that they are finite in extent and radiate in all directions. Thus, each radiating atom or molecule emits randomly in any direction, independent of any of the other radiating parts. As a result, the multiplicity of spherical waves that emanate from various parts of the source cannot be effectively gathered to concentrate the radiation. Thus, if a lens is used to focus the radiation from the source, it is found that the best that can be done is the formation of an image of the source (Fig. 1-3). Only a small fraction of the radiated power is captured by the lens and brought into the image, because power is being radiated in all directions.

Image size is inversely related to the distance from the source; thus, the farther the source, the smaller the image that results. It appears, then, that a higher concentration of power may be obtained. However, in receding from the source, a proportionally smaller fraction of the radiated power is being captured by the lens, so the power density of the image stays the same. Eventually, at a sufficiently distant location, a diffraction-limited spot, or the smallest possible image size, will be obtained at the focus of the lens.

A fundamental limitation of natural sources apparent from this description is that the power density of an image cannot be made higher than that of the source. It is this limitation that makes it impossible to obtain small photocoagulation exposures for short times with conventional light sources, such as the xenon arc bulb.

Coherence

The two aspects of radiation from natural sources, when extended to their limit, are related to two aspects of coherence.

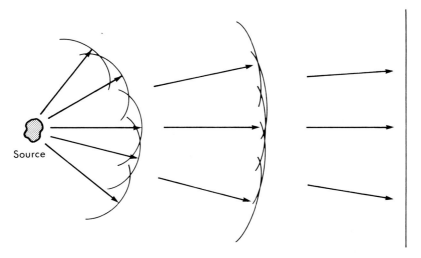

Fig. 1-4. Spatial coherence.

The first type of coherence is spatial coherence, which is associated with the relationship of one part of a wave with another part of the wave in space; thus it is a description of the character of the phase front of a wave.

Various parts of a light source radiate independently. Each atom of the source radiates a photon in a random direction and with a random phase. Thus, each infinitessimal part of the source can be thought to emit a spherical wave. Near the source, the total radiation field will consist of innumerable spherical waves coming from various directions and distances. As one moves away from the source, however, these waves approach each other more and more and ultimately begin to merge into a single plane wave (Fig. 1-4). This process of the gradual merger of the wavefronts of the wavelets into one is a representation of the process of increasing spatial coherence of the composite wave. It is apparent, and it can be shown with mathematical rigor, that the spatial coherence of any source increases with increasing distance from the source. Spatial coherence is important because a spatially coherent wave can be focused down to a diffraction-limited small spot.

Stars are familiar natural sources whose radiation on the earth is spatially coherent. The waves that reach the earth from these bright sources are plane waves, because the sources are at such a large distance from the earth. Consequently, the waves have high spatial coherence and, when observed with the eye or telescope, appear as points of light, because they are focused to very small spots on the retina or on photographic plates.

Spatial coherence is quite important in application to ophthalmology, because radiation having this property can be focused down to very small spot sizes; in addition, a beam that is spatially coherent diverges very slowly.

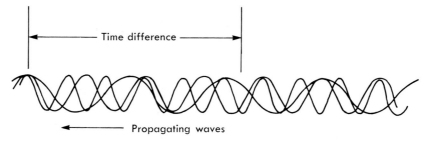

Fig. 1-5. Temporal coherence.

The second kind of coherence is temporal coherence, which relates a wave with itself at a later time; thus it is an indication of the correlation of the wave with itself. Radiation from a natural source consists of waves of many different wavelengths (Fig. 1-5). Indeed, natural sources emit radiation over all parts of the electromagnetic spectrum; thus the total radiation is a summation of innumerable waves of different lengths. As a result, there is virtually no relationship between one part of the wave and another at a later time, and time coherence is said to be poor.

If, however, a small part of the spectrum is limited by use of selective filters, prisms, or gratings, the radiation will consist of fewer waves of different lengths. It follows that the relationship of one part of the wave with itself at a later time will be better correlated. As the spectrum is narrowed further, the correlation of the wave at two different times will increase. At the limit, there is virtually only a single wavelength. The wave is now essentially a single pure wave, and the relationship of one part to the other is excellent and the temporal coherence is very long. It is apparent that temporal coherence is associated with the width of the spectrum of radiation.

This type of coherence is extremely important in certain applications, such as holography and optical data processing. However, for interactions with biologic material (e.g., the eye) the absorption characteristics of the tissues are relatively broad. Therefore, the radiation used need not have a very narrow spectral width in order to achieve optimum interactions with the tissues.

Units

Minimum discrete amounts of energy in the radiation field are called photons. There are a large number of photons in a typical interaction between light and matter.

The magnitude of the interaction can be measured in terms of the total number of photons, which in turn is related to the energy. Energy, U, is usually measured in joules. A joule is a unit that is related to the familiar gram-calorie, also a measure of energy or heat. There are about 4.18 J in 1 gram-calorie. For example, a dose of 40 mJ is equivalent to

$$U = 40 \text{ mJ} = 0.04 \text{ J} \cong 0.01 \text{ cal} \cong 0.00001 \text{ kcal}$$

Another important unit is the power of a wave. Power, P, is the rate at which energy is delivered:

$$P = U/T$$

where T is time of the exposure. Thus, power is a number of photons arriving per unit time. The unit for power is the watt, W, which is related to the joule:

$$1 \text{ W} = 1 \text{ J/sec}$$

Because power is the rate at which energy is being delivered, it is a very convenient term to use in photocoagulation, particularly for continuous-wave (cw) lasers using longer exposures. For example, if the power setting is 200 mW and the length of time of the exposure is 0.1 sec, the energy in the exposure is

$$U = PT = 200 \times 0.1 = 20 \text{ mJ}$$

Another important way of specifying or indicating interaction parameters is to refer to the power density of the laser beam at the area of interaction. The power density is an indication of the concentration of photons in a given area. In order to calculate the power density, the power in the beam is divided by the area of the spot size that the beam covers:

$$\text{Power density} = P_d = P/A = 4P/\pi D^2$$

where A is the area and D is the diameter of the spot. Thus, the power density depends on the size of the beam and the power being used.

All of these terms are interrelated and are useful in discussions of photocoagulation. In order to fully specify an exposure, the beam diameter and either the energy and the time of exposure or the power and the time of exposure must be specified.

CHARACTERISTICS OF LASERS
Interaction of radiation and matter

Radiation energy is measured in discrete quantities called photons. This, plus the observation that emission and absorption spectra of gases display narrow spectral lines, led to the development of the quantum theory and a better understanding of the atomic world.

In order to explain the experimental observations, in 1913 Bohr postulated the quantization of the energy levels of atoms.[1] According to his theory, the atom cannot exchange energy with its environment in a continuous manner, because it can only exist in certain specific stationary or quantum states, each having a specific energy associated with it. Thus an atom or molecule can change internal energy only by jumping from one state to another. During such transition, the atom must either gain or lose energy by absorbing or emitting a photon or by exchanging energy by collision, for example. In addition, the lowest energy state, called the ground state, is stable, and an atom in this state can no longer radiate.

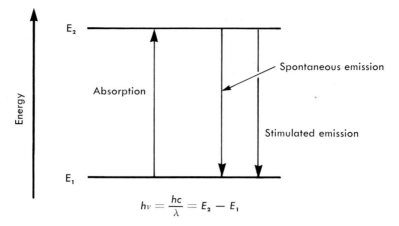

Fig. 1-6. Interaction of light and matter.

A simple atom

An atom can exist in innumerable states, each associated with a specific quantized internal energy. In order to understand the interactions that are possible with photons, consider a hypothetical atom that has only two energy levels (Fig. 1-6); the lower level, E_1, is the ground state, and the upper level, E_2, is the excited state.

An atom is usually in the ground state, where it naturally acquiesces and is stable. If an atom is in the ground state, and a radiation field containing photons of the appropriate wavelength is incident on it, the atom can absorb a photon and transit to the excited state. The energy of the photon required will be related to energy difference between the two levels of internal energy; that is, the energy of the photon is

$$h\nu = hc/\lambda = E_2 - E_1$$

Thus a photon of a particular energy, or related wavelength, is specified by the energy difference. After some random time in the excited state, the atom will spontaneously emit a photon of the same energy (wavelength) and return to the stable ground state. By carefully examining the basic processes of emission and absorption by atoms in equilibrium, Einstein[2] in 1917 showed that there had to be an additional way for an excited atom to return to the ground state. If an atom in the excited state is in a radiation field of photons of correct energy (wavelength), the atom can be induced or stimulated to emit a photon and thus return to the ground state. Although spontaneous emission is emitted randomly in any direction, Einstein showed that the photons radiated by stimulated emission are in phase and coherent with the incident radiation wave. Stimulated emission from atoms and molecules makes the laser possible.

Laser operation

General considerations. Atoms or molecules naturally decay and eventually settle on the lowest internal energy level available. Because of temperature, however, there will always be thermal agitation. Consequently, atoms will constantly fluctuate to higher excited levels; thus they will not all be in the ground state. The distribution of the number of atoms in each state depends on the temperature and is described by Boltzmann's distribution. This distribution is such that a higher level always has less atoms populating it than does a lower level, and the predominant population is in the lowest levels.

When a beam of radiation whose photon energy is equal to the energy separation between two states is incident on an atom, it can cause it to change state. If the atom is in a lower state, it can absorb a photon and go to an upper level; if it is in an upper level, it can be stimulated to emit a photon and return to a lower level. Thus, when a light beam is incident on a large population of atoms, the atoms in the lower state will absorb energy from the beam, and those in the upper level will emit energy to the beam. The net loss (or gain) to the beam will depend on whether there are more (or less) atoms in the lower level than in the higher level. In nature there are usually more atoms in a lower level than in a higher level; thus a light beam traversing a medium of atoms will be attenuated. However, if by some artificial means one could arrange for more atoms to be in an upper level than in a lower level, introduction of a light beam into the medium would amplify the beam.

The basic requirements for laser operation are now clear. First, a population inversion must be established: more atoms must be placed in an upper or excited state than in a lower state. Second, a light beam of the correct wavelength must

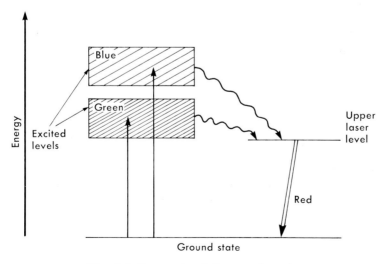

Fig. 1-7. Energy level diagram for ruby.

be introduced, to stimulate the excited atoms to emit light coherent with the incident beam, thus amplifying it.

A number of methods are used to obtain population inversion, depending on the material used. Two of these methods will be described in the laser examples below.

Ruby laser. The ruby laser is an optically pumped laser. Historically, it was the first to be operated, as demonstrated by Maiman[9] in 1960. Ruby is a sapphire crystal with a very small percentage of impurity, in the form of chromium. Chromium ions in the lattice absorb strongly in the green-blue part of the spectrum, thus giving the ruby its pink to red appearance, depending on the concentration of chromium. Ruby fluoresces in the red part of the spectrum at 694 nm when flashed with white light.

A simplified energy-level diagram for ruby is shown in Fig. 1-7. Ruby has such a large number of excited levels that they merge into whole bands of absorption in the green, blue, and ultraviolet parts of the spectrum. Thus, if white light, containing all wavelengths, impinges on ruby, large bands of radiation are absorbed very readily. Usually the ruby is excited or prepared for laser action by pulsing it with xenon flash lamps, which emit intense radiation at all useful wavelengths.

Chromium ions that absorb photons from the flash lamps are excited to the upper-level states. From these states, they lose some energy nonradiatively and relax to a lower level, that is, a metastable level, which has a long lifetime compared with other transition lifetimes. In this way, the number of ions in an upper level is made greater than the number in the ground state, and a population inversion is obtained.

Argon laser. The argon laser is one of a large number of gas lasers that have been successfully operated. As in all gas lasers, an electric current discharge is initiated and sustained in the argon gas. In this discharge, a number of collisional processes are responsible for generating the population inversion. The argon gas is first ionized by collisions with the electrons in the discharge. The singly ionized argon ions are then further excited to upper levels by additional collisions with electrons.

A simplified schematic diagram of the energy levels of the argon ion is shown in Fig. 1-8. When some of the argon ions have been excited to the higher energy levels, they will gradually decay to lower levels by spontaneous processes. In some of these excited levels, ions can accumulate; at the same time, some of the lower excited levels are virtually empty of ions, because of their extremely short lifetimes. Thus, laser action can occur between the upper states that are above the ground state. From these levels the ions quickly return to the ground state, thus completing the cycle.

The argon ion laser operates as a four-level system: (1) ions begin the cycle in the ground state; (2) the ions are then excited to the high-excitation levels, which may be grouped as the second effective level; (3) they then decay to the upper

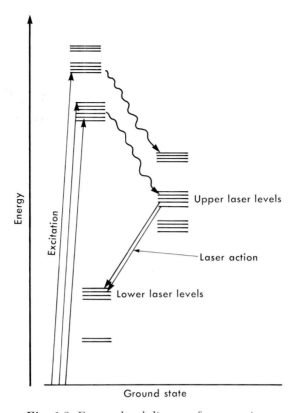

Fig. 1-8. Energy level diagram for argon ion.

laser levels; and (4) the ions then emit radiation through laser action and jump to the lower laser levels. From the fourth level, the ions quickly return to the first, or ground, level and again are available to begin the cycle. This four-level closed cycle facilitates operation of the argon laser in a continuous mode.

The argon laser can lase between several of the excited levels, thus emitting radiation at several wavelengths. All of these wavelengths are fairly close together in the blue-green part of the spectrum and all are effective and useful in photocoagulation.

Laser cavity

The second requirement for the operation of a laser is that there must be a way of providing radiation whose photons have an energy equal to the energy separation of the atomic states. The method that is used to provide radiation of the correct wavelength is placement of the laser material in an optical cavity, which acts as a resonator.

The salient features of a laser cavity are shown in Fig. 1-9. The resonant cavity consists of a mirror on either side of the laser material. The mirrors are carefully

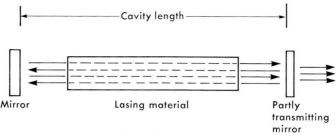

Fig. 1-9. Laser cavity.

aligned with each other, so that light bounces back and forth between them. One of the mirrors is partly transmitting, so as to allow some of the radiation out of the cavity. The buildup of oscillations in the cavity occurs as follows. First, some of the excited atoms in the laser material will emit spontaneously in random directions. The radiation that is emitted spontaneously is exactly the correct wavelength for interacting and stimulating the material, because the material itself radiated it. Some of this spontaneous radiation will hit one of the mirrors perpendicularly and thus be reflected back through the material. This radiation that is now reentering the material is of the correct wavelength to stimulate some of the excited atoms to emit radiation in phase with the beam, thus amplifying the beam. The beam that transits through the laser material in this way is reflected from the second mirror, and as it passes through the material, it is again amplified. Note that there is transit of many waves in this initial phase of oscillation buildup; however, the ones that are not in exactly the correct direction to reverberate between the two mirrors will be reflected at angles that do not allow repeated passage through the laser material. The amplified wave will gain in strength very rapidly, because as the intensity of the beam increases, the probability of stimulating additional atoms increases. By this regenerative mechanism a coherent beam is quickly built up, stimulated emission becomes a dominant mechanism of deexcitation of the atoms, and laser operation is possible. It is apparent that a laser is really an oscillator.

The beam that is generated by the laser cavity is spatially coherent, by virtue of the reflecting geometry as described above and because stimulated emission is radiated in phase with the exciting beams. The laser beam is also relatively monochromatic, because the internal energy of the atoms, as depicted by the energy levels, are specific and quantized.

Other laser characteristics

Some additional details of the resonances of lasers should be mentioned. Energy levels of atoms are distinct, quantized, and sharp values. Although they are sharp, they have a finite width, and consequently the resonance line associated with the transition between two states is broadened.

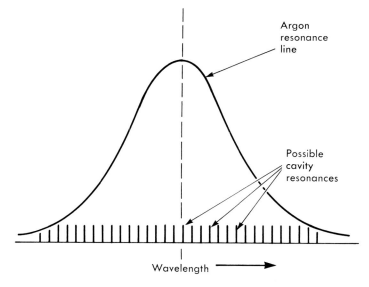

Fig. 1-10. Laser cavity resonances.

There are numerous broadening mechanisms; however, the dominant cause in an argon ion laser is the Doppler effect. Because the ions are moving in all directions, when an ion emits a photon its exact wavelength will be somewhat shifted from the norm, depending on whether it is moving toward or away from the direction in which it emits. A Gaussian, or bell-shaped, curve represents the radiation in one of the resonance lines of the argon ion (Fig. 1-10). The width of the resonance line is on the order of 0.001 nm.

In addition to this resonance, due to the argon ions in the discharge, there are resonances associated with the laser cavity and the light waves that are traveling back and forth in the cavity. These waves, which in the process of traveling back and forth propagate along the length of the cavity, set up standing waves that have resonances, in the same way that a piano wire that is struck has resonances. This type of resonance is associated with the number of half-wavelengths along the length of the cavity and are referred to as longitudinal modes. In order to resonate, there must be an exact integer number of half-wavelengths of the radiation in the cavity. Because the wavelength of light is so short (about 0.5×10^{-4} cm for argon) and cavity length is long (about 1 m), there are a very large number of half-wavelengths in a typical resonance condition. For example, for a cavity length of 100 cm and a wavelength of 0.5×10^{-4} cm, there are 4×10^{6} half-wavelengths along the cavity axis. Because of the small but finite width in the argon line, however, another resonance could occur with 1 more half-wavelength along the axis, and so on. In this way, there can be a number of longitudinal modes that can and do lase simultaneously (Fig. 1-10). Depending on the length

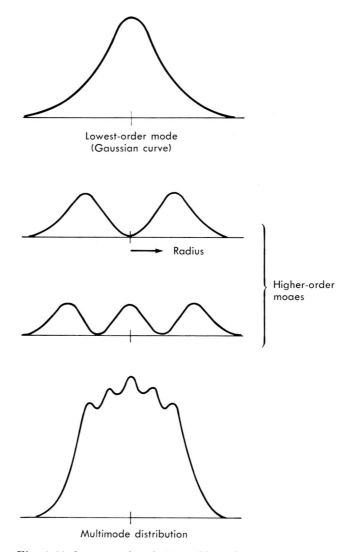

Fig. 1-11. Intensity distribution of laser beam cross section.

of the cavity, there can be on the order of 20 modes lasing within an argon laser line.

Another aspect of laser cavity resonances that needs to be considered is the transverse modes. These determine the profile of the intensity across the laser beam. Ordinarily, the cavity can be forced by restrictions to lase so that only the simplest distribution exists, or the lowest-order transverse mode, which has a profile of a Gaussian, or bell-shaped, curve (Fig. 1-11). However, there are many higher-order modes possible. Each is associated with a different intensity distribution across the beam (Fig. 1-11). By design, a laser can be operated so that a few of the lowest-order modes are allowed to oscillate. When a laser is allowed to lase in a number of low-order modes, it is termed a multimode laser. When this is done, the profile of the beam is a summation of the various modes (Fig. 1-11). In most argon laser photocoagulators, the argon laser operates in a multimode configuration that includes only a few lower-order modes. In contrast, most ruby lasers invariably lase in a very large number of modes.

In photocoagulation, multimode operation is not detrimental unless it is excessive. If a laser has too many higher-order modes, the divergence of the beam is large (coherence is lower), and the beam cannot be focused to as small a spot as might be desired, as is the problem with most ruby lasers. However, because the number of modes is low in the argon laser, this is not a limitation in argon laser photocoagulation.

PHOTOCOAGULATION
Interaction of radiation with molecules

In simple atoms, the possible energy levels associated with electron orbits are numerous. As a result, transitions from one level to another are innumerable. When molecules are considered, the situation is even more complicated by the vibrational, rotational, and bending energy levels that are possible.

Depending on the wavelength of the radiation, different types of transitions and interactions will take place. Thus the primary interactions involving radiation in the ultraviolet and visible parts of the spectrum are associated with electron orbit changes, if the photons are not energetic enough to lead to ionization or dissociation of the molecule. In radiation at infrared and longer wavelengths, the interactions involve vibrational, rotational, and bending types of changes.

Once a molecule has absorbed a photon and reached an excited state, the energy is converted in a number of independent and sometimes competing ways. Aside from spontaneous and stimulated emission of a photon and return to the ground state, the molecule may be deactivated by collisions with other molecules. Thus the energy may be converted totally to heat, or part may be converted to heat and part may be reradiated by fluorescence or by phosphorescence. Finally, the absorbed energy may be used to provide energy of activation for a chemical reaction, thus making possible the formation of new molecules.

Interaction with biologic systems

The molecules involved in biologic systems are extremely complex and, although extremely stable under certain conditions, maintain their vital effectiveness only in very specific configurations and environments.

The energy of a photon varies in inverse proportion to the wavelength. It is not surprising, therefore, that interactions associated with biologic material are quite different, depending on the wavelength. In the ultraviolet part of the spectrum, the photons are so energetic that interactions can be totally disruptive. Thus the absorption of a single photon by DNA, RNA, or a protein molecule can change them to abiotic (incompatible with life) forms, and cell death follows very quickly. In the visible part of the spectrum, primarily two types of interactions can take place. Photons in this range provide energy for photochemical reactions, such as in photosynthesis and in the chemistry of vision. The second method whereby biologic material is altered with this radiation is thermal. The radiation that is absorbed and not reradiated is converted into heat by nonradiative processes and leads to a gradual heating of the irradiated specimen. Because temperature is an extremely critical parameter for the normal operation of a cell, even a small increase can damage a cell irreparably.

Thermal damage is caused by the denaturation of proteins or the inactivation of enzymes in the cells. The temperature rise associated with this type of damage is not very high. A rise of 10 C to 30 C in temperature is sufficient to cause severe damage to the irradiated area. Radiation in the infrared part of the spectrum also can lead to this type of thermal damage to biologic systems.

Applications to the eye

Characteristics of the eye. In order to determine which wavelengths are most appropriate for use in photocoagulation of the fundus of the eye, the characteristics of the eye must be examined. Fig. 1-12 shows the transmission characteristics of the ocular media for radiation entering the eye and proceeding to the retina. Also shown is the absorption of the radiation by the pigment epithelium and choroid, in terms of the radiation incident at the cornea. These curves are based on in vitro measurements of human eyes.[3]

Note that transmission of radiation to the retina is good over a broad region, including the visible and near-infrared parts of the spectrum. Thus, in this limited

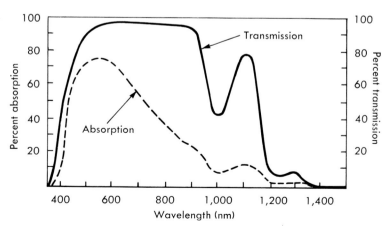

Fig. 1-12. Ocular transmission and absorption of pigment epithelium and choroid.

spectral region the ocular media are very transparent and effective in getting radiation to the area where interaction is to take place, the retina. In the infrared region, however, the transmission becomes increasingly poorer, primarily because of the absorption characteristics of water in the media, and eventually falls off completely.

The absorption characteristics of the melanin granules are responsible for the major part of the absorption in the pigment epithelium and choroid, and it is noted that the absorption falls off more rapidly. Thus, for heating the pigment epithelium, the blue-yellow part of the visible spectrum is most effective. The falloff of the curve on the long wavelength side is due to the decreasing absorption of the melanin granules, and the falloff on the short wavelength side is due to the decreased transmission of the ocular media rather than to a decrease in absorption by the granules.

The absorption of hemoglobin is an important consideration in interactions with vessels. Fig. 1-13 shows the absorption characteristics of hemoglobin in a 100-μm thickness of blood.[6] It is apparent that the shorter wavelengths, particularly the blue-yellow part of the spectrum, are far more effective than the red or infrared parts of the spectrum. Therefore, a red laser, such as ruby, for example, which emits radiation at 694 nm, is almost totally unabsorbed by hemoglobin. Thus, for effective interaction with vessels, radiation with wavelength shorter than 550 nm must be used.

It is of interest to compare the output of the argon laser with the output of the xenon arc photocoagulator. Fig. 1-14 shows the output of the xenon arc pho-

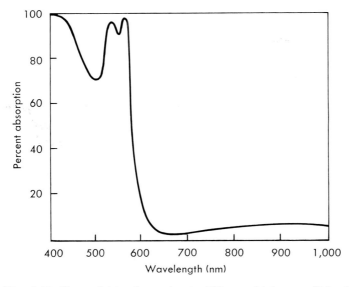

Fig. 1-13. Hemoglobin absorption in 100-μm thickness of blood.

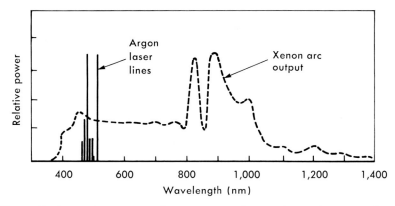

Fig. 1-14. Spectral emission of xenon arc and argon laser photocoagulators.

tocoagulator and the various lines that an argon laser photocoagulator usually emits when running on all lines. All wavelengths of the argon laser are fairly well located within a relatively narrow part of the spectrum in the blue-green region. As noted from the previous figures, the absorption characteristics of the important absorbers in the eye are spectrally broad; thus all argon wavelengths are almost equally effective. In contrast, the majority of the radiation of the xenon arc is in the near-infrared and infrared parts of the spectrum and consequently is not as effective. Calculations show that for interactions with the pigment epithelium and choroid, the argon laser, in terms of power entering the eye, would be 2.2 to 3.5 times more effective (on the basis of raising the temperature of the pigment epithelium) than the xenon arc. In interactions with vessels, the argon laser is calculated to be at least five times more effective than the xenon arc, insofar as absorption by hemoglobin is concerned.

These calculations are corroborated by experiments in vitro by L'Esperance,[7] which showed a difference of a factor of 5 between argon and xenon arc, and at Stanford Research Institute by in vivo experiments on monkeys,[8] which showed that a factor of about 10 is more applicable to vessels with flowing blood. It is apparent that the wavelengths in the blue-green region of the argon laser are most effective for photocoagulation of both the pigment epithelium and choroid and for interactions with vessels.

Thermal processes. Most of the radiation that reaches the retina will be transmitted by the sensory retina, and a large fraction of it will be absorbed by the pigment epithelium and the choroid. Because of the high density of melanin granules, the pigment epithelium is the layer where the highest absorption per unit volume takes place. It follows that the highest temperature reached during an exposure will be in or near the pigment epithelium layer.

During an exposure, the temperature of the exposed area will begin to increase.[11] At the same time, because of the increasing temperature difference,

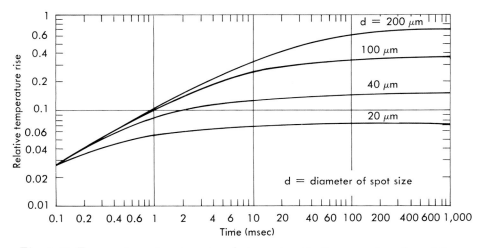

Fig. 1-15. Temperature rise at center of pigment epithelium as a function of time.

thermal conduction away from the exposed site will begin. Thus the geometry of the interaction volume, and particularly the area of the exposure, plays a very important role in temperature rise and decay. For example, consider a beam size of 50-μm diameter at the retina, so that we are dealing with a small absorbing area. As the light is absorbed and the temperature rises, there is thermal relaxation, or conduction of heat away from the site. The thickness of the pigment epithelium layer is 10μm, and the melanin granules are clustered in the anterior half of this thickness. Thus, to a first approximation, the absorbing volume is a thin disc. The center part of this absorbing volume gets the hottest, and because it is so small in diameter it can cool off radially in all directions. Thus the cooling of a small spot is quite effective. However, in a 500-μm diameter spot, all parts of the area heat up simultaneously. The center cannot cool off as effectively, because the surrounding areas are heated. Thus, it takes less photons per unit area to generate a certain temperature rise in a large spot than it does in a small one, in exposures that are long enough for thermal conduction to play a role in cooling the irradiated area.

This effect can be demonstrated by examining the results of some theoretical calculations based on a simple thermal model. The calculated temperature rise[12] at the center of the pigment epithelium layer is shown as a function of time in Fig. 1-15. This illustration shows the temperature rise for various spot-size diameters for the same power density at the retina. For a small spot size, the temperature quickly rises and reaches a constant value; that is, thermal equilibrium is reached: the amount of heat being introduced into the material is equal to the amount being conducted away to the surrounding tissues. For larger spot sizes, it is apparent that it takes longer for equilibrium to be reached, and the

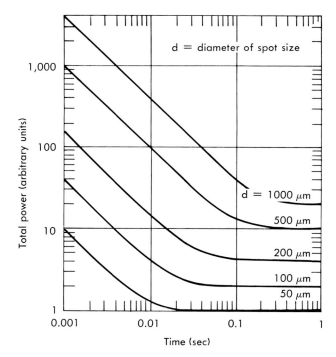

Fig. 1-16. Power required for equal temperature rise. Graph shows idealized theoretical curves.

temperature rises to a much higher value even though the power density has been kept constant.

In photocoagulation it is desirable to generate the same temperature at the center of the lesion (for the same exposure time); therefore it is necessary that the power density be reduced as the spot size is increased. The effect of spot size can be examined better by replotting the theoretical data in a different form. Fig. 1-16 shows the total beam power that is required to cause the same temperature rise for each spot size, as a function of time of the exposure. At very short exposures, the tissues heat up in a short time, compared with the thermal relaxation time; that is, no cooling takes place during the exposure. The power required varies in proportion to the area. Thus, if the spot size is increased by a factor of 2, the area correspondingly increases by a factor of 4, and four times as much power is required to reach the same temperature. At relatively long exposure times (e.g., 1/20, 1/10, 2/10 sec), however, where most clinical applications take place, thermal conduction does play a role, and the dynamics are totally different. At long exposure times, after the curves level off, the power requirement varies in proportion to the diameter, *not* the area. Thus, if the spot size is increased by a factor of 2, only twice as much power is required to reach the same temperature, because

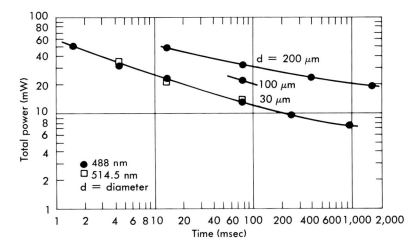

Fig. 1-17. Threshold retina damage in rhesus monkey for argon laser. Total power into eye for 50% probability of damage.

the smaller spot can cool to the temperature of the surrounding tissues more effectively.

Actual experimental data obtained by using argon laser in rhesus monkeys[12] are shown in Fig. 1-17. The curves represent threshold damage data, and each point represents a large number of exposures that have been averaged. One feature of the data is of special interest: the curves continue to decrease as a function of the time of the exposure, even though thermal equilibrium has been reached.

Fig. 1-18 compares the 30-μm diameter data with theoretical calculations for simple thermal models.[13] The curves have been arbitrarily shown to coincide at the 1-sec exposure. The theoretical models respectively include a simple pigment epithelium and a choroid. In both, the experimental data show considerably more variation in time than would be expected from simple thermal models, which assume that an equal temperature rise is required for damage, independent of exposure time.

It is apparent that consideration of damage as dependent on a single critical temperature is not adequate. The denaturation of proteins and the inactivation of enzymes must be analyzed as a rate process; as in any chemical reaction, the rate critically depends on the temperature. Coagulation, however, is more related to a survival fraction criterion. Therefore, an analysis that uses such a criterion would represent the physical situation more accurately. Such an analysis was carried out approximately, and an excellent fit with the experimental data was obtained for an activation energy of 70,000 cal/mole, which is well within the range for proteins and enzymes (Fig. 1-19). Although this is only an approximation, it gives confidence in the thermal damage model and the denaturation of protein theory.

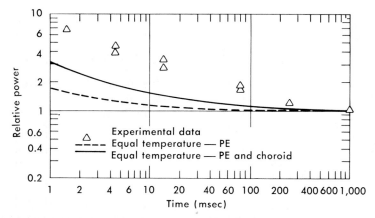

Fig. 1-18. Comparison of relative shape of threshold variation for simple model with actual data, assuming (1) only pigment epithelial layer absorbing and (2) pigment epithelium and choroid equally absorbing.

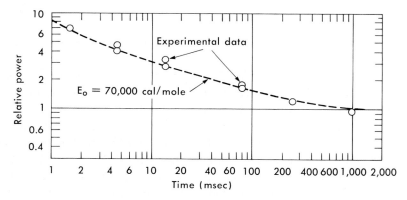

Fig. 1-19. Comparison of relative shape of threshold variation for inactivation thermal model with experimental data. Pigment epithelium and choroid assumed equally absorbing.

Other considerations. A number of important observations must be made in order to deliver effective photocoagulation.

For photocoagulation of the fundus, it is essential at the outset that an estimate of ocular media clarity be obtained. The aiming beam of the argon laser photocoagulator can be used effectively for this purpose by always setting it at the same value before treatment and observing the spot on the fundus. Additionally, careful examination should be made of the lens and the cornea.

Careful examination and consideration must then be given to the area where treatment is to be administered. Note must be made of the amount of pigmentation in the area, because the temperature rise during the exposure will depend on

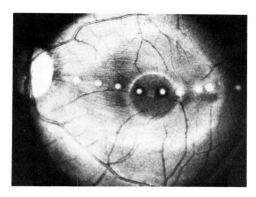

Fig. 1-20. Identical exposures across rhesus monkey macular area. Difference in response is due to variation in pigmentation.

the fraction of the beam that is absorbed. Even in a normal eye, pigmentation varies with different locations, and power adjustments must be made accordingly. As an example, Fig. 1-20 shows identical exposures made across the macular area of a rhesus monkey; it is seen that the lesions near the fovea are appreciably heavier than the more distant ones. Attention should also be paid to the presence of edema or fluid in the area being treated, because as one moves out of the area with fluid, much heavier lesions will result unless the power is reduced.

The response of the tissues depends radically on the temperature rise; there is a very small temperature difference between a very minimal and a heavy lesion. Inasmuch as temperature rise is proportional to power, it takes a very small power increase to progress from a very light lesion to a very heavy response; thus, increases in power should be made in small steps. It must also be remembered that the heat is conducted away from the exposed area; thus, if the power is increased beyond the point where a heavy lesion is obtained within the spot size, the lesion will expand to a size larger than the exposed area. This is particularly true of small lesions.

Changing the spot size with argon laser photocoagulators requires different considerations than with the xenon arc photocoagulator. If the spot size is decreased, the power must be decreased proportionally. Thus, if the spot is decreased by a factor of 2, the power must also be decreased by a factor of 2. If one increases the spot size by a factor of 2, for safety the power should be increased by a factor of 1.5 and then adjusted in small increments to the required level.

The kind of interaction that is desired for effective treatment depends on the disease that is being treated. If a minimal extent of damage away from the pigment epithelium is the correct approach, that is, if longitudinal damage is to be kept to a minimum (e.g., in the treatment of central serous retinopathy), very short exposures should be used, so that heat will not spread very far, as well as very small spot sizes, because the smaller the spot size the smaller the extent of damage in the longitudinal direction. In contrast, if a coagulation deep into the choroid or into the retina is desired (e.g., in the treatment of histoplasmosis), the best approach is to use long exposure times and large spot sizes, because both increase the depth of damage in all directions.

REFERENCES

1. Born, M.: Atomic physics, New York, 1962, Hafner.
2. Einstein, A.: Physik Z, **18:**121, 1917.
3. Geeraets, W. J., and Berry, E. R.: Ocular spectral characteristics as related to hazards from lasers and other light sources, Am. J. Ophthalmol. **66:**15, 1968.
4. Kapany, N. S., Peppers, N. A., Zweng, H. C., and Flocks, M.: Retinal photocoagulation by laser, Nature **199:**146, 1963.
5. Koester, C. J., Snitzer, E., Campbell, C. J., and Rittler, M. C.: Experimental laser retina coagulator, J. Opt. Soc. Am. **52:**607, 1962.
6. Lemberg, R., and Legge, J. W.: Hematin compounds and bile pigments, New York, 1949, Interscience Publishers.
7. L'Esperance, F.: An ophthalmic argon laser photocoagulation system: design, construction and laboratory investigations, Trans. Am. Ophthalmol. Soc. **66:**827, 1968.
8. Little, H. L., Zweng, H. C., and Peabody, R. R.: Argon laser slit lamp retinal photocoagulation, Trans. Am. Acad. Ophthalmol. **74:**85, 1970.
9. Maiman, T. H.: Stimulated optical radiation in ruby, Nature **187:**493, 1960.
10. Meyer-Schwickerath, G.: Light coagulation, St. Louis, 1960, The C. V. Mosby Co.
11. Vassiliadis, A.: Ocular damage from laser radiation. In Wolbarsht, M. L., editor: Laser applications in medicine and biology, vol. 1, New York, 1971, Plenum Publishing Corp.
12. Vassiliadis, A., Rosan, R. C., and Zweng, H. C.: Research on ocular laser thresholds: final report, SRI Project 7191, Menlo Park, Ca., 1969, Stanford Research Institute.
13. Vassiliadis, A., Zweng, H. C., and Dedrick, K. G.: Ocular laser threshold investigations: Final report, SRI Project 8209, Menlo Park, Ca., 1971, Stanford Research Institute.
14. Zaret, M. M., Ripps, H., Siegel, I. M., and Breinin, G. M.: Laser photocoagulation of the eye, Arch. Ophthalmol. **69:**97, 1963.
15. Zweng, H. C., Flocks, M., Kapany, N. S., et al.: Experimental laser photocoagulation, Am. J. Ophthalmol. **58:**353, 1964.

2
ARGON LASER PHOTOCOAGULATORS

HISTORY

The usefulness of the argon laser photocoagulator can best be understood by considering its predecessor, the xenon arc photocoagulator. Although the laser is the logical sequel to the original photocoagulator, the xenon arc instrument still is used extensively by many ophthalmologists. This speaks highly for an instrument that was conceived and developed in the early 1950s.

The first successful use of photocoagulation was demonstrated by Meyer-Schwickerath[8] in pioneering work that began in 1946. In his early experiments, Meyer-Schwickerath used the sun as the light source to obtain coagulation in the retina for the prevention of retinal separation from retinal tears. Shortly thereafter, the Zeiss Optical Company developed a photocoagulator, using a xenon arc lamp as the source, based on collaborative effort of Meyer-Schwickerath and Littman.[6]

The Zeiss xenon arc photocoagulator permitted treatment of a number of diseases that could not be helped previously. In addition to peripheral retinal degenerations, such conditions as Coats' disease, Eales's disease, and diabetic retinopathy were treated successfully.

Although the xenon arc photocoagulator is a useful instrument, it has limitations as well as difficulties associated with its use. Major difficulties are—

1. A retrobulbar anesthetic must be used nearly always.
2. The exit beam is large; thus the iris is often exposed to the beam, contracting the pupil.
3. A very small retinal field is seen.
4. Macular pucker or microcystic macular edema can occur from extensive treatment of peripheral areas.

The limitations of the instrument that derive from its incoherent white-light source, however, present even stronger arguments for development of a laser photocoagulator. Because of the nature of the incoherent source, small retinal areas cannot be photocoagulated, nor can there be effective photocoagulation at very short time exposures. In addition, because radiation from the xenon arc bulb extends from the ultraviolet to the infrared spectrum, an appreciable fraction of the radiation is relatively ineffective in the target area.

EARLY LASER PHOTOCOAGULATION

By the time the laser was first proposed in 1968 by Townes and Schlawlow,[9] there was worldwide acceptance of photocoagulation. It is not surprising, therefore, that very shortly after Maiman[7] reported the first successful operation of a laser in 1960 ophthalmologists immediately began exploring its possible use in photocoagulation.

The laser offers the attributes of coherence and high intensity. With temporal coherence (see Chapter 1), radiation is relatively monochromatic; thus, by selecting an appropriate wavelength, maximal effect at the target and minimal effects elsewhere can be achieved. Spatial coherence allows focusing of the beam to very small spot sizes at the retina or elsewhere, thus making possible the treatment of macular diseases and other ocular disorders. With high intensity, interactions can be obtained at relatively short times; thus less energy is required for a significant interaction. In addition, because laser instruments require preselection of energy, quantitative photocoagulation is possible.

The first laser successfully demonstrated was the pulsed ruby, and it was with this laser that researchers on both coasts of North America began work in 1961-1962.[2,3,10] As a result of this pioneering work two commercial instruments were introduced. The instrument developed by Optics Technology, Inc., in cooperation with Zweng and his colleagues (1964), made use of a direct ophthalmoscope delivery system; that developed by the American Optical Co., in cooperation with Campbell and his colleagues (1965), used a modified indirect delivery system.

In the first few years of ruby laser photocoagulation, hundreds of patients were treated for peripheral retinal pathologic conditions, such as retinal tears and holes.[11,12] Zweng in 1965 was the first to use the ruby laser in treating a patient with macular disease; since then, it has been applied clinically in the treatment of such disorders as persistent central serous retinopathy, detachments of the retinal pigment epithelium, some forms of senile macular degeneration, aphakic macular edema, and macular edema secondary to diabetic retinopathy.[1,11,13]

PROTOTYPE ARGON LASER PHOTOCOAGULATOR

It became apparent in the mid-1960s that ruby laser photocoagulation was an effective mode of treatment of a number of ophthalmic disorders. The delivery systems used, however, had a number of limitations. The direct ophthalmoscope delivery system offered adequate magnification and viewing of the posterior pole; however, in the far periphery it was very difficult to view the fundus, and the laser spot was badly distorted. The modified indirect delivery system could reach farther into the periphery, but did not offer sufficient magnification for treatment of the macular area.

The instrument that offers the best view of the fundus is a slit lamp used in conjunction with a Goldmann diagnostic corneal contact lens. The slit-lamp–Goldmann lens combination provides a clear, binocular view of the fundus, from fovea to ora serrata. This view can be obtained under high illumination and high magnification, which is especially important in the treatment of macular disease, with any form of photocoagulation. For these reasons the prototype instrument was developed around a slit-lamp delivery system.

In addition to the shortcomings of the delivery systems used, there were limitations due to the ruby laser light. The red wavelength of the ruby was almost totally ineffective in vascular problems, because of the negligible absorption of radiation by hemoglobin. The output energy was not reproducible accurately, and the beam could not be focused down to a sufficiently small retinal spot. Thus, a more coherent and more stable source was required.

For these reasons animal experiments, using a continuous-wave (cw) argon laser, were undertaken in 1967 at the Stanford Research Institute (SRI) by Zweng, Little, Vassiliadis, Peppers, and Peabody,[5] and by L'Esperance[4] in New York, who first reported the application of the argon laser to humans in 1968.

The success of the animal experiments, which demonstrated the effectiveness of the argon laser in occluding retinal vessels and creating small spot sizes in retinal photocoagulations, made the argon laser the light source of choice in the prototype laser photocoagulator, described in the next section.

Design and construction of photocoagulator

Because the argon laser offered the greatest potential as a light source for treating not only macular but also vascular diseases, and because the slit-lamp delivery system appeared to be the best method of delivering the light to the retina, it was decided by the SRI team that they would design and construct an argon laser slit-lamp photocoagulator.

The subsequent instrument had a number of important features:
1. The laser beam could be manipulated on the fundus, independently of the viewing optics.
2. The laser beam was coaxial with the viewing light.
3. The focus of the laser beam was always parfocal with the viewing optics.
4. The size of the beam on the fundus could be varied.
5. The power level was continuously monitored.
6. The laser beam could be shuttered at preset times or could be run continuously.
7. An aiming beam was provided that was an attenuated part of the laser beam itself.
8. The power level of the beam could be varied continuously.
9. The aiming-light intensity could be varied independently.

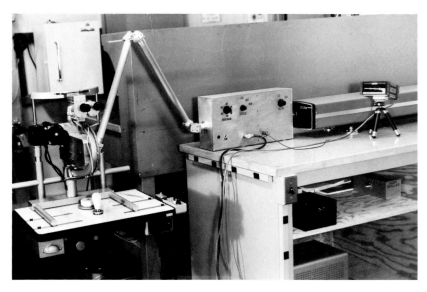

Fig. 2-1. Prototype argon laser photocoagulator. Head of the argon laser is at far right. Rectangular box to left of laser contains electronic shutter and controls to regulate beam. Laser beam is brought to slit lamp by way of articulating arm. Beam then passes through a series of optics and exits slit lamp coaxial to the viewing light. Details of slit-lamp optics are shown in Fig. 2-2. (From Zweng, H. C., et al.: Laser photocoagulation and retinal angiography, St. Louis, 1969, The C. V. Mosby Co.)

   10. All functions and adjustments of the slit lamp were left intact.
   11. Individual wavelengths of the argon laser could be selected or all the wavelengths could be used simultaneously.
   12. A protective filter came down over the viewing optics, to allow continuous viewing during the interaction of the beam and the ocular tissue, without dazzling the operator, but was not present during other viewing of the fundus.

The argon laser slit-lamp photocoagulator was designed and constructed in the Electromagnetic Techniques Laboratory of Stanford Research Institute, under the direction of A. Vassiliadis and with major contributions by N. A. Peppers, L. Alterton, and R. E. Meyers.[5]

The prototype system is shown in Fig. 2-1. The laser shown on the right is a Coherent Radiation Model 52 argon laser. Immediately to the left of the laser head is a control box, where the beam was expanded through a telescope and then passed through an adjustable iris. A part of the beam was reflected by a pellicle beam splitter, to provide a sample of the beam. This beam bypassed the electronic shutter that controlled the main beam and thus provided an aiming beam for the instrument. In addition, a small portion of the bypassed beam was directed into a photodiode whose output was displayed on a digital meter. The cir-

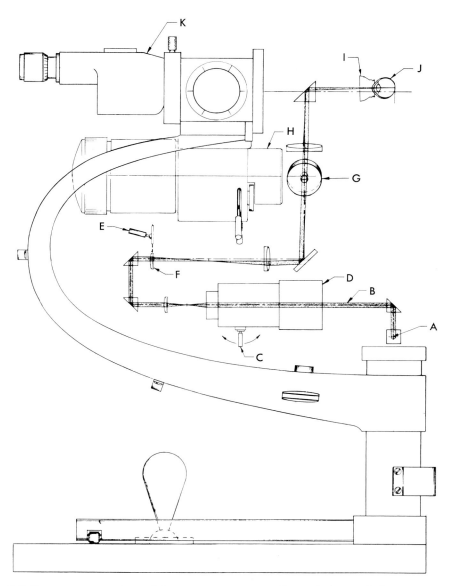

Fig. 2-2. Prototype argon laser delivery system using a Zeiss slit lamp. *A*, Beam entrance prism; *B*, laser beam; *C*, zoom control; *D*, zoom lens for changing spot size; *E*, beam lateral deflection control; *F*, moveable lens for prismatic deflection; *G*, full reflecting mirror with central hole for laser beam; *H*, modified slit-lamp illumination source; *I*, contact lens; *J*, patient's eye; *K*, slit-lamp viewing optics. (From Zweng, H. C., et al.: Laser photocoagulation and retinal angiography, St. Louis, 1969, The C. V. Mosby Co.)

cuit was adjusted so that the meter read the power delivered into the eye in milliwatts, as calibrated by an Eppley thermopile placed at the locus of the eye. The aiming beam was passed through neutral-density step filters, so that its intensity could be adjusted. The aiming beam was then made coaxial with the main beam by another pellicle. The power of the main laser beam could be adjusted by varying both the laser power supply and the iris diameter.

The beam passed through the control box and entered an articulating arm that contained six prisms. The parts of the arm were connected with ball-bearing joints, which provided sufficient freedom of motion that the slit lamp could be moved freely in any direction. The articulating arm connected to a Zeiss slit lamp, as seen on the left in Fig. 2-1, where the controls for the beam adjustment were located.

A schematic of the optics in the slit-lamp mount is shown in Fig. 2-2. The beam from the articulating arm entered at point A and was deflected by two prisms into a zoom lens, D. By manipulating dial C, the spot-size diameter at the back of the eye could be adjusted to vary from 70 to 350 μm in five steps. The optics were so adjusted that the laser beam remained in focus at the same plane as the slit-lamp binocular viewing optics, K; whatever structures were in focus to the viewer were in focus to the laser beam. The beam was then bent and passed through lens F, which could be translated laterally in any direction by lever E. Movement of this lens moved the beam at the focus in the back of the eye. Freedom of beam motion independent of the viewing optics was afforded by this manipulator. The beam was passed through a small hole in mirror G, which made the laser beam coaxial with the illumination light for viewing from lamp source H.

The delivery of the beam was additionally controlled by selection switches on the right of the slit-lamp table, so the experimenter could preselect the duration of exposure. The actual delivery of the treating beam was accomplished by depressing a foot switch. When the foot switch was pressed, a color filter dropped in front of the slit-lamp optics, in order to protect the operator from the bright glare of the beam reflected and scattered from various surfaces and from the fundus and still allow an adequate view of the tissue being treated during the exposure. Although shutter lengths could be preselected from 1/125 to 4 sec or even continuous, the foot switch could override the preselection; thus an exposure could be interrupted by releasing the foot switch.

Use of argon laser slit-lamp photocoagulator

The argon laser photocoagulator was constructed in 1968 and was first used in rhesus monkey experiments in early 1969. The instrument performed completely as had been specified, providing satisfactory exposures in both retinal and vascular experiments.

Because animal experiments had produced highly positive results, clinical experimentation was begun. Accordingly, Zweng treated the first patient in May

1969. The immediate success of the prototype instrument in numerous retinal applications led to the development of commercial instruments.

COMMERCIAL ARGON LASER PHOTOCOAGULATORS
General remarks

All of the argon laser photocoagulators currently available deliver the argon laser beam through a slit-lamp delivery system, and they all encompass the major features of the SRI prototype. The various instruments combine a variety of features; thus each has its own set of advantages and disadvantages in comparison with other systems.

One feature of the prototype that developed into a problem was the use of a single-mode laser. With the laser operating in the lowest-order mode, the physics of Gaussian beam propagation are such that the laser beam diameter was small at the plane of the cornea and the lens. Consequently, corneal and lenticular damage was observed in some instances, because of the high power densities at those tissues. This complication was easily corrected by operating the laser multimodally and by obtaining larger beam sizes by defocusing the 100-μm spot diameter beam. With the exception of the Medical Instrument Research Associates (MIRA) instrument, all commercial argon laser systems are multimodal, giving a beam diameter at the cornea large enough that the power density is below that which gives corneal and lenticular damage while treating retinal problems.

A related phenomenon, observed on occasion in patients with nuclear sclerosis of the lens, is that the beam spot expands during an exposure. This expansion of the beam, or thermal blooming, occurs because a very small fraction of the beam is absorbed by the tissues it traverses. The lens tissue at the center of the beam is heated more than that at the edge of the beam, resulting in greater expansion of the lens tissue at the center of the beam. The thermal effect of expansion of the tissues makes the index of refraction of tissue less at the center than at the edges of the beam, giving the same effect as a negative lens expanding the beam diameter at the retina. This effect has been seen with the Coherent Radiation Model 800 and would probably be seen in the MIRA unit. However, because the diameter of the beam is much larger when it traverses the lens in the other argon photocoagulators, the effect of thermal blooming is minimal.

Argon laser photocoagulators are currently supplied by four American manufacturers: Britt Corporation, Coherent Radiation, Inc., Medical Instrument Research Associates, Inc., and Optics Technology, Inc. The basic characteristics and features of these argon laser photocoagulators are summarized in Table 2-1 and discussed on the following pages. It is not the intent here to evaluate the technical merits of the various instruments or to identify the superior instrument. Other factors that bear on the selection of one instrument over another, such as quality of manufacture and reliability of operation and service, are also beyond the scope of this discussion but should also weigh heavily in evaluating the instruments for purchase.

Table 2-1. Currently available argon laser photocoagulators

	Britt Corporation	Coherent Radiation, Inc.		MIRA, Inc.	Optics Technology, Inc.	
Model	150	800	900	MF2,000	V-A	VI
Argon laser	Pulsed at 3,000 pps	Continuous wave	Continuous wave	Continuous wave	Continuous wave; electronically on-off	Continuous wave; electronically on-off
Laser cooling	Air	Water	Water	Water	Water	Air
Electrical requirements	1-phase, 220 V	3-phase, 220 V	3-phase, 220 V	3-phase, 220 V	3-phase, 220 V	1-phase, 220 V
Laser beam coaxial with viewing light	No	Yes	No	No	Yes	Yes
Articulation of laser beam	4 mirrors	7 mirrors	Quartz fiber	3 mirrors	Quartz fiber	Quartz fiber
Parfocal with viewing light (spot diameter in μm)	50, 100, 200	50, 100	50, 100	50	50, 100	50, 100
Spot-size diameters available (μm)	50, 100, 200, 400, 700	50, 100, 200, 500, 1,000	50, 100, 200, 500, 1,000, 2,000	50, 100, 200, 500, 750, 1,000	50, 100, 200, 500, 1,000, 2,000	50, 100, 200, 500, 1,000, 2,000
Time settings available (sec)	0.02, 0.05, 0.1, 0.2, continuous	0.01, 0.02, 0.05, 0.1, 0.2, 0.5, 1, 2, 5, continuous	0.02, 0.05, 0.1, 0.2, 0.5, 1.2, 5, continuous	0.05, 0.1, 0.2, 0.3, 0.5, 0.8, 1, 2.5	0.02, 0.05, 0.1, 0.2, 0.5, 1, 2, 5, continuous	0.02, 0.05, 0.1, 0.2, 0.5, 1, 2, 5, continuous
Power output (watts)	>1.5	>2	>2	> 0.55 @ 488 nm; > 0.65 @ 514.5 nm; > 1, all lines	>2	>2

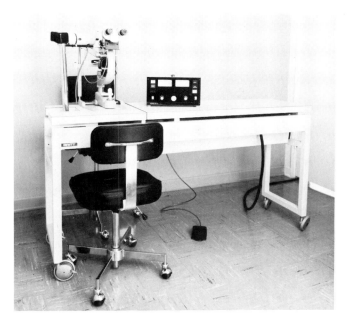

Fig. 2-3. Britt Corporation Model 150 argon laser photocoagulator. Air-cooled argon laser is located in desk console. Laser beam is brought to Zeiss slit lamp by way of four-mirror articulating arm. Control box on console contains controls for laser beam. (Courtesy Britt Corporation, Los Angeles, Calif.)

Britt Corporation

The Britt Corporation photocoagulator uses a high repetition rate, pulsed-argon laser. In the standard model (Model 150), each pulse is 30μm in length in a 3,000-pps beam. Britt also offers Model 152, which uses pulses of about 120μm delivered at a rate of 750 pps, as an experimental photocoagulator. At these high repetition rates, the thermal effect of radiation on the retina at normal photocoagulation levels is essentially equivalent to the effect of a continuous-wave (cw) laser. If the energy per pulse were made sufficiently high, a single pulse could give a burn.

The Britt system is designed to deliver the beam only with a Zeiss slit lamp (Fig. 2-3). The laser beam is delivered into the eye at an angle that blocks an appreciable fraction of the viewing light. This may result in poor viewing of the target sites in the periphery. A four-mirror articulating arm, which brings the beam from the console to the slit lamp, allows sufficient freedom to manipulate the beam within the eye. Selection of power, time of exposure, and aiming-beam intensity is made at a movable control box, which also has a resettable counter that indicates the number of exposures.

The spot-size diameter can be varied in steps, from 50 to 700μm in the latest model. To create such lesions, the available maximum power of 1.5 W is ade-

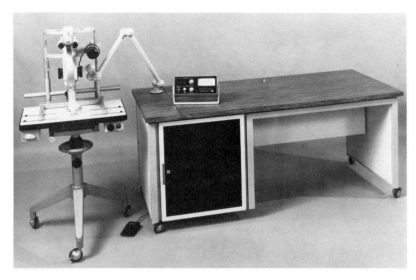

Fig. 2-4. Coherent Radiation Model 800 argon laser photocoagulator. Water-cooled laser and power supply are in console. Laser beam is brought to the slit lamp by way of seven-mirror articulating arm. Photograph shows Zeiss slit lamp used for delivery of beam. (An American Optical Co. slit-lamp delivery system is also available.) Moveable control box on console provides main controls for laser beam. (Courtesy Coherent Radiation, Inc., Palo Alto, Calif.)

quate. The laser is air-cooled and operates on a single-phase power connection, which are advantages in certain situations. The laser beam focus is parfocal with the viewing optics for the 50-, 100-, and 200-μm settings.

Coherent Radiation, Inc.

Coherent Radiation was the first company to market an argon laser photocoagulator, Model 800, which was a direct development of the SRI prototype. This instrument was introduced at the American Academy of Ophthalmology meeting in October 1970 and initially was used in treating patients by Zweng and Little in November 1970.

The basic Model 800 argon laser photocoagulator is shown in Fig. 2-4. Essentially, it has all but two of the features of the SRI prototype, with slight modifications. Because experiments on monkeys, carried out by the authors with the prototype model, demonstrated no essential difference in the effect on the retina or its vasculature from the two main argon laser wavelengths, this photocoagulator is operated with all lines simultaneously. The second variation, which has to do with the beam diameter entering the eye, will be discussed later. The water-cooled continuous-wave laser, located in the desk console, requires three-phase electrical connections. For stable and safe operation, the quartz-graphite laser tube must be warmed up for 15 minutes before use, and water must be left circu-

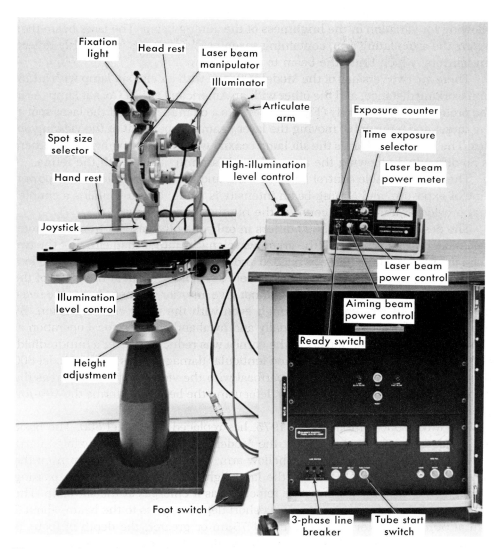

Fig. 2-5. Coherent Radiation Model 800 laser control details. Laser beam adjustment of power and time of exposure is made on control box; spot-size diameter selection and manipulation of beam are made on slit lamp. Adjustment of aiming beam intensity is also made on control box.

lating for 15 minutes after the laser is turned off. The laser beam is passed through an electronic shutter that permits only a very small fraction of the laser power to be transmitted as an aiming beam. The fraction of the beam that is transmitted can be varied by placing different attenuators in the path of the beam, allowing for variation in the brightness of the aiming beam. The laser beam then enters the articulating arm, containing seven precision joints with highly reflecting mirrors, which bring the beam to the slit lamp.

There are two versions of the Model 800: one with a Zeiss slit lamp with a 125-mm working distance, and the other with an American Optical Co. slit lamp. As in the prototype, the assembly (Fig. 2-5) permits a change in size of the laser spot at the target and a means of moving the laser beam independent of the viewing optics. The laser beam leaves the slit lamp coaxial with the viewing light; thus there is no difficulty in viewing the area of laser beam interaction with the retina.

There is a movable control box (Figs. 2-4 and 2-5), where selection of power, time of exposure, and aiming-beam intensity is made. It also contains a counter that provides a cumulative count of the number of exposures.

The design of the Model 800 differs in only one other aspect from the prototype model (besides using all the argon wavelengths rather than either of the two main lines). A modification was needed and made because some corneal and lenticular damage occurred, caused by the very small laser beam at the plane of the cornea and the lens. The prototype did not give anterior segment burns, because its power output was not high enough even with the small entering beam. By operating the laser cavity multimodally and by abandoning parfocal operation at *all* spot sizes, the power density at the cornea was reduced by over a hundredfold, eliminating the danger of corneal and lenticular damage. Thus, in the Model 800 the 50- and 100-μm spot sizes are parfocal with the viewing optics, whereas the remaining spot sizes are obtained by defocusing the beam that forms the 100-μm spot diameter.

The Model 900, introduced in 1975, has replaced the Model 800. The basic difference between the two is that the Model 900 uses a single flexible quartz fiber, rather than the articulating hollow arm, to bring the laser beam from the console to the slit lamp. Because the laser light loses its coherence in passing through an optical fiber, it must be refocused as it emerges at the slit lamp. The net effect of the refocusing is to give a short depth of focus to the beam, about 2 mm at 50μm diameter. At diameters of 75μm or greater, the depth of focus is similar to that with the Model 800. The Model 900 is available with both the American Optical Co. slit-lamp delivery system (Fig. 2-6) and the Zeiss slit lamp. Because the slit lamp is not modified, the illumination light and the laser beam are no longer coaxial but are at a slight angle to each other. The viewing in the far retinal periphery is not as good, therefore, as with the Model 800.

The Model 900 has spot-size diameters available in infinite gradation from 50 to 2,000μm; the Model 800 had spot-size diameters in steps from 50 to 1,000μm. In both models the 50- and 100-μm spots are parfocal with the slit-lamp optics,

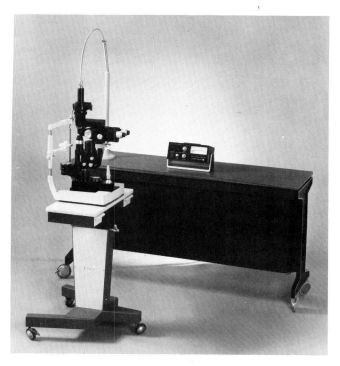

Fig. 2-6. Coherent Radiation Model 900 argon laser photocoagulator. Laser and power supply are located in console. Laser beam is brought to slit lamp by flexible quartz fiber. Photograph shows American Optical Co. slit lamp being used for beam delivery. Beam controls are contained in moveable box on console. (Courtesy Coherent Radiation, Inc., Palo Alto, Calif.)

whereas the larger spot sizes are obtained by defocusing the laser beam. The maximum power of both models is 2W.

Medical Instruments Research Associates, Inc.

The Medical Instruments Research Associates (MIRA) photocoagulator uses a continuous-wave argon laser delivered through a Zeiss slit lamp (Fig. 2-7), an operating microscope, or a monocular indirect ophthalmoscope. This instrument allows the operator to select either of the two main wavelengths of the argon laser, the 488- and 514.5-nm lines. Inasmuch as our experiments did not show any significant advantage of one wavelength over the other for specific photocoagulation applications, there seems no justification for the complexity and the inconvenience of changing laser operation from single-line to multiline operation. Because the power available in a single line is insufficient to photocoagulate at the larger spot sizes, it is necessary when using them to change from single-line to multiline operation by changing the laser cavity. The change is accomplished by replacing a prism with a mirror, which reflects all wavelengths equally.

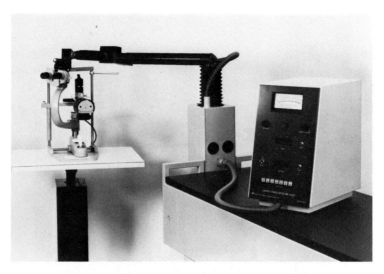

Fig. 2-7. Medical Instruments Research Associates argon laser photocoagulator. Water-cooled laser and power supply are in console, and beam is brought to slit lamp by way of three-mirror articulating arm. Beam parameters are adjusted on control panel on console. (Courtesy Medical Instruments Research Associates, Boston, Mass.)

In this system also, the laser beam is delivered at an angle with the viewing light, which may make peripheral exposures difficult. The blocking filter to protect the operator from glare is in place at all times, which requires that the intensity of the aiming beam be high so that the operator can see the beam through the filter. In fact, the power of the aiming light at certain settings may be marginal, with regard to safety. The foot switch used is a two-position switch: the first position (partial depression) initiates the aiming beam, and the second (full depression) switches on the full beam. This mode of control is inherently dangerous because of the constant danger of triggering the full beam by too much initial depression of the switch.

The MIRA unit provides a spot-size diameter variation in steps from 50 to $1,000\mu$m. The maximum power available is 550 mW at 488 nm and 650 mW at 514.4 nm; for all lines it is over 1 W. The 50-μm size diameter is parfocal with the viewing optics, and the others are obtained by defocusing.

Optics Technology, Inc.

Optics Technology has been manufacturing photocoagulators since the early 1960s; it was the first company to develop and market a ruby laser photocoagulator, and it developed and offered an argon laser slit-lamp photocoagulator in 1973.

The original model was unique in that it could be adapted to all popular slit lamps without modifying them, using three-glass fibers to couple the laser beam to the slit lamp. The two recent models, V-A and VI, use a single flexible-quartz

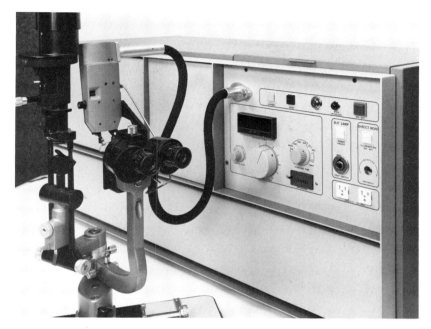

Fig. 2-8. Optics Technology, Inc., Model V-A argon laser photocoagulator. This model uses water-cooled laser located in console. Laser beam is brought to slit lamp by way of flexible quartz fiber. Attachment can be made to all popular slit lamps. Beam parameters are adjusted by controls on console. (Courtesy Optics Technology, Inc., Redwood City, Calif.)

fiber. Both models allow the slit lamp to move independently of the illumination. The company also offers a direct ophthalmoscope delivery system.

Model V-A (Fig. 2-8) uses a water-cooled laser with a beryllium oxide laser tube, which may be switched on and off without warmup or cooldown time necessary. The laser tube is idled to provide the aiming beam. A foot switch electronically turns on the tube to high power for the duration of the preset exposure time. The power setting is adjusted at the console, where the power in milliwatts is indicated by a digital meter. The time exposure is selected on the console also, and a resettable counter totals the number of exposures that are made. The simple attachment to the slit lamp allows the laser beam to leave the slit lamp coaxially with the viewing light.

Model VI (Fig. 2-9) is similar to Model V-A, except that the laser is air-cooled, requiring only a single-phase electrical connection. The Model VI console is also slightly smaller than that of the Model V-A.

Both models have spot-size diameter selection in a step from 50 to 100μm and then continuously variable up to 2,000μm. The 50- and 100-μm spots are parfocal with the viewing optics of the slit lamp, whereas the larger spots are obtained by

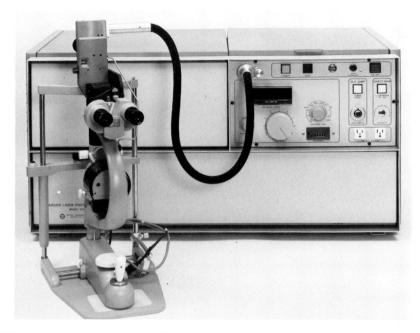

Fig. 2-9. Optics Technology, Inc., Model VI argon laser photocoagulator. This model uses an air-cooled argon laser located in console. The laser beam is brought to slit lamp by use of a flexible quartz fiber. Beam parameters are adjusted by controls on console. (Courtesy Optics Technology, Inc., Redwood City, Calif.)

defocusing the 100-μm beam. The maximum power available in both models is 2 W.

Ferlux Instruments (France)

This instrument uses a water-cooled continuous-wave argon laser, with the laser beam brought to the slit lamp by a flexible fiber. The slit lamp is a Zeiss 125/16. The retinal spot sizes range in steps from 50 to 1,000 μm and the exposure times in steps from 0.01 to 1 sec and continuous. All the controls for the beam are fixed on the main console that contains the laser and power supply.

Lasertek Oy (Finland)

This system uses two water-cooled lasers, an argon laser providing output in the blue-green part of the spectrum and a krypton laser providing red wavelength radiation (647 nm).

The laser beam is attached to the slit lamp by a four-mirror articulating arm. It is attached to either a Haag-streit Model 900 or a Zeiss Model 100 slit lamp. The retinal spot sizes vary continuously from 50 to 1,000 μm and exposure times from 0.02 to 9.99 sec in 0.01-sec steps. The adjustments are made on a moveable control box on the console.

REFERENCES

1. Campbell, C. J., Rittler, M. C., and Koester, C. J.: Laser photocoagulation of the retina, Trans. Am. Acad. Ophthalmol. Otolaryngol. **70:**939, 1966.
2. Kapany, N. S., Peppers, N. A., Zweng, H. C., and Flocks, M.: Retinal photocoagulation by laser, Nature **199:**146, 1963.
3. Koester, C. J., Snitzer, E., Campbell, D. J., and Rittler, M. C.: Experimental laser retina coagulator, J. Opt. Soc. Am. **52:**609, 1962.
4. L'Esperance, F. A., Jr.: An ophthalmic argon laser photocoagulation system: design, construction, and laboratory investigations, Trans. Am. Ophthalmol. Soc. **66:**827, 1968.
5. Little, H. L., Zweng, H. C., and Peabody, R. R.: Argon laser slit lamp photocoagulator, Trans. Am. Acad. Ophthalmol. Otolaryngol. **74:**85, 1970.
6. Littmann, H.: The Zeiss light coagulator after Meyer-Schwickerath with xenon high pressure lamp, Bericht über die 61. Zusammenkunft der Deutschen Ophthalmologische Gesellschaft in Heidelberg, 1957, p. 311.
7. Maiman, T. H.: Stimulated optical radiation in ruby, Nature **187:**493, 1960.
8. Meyer-Schwickerath, G.: Light coagulation, St. Louis, 1960, The C. V. Mosby Co.
9. Schlawlow, A. L., and Townes, C. H.: Infrared and optical lasers, Physiol. Rev. **112:**1940, 1958.
10. Zaret, M. M., Ripps, H., Siegel, I. M., and Breinin, G. M.: Laser photocoagulation of the eye, Arch. Ophthalmol. **69:**97, 1963.
11. Zweng, H. C.: Laser photocoagulation of the peripheral retina and macula, Proceedings of the Twentieth International Congress of Ophthalmology, Amsterdam, 1967, Excerpta Medica Foundation.
12. Zweng, H. C., and Flocks, M.: Retinal laser photocoagulation, Trans. Am. Acad. Ophthalmol. Otolaryngol. **71:**39, 1967.
13. Zweng, H. C., Little, H. L., and Peabody, R. R.: Laser photocoagulation and retinal angiography, St. Louis, 1969, The C. V. Mosby Co.

3
HISTOPATHOLOGY

LIGHT SOURCES AND RETINAL LESIONS

Light emitted by the argon laser photocoagulator is maximally absorbed by the red pigment of hemoglobin and of melanin-containing cells of the retinal pigment epithelium and the choroid. Through the absorption of light by these pigments, heat is produced. The resulting histopathologic changes are directly related to the amount of heat produced in the lesion. Tissue response to heat generated by any light source, whether it be xenon arc, ruby laser, or argon laser, is similar. The variable factors influencing the kind of lesion produced are—

1. Power of light source (photons per sec)
2. Duration of exposure
3. Diameter of light beam
4. Wavelength of light source
5. Clarity of ocular media
6. Pigment of tissue exposed to light source
7. Heat conductive properties of surrounding tissues

In different areas of the retina, the intensity of the coagulation point can vary for the same power, exposure time, and spot-size settings. Because of greater pigmentation in the macula, settings that give a minimal lesion in the paramacular region will produce a moderately heavy lesion in the parafoveal area (Fig. 3-1). Lesions in the far periphery are heavier than those produced with similar settings in the midperiphery. In treating a more heavily pigmented region, as compared with a less pigmented area, the power must be reduced to produce a similar lesion.

With the same spot-size diameter and time settings, a lesion produced with higher power will be larger than one produced with lower power.[1] A lesion produced with a 50-μm spot, 200 mW of power, and 0.1 sec will be larger than one made with a 50-μm spot produced at 50 mW at 0.1 sec (Fig. 3-2). For similar spot-size and power settings, a lesion produced with a longer exposure time will be larger than a lesion produced with a minimal time setting. Thus a lesion produced with a 50-μm spot at 1 sec and 100 mW will be larger than one produced by a 50-μm spot at 0.1 sec and 100 mW.

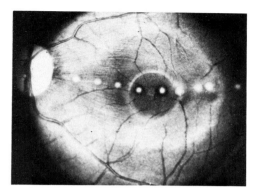

Fig. 3-1. Without changing settings of photocoagulator, more intense photocoagulation lesions are produced in parafoveal region than in paramacular area, because of increased absorption by xanthophil and pigment epithelial pigment granules in parafoveal area of the rhesus monkey retina.[1]

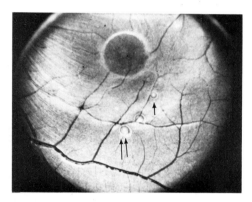

Fig. 3-2. Without changing diameter setting of laser beam, diameter of photocoagulation lesion is increased (*double arrow*) by either increasing power or duration of exposure to the rhesus monkey retina.[1]

Ophthalmoscopically and histopathologically similar retinal lesions can be made with xenon arc, ruby laser, and argon laser photocoagulation (Figs. 3-3 and 3-4). However, there are certain characteristic features of lesions made by the three light sources that should be noted. First, because of the infrared component of the xenon light, which is not absorbed well by hemoglobin or melanin pigment, more energy (power × time) is required to produce a retinal lesion with xenon arc than with argon laser photocoagulation.

Second, the exposure times required to produce a retinal lesion differ between the three modalities: ruby laser coagulation is produced in milliseconds; argon laser burns require from 0.05 to 0.2 sec; and xenon arc retinal burns require from 0.2 to 2 sec. Moderately intense photocoagulation of vascular tissue is more likely to be complicated by hemorrhage when exposure times are less than 0.1 sec. Because there is not sufficient time for heat to be conducted from the center of

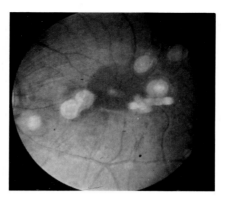

Fig. 3-3. Ophthalmoscopically similar lesions are produced with ruby laser and xenon arc photocoagulators. Laser lesions are made between disc and macula with Optics Technology, Inc., ruby laser. Xenon lesions are made temporally in macula with Zeiss instrument. Ruby laser lesions are made with 15 mJ power, whereas xenon lesions require approximately 200 mJ. Rhesus monkey retina.[5]

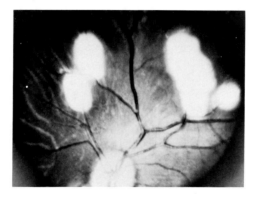

Fig. 3-4. Ophthalmoscopically similar lesions are produced with argon laser on the left and xenon arc on the right in a rhesus monkey retina.

the lesion, vaporization of tissue and disruption of blood vessels occur more readily in very short exposure times; that is, long-pulsed and Q-switched ruby laser lesions, produced in milliseconds and nanoseconds respectively, have a much higher incidence of hemorrhage than do lesions made by argon laser or xenon arc photocoagulation.

Third, because the three lights sources used in photocoagulation have different wavelengths, they are not equally well absorbed by hemoglobin and melanin pigment. Light emitted by the argon laser is the best source for obliterating retinal vessels. Inasmuch as both xenon and argon light are absorbed by malanin, both are effective sources for coagulating choroidal vessels. Light emit-

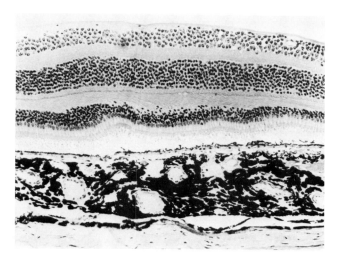

Fig. 3-5. Immediate histopathologic changes in retina of rhesus monkey following ruby laser photocoagulation show pyknotic nuclei of outer nuclear layer, edema of rods and cones, and slight dispersion of retinal pigment epithelium. Inner retinal layers are well preserved.[5]

ted by the ruby laser is absorbed poorly by hemoglobin; thus, the ruby laser is a poor light source for coagulating blood vessels.

HISTOPATHOLOGIC CHANGES
Ruby laser

Histopathologic changes observed immediately following ruby laser photocoagulation consist of pyknotic nuclei of the outer nuclear layer, edema of the rods and cones, slight pigment dispersion of the retinal pigment epithelium, and reduced basophilic staining of the retinal pigment epithelium with the periodic acid-Schiff, alcian blue, and toluidine blue preparations (Fig. 3-5).[5] The inner retinal layers are undisturbed. Bruch's membrane is usually well preserved. The choriocapillaris is difficult to evaluate in the rhesus monkey when the specimen is unbleached, and it is obliterated in lesions in humans (Fig. 3-6). Furthermore, there is a focal choroiditis, but the large choroidal vessels remain patent. The choriocapillaris is affected by the heat produced when the light of the ruby laser is absorbed by the overlying retinal pigment epithelium. In some lesions, the retinal pigment epithelium is adherent to the sensory retina; in the adjacent untreated areas, there is an artifactual detachment of the retinal pigment epithelium from the overlying sensory retina, as usually occurs in preserved specimens (Fig. 3-7).[4]

A ruby laser lesion 3 weeks after photocoagulation shows thinning of the outer nuclear layer, with pyknotic nuclei, destruction of the rods and cones, and

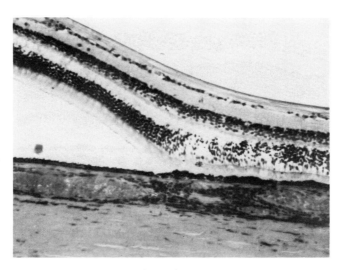

Fig. 3-6. Human retina 92 hours after exposure to ruby laser shows lesion with distinct margin, dispersion and pyknosis of outer nuclear layer, edema of rods and cones, edema of retinal pigment epithelium, and occlusion of choriocapillaris.[4]

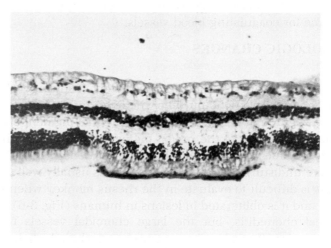

Fig. 3-7. Adhesion of retinal pigment epithelium to sensory retina noted at site of lesion.[4]

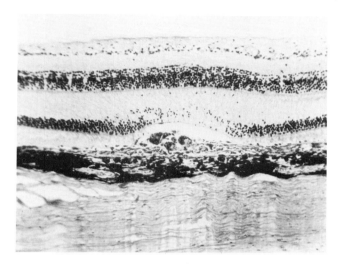

Fig. 3-8. Lesion 3 weeks after ruby laser photocoagulation of rhesus monkey retina shows thinned outer nuclear layer with pyknotic nuclei, destruction of rods and cones, and hyperplasia of retinal pigment epithelium.[5]

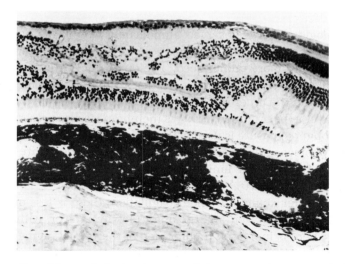

Fig. 3-9. Immediate histopathologic changes of rhesus monkey retina following Zeiss xenon arc photocoagulation show marked pyknosis of outer nuclear layer, edema, and disruption of rods and cones, outer nuclear layer, outer plexiform layer, and inner nuclear layer.[5]

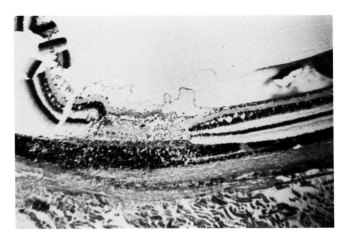

Fig. 3-10. Histopathologic appearance of rhesus monkey retinal lesion, seen immediately after xenon arc photocoagulation with exposure time 1 sec longer than lesion in Fig. 3-9, shows disruption of all retinal layers.[5]

hyperplasia of the retinal pigment epithelium (Fig. 3-8).[5] There is no inflammation, and the inner retinal layers are preserved.

Xenon arc

Histopathologic changes observed immediately after xenon arc retinal photocoagulation, where ruby- and xenon-produced lesions were comparable ophthalmoscopically, are more pronounced. The outer nuclear layer shows marked pyknosis. There is edema of the rods and cones, the outer nuclear layer, the outer plexiform layer, and the inner nuclear layer (Fig. 3-9). The nerve fiber layer and ganglion cell layer appear normal. Bruch's membrane is also preserved. However, when a 1-sec longer exposure is used without changing the power or the spot size of the xenon photocoagulator, marked destruction of the entire retina occurs with rupture of the internal limiting membrane and probable heating of the overlying vitreous (Fig. 3-10).[5]

Three weeks after xenon arc photocoagulation, there is loss of the rods and cones, the outer nuclear layer, and the outer plexiform layer, with resultant retinal thinning. There is increased proliferation of the retinal pigment epithelium, which extends into the remnants of the outer plexiform layer (Fig. 3-11).[5]

Argon laser

Argon laser photocoagulation lesions were applied to normal human retina in an eye to be removed for melanoma. Lesions were made with settings of 500-μm diameter, 500 mW of power, and 0.1 sec; and 50 μm, 100 mW, 0.2 sec. The settings selected are frequently used in laser photocoagulations. Photocoagulation was performed both 1 week and 72 hours prior to enucleation, to observe early

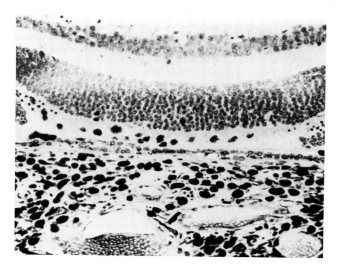

Fig. 3-11. Three weeks after xenon arc photocoagulation, lesion of rhesus monkey retina shows loss of outer retinal layers, with proliferation of retinal pigment epithelium extending into remaining outer plexiform layer.[5]

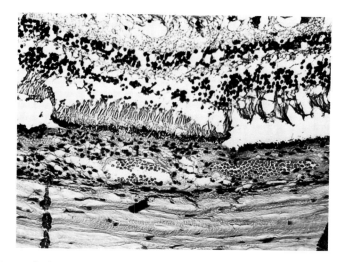

Fig. 3-12. Histopathologic appearance of human retina 72 hours after argon laser retinal photocoagulation with 500-μm spot, 500 mW, and 0.1 sec shows adhesion of retinal pigment epithelium to sensory retina, edema and disruption of outer nuclear and of rod and cone layers, and focal choroidal invasion of choroid. Inner retinal layers are undisturbed.[1]

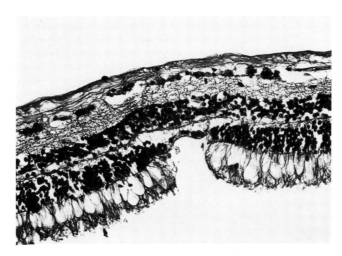

Fig. 3-13. Histopathologic appearance of human retina 1 week after argon laser photocoagulation with settings of 50-μm spot, 100 mW, and 0.2 sec shows focal loss of outer nuclear layer and of rods and cones, with intact inner retinal layers.

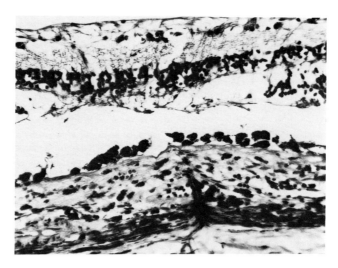

Fig. 3-14. Histopathologic appearance of human retinal lesion 1 week after argon laser photocoagulation with 500-μm spot, 500 mW, and 0.1 sec shows loss of outer retinal layers; hyperplasia of retinal pigment epithelium is artifactual. Inner retinal layers are normal.[1]

and moderately late histopathologic changes. In the early lesion, there is disruption of the outer nuclear layer, edema of the rods and cones, and adherence of the retinal pigment epithelium to the sensory retina (Fig. 3-12).

After 1 week, the outer nuclear layer and the rods and cones have disappeared, and there is hyperplasia of the retinal pigment epithelium. The inner retinal layers are preserved. The choriocapillaris is obliterated, and the choroidal infiltrate of the inflammatory cells is resolved (Figs. 3-13 and 3-14). Lesions observed in an autopsy specimen 2 years after panretinal photocoagulation for proliferative diabetic retinopathy do not differ significantly from the one described 1 week after treatment (Fig. 3-15).

Even though the argon laser is best suited to treating retinal vessels, the obliteration of retinal vessels is difficult. As shown in Fig. 3-16, a major vessel remains patent 1 month after attempting to occlude it with four-times-threshold energy. (A threshold lesion is one with minimally perceptable retinal edema 1 hour after photocoagulation). Note the migration of retinal pigment epithelium into the perivascular zone. With ten-times-threshold energy, a retinal vessel is obliterated (Fig. 3-17).

The obliteration of retinal vessels and of choroidal vessels is achieved with different photocoagulation techniques. In order to occlude a retinal vessel, a 50-μm spot diameter is used, with 100- to 200-mW power at 0.2 sec. In order to avoid creating a choroidal hemorrhage, which can occur with these settings, particularly in a monkey, the surgeon should first place large-spot-size lesions (200 μm,

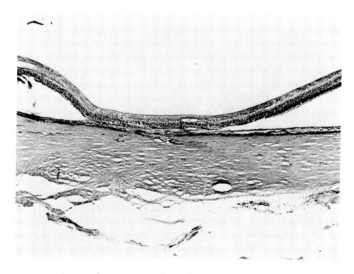

Fig. 3-15. Autopsy specimen shows argon laser lesion in human retina 2 years after panretinal photocoagulation. Histopathologic appearance is similar to that described in Fig. 3-14, in which the lesion was observed 1 week after photocoagulation.

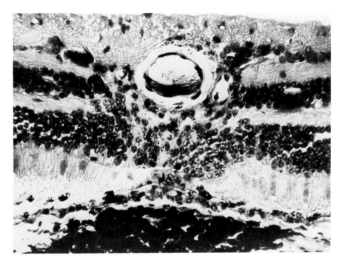

Fig. 3-16. Major retinal vessel in rhesus monkey remains patent 1 month after attempted closure with a four-times-threshold argon laser burn.[3]

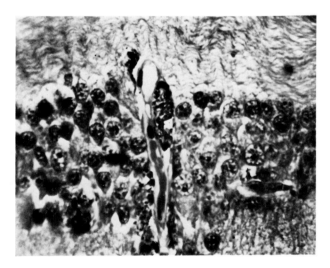

Fig. 3-17. Histopathologic appearance of retinal vessel in rhesus monkey, seen 2 weeks after photocoagulation with a ten-times-threshold lesion, shows migration of pigment epithelial cells around occluded vessel.[3]

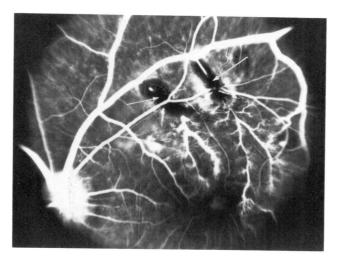

Fig. 3-18. Fluorescein angiogram taken 3 weeks after experimentally induced branch retinal venous occlusion in rhesus monkey shows two obstructed venules *(arrows)* with venous distension and capillary dilation that extends into fovea. Note early collateral channel temporal to macula.[2]

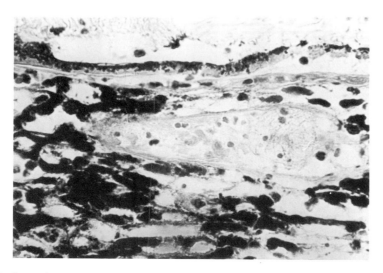

Fig. 3-19. Coagulative necrosis of choriocapillaris and large choroidal vessel in rhesus monkey is present immediately after intense argon laser photocoagulation burn made with 500 μm, 400 mW, and 4 sec.[2]

with 200 mW at 0.1 sec; or 500 μm, with 400 mW at 0.1 sec) along the vessel where it is to be treated. This is done to create a reflecting white background, produced by the retinal edema from photocoagulation. This procedure minimizes coagulation of the choroid and choroidal hemorrhage. Thereafter, the 50-μm spot can be focused on the retinal vessel to be occluded. An experimental branch retinal vein occlusion is produced by this technique (Fig. 3-18).[2]

When obliterating choroidal vessels, large spot sizes are recommended, with high power and long exposure times. Typical settings include 200 μm, 400 to 500 mW, 0.2 to 0.5 sec; or 500 μm, 700 to 800 mW, 0.2 sec. With similar settings, coagulative necrosis of the choriocapillaris and of the large choroidal vessels can be produced (Fig. 3-19).[2] These settings are applicable when treating subretinal neovascular membranes, as occur in presumed histoplasmic choroiditis and senile choroidal macular degeneration.

In conclusion, one should select the energy source for photocoagulation and the instrument settings (spot size, power, and exposure time) that will produce the desired histopathologic lesion. Hence, understanding of histopathology should improve the treatment techniques of the photocoagulator.

REFERENCES

1. Little, H. L. In Francois, J., editor: Symposium on light-photocoagulation, Ghent, June 15-16, 1972, The Hague, 1973, W. B. Junk.
2. Little, H. L., and Zweng, H. C. In L'Esperance, F. A., Jr., editor: Current diagnosis and management of chorioretinal diseases, St. Louis, 1977, The C. V. Mosby Co.
3. Rosan, R. C., Zweng, H. C., et al.: Pathology of retinal argon laser lesions, Inv. Ophthalmol. **6:**669, 1967.
4. Zweng, H. C., Flocks, M., and Peabody, R. R.: Histopathology of human ocular laser coagulations, Arch. Ophthalmol. **76:**11, 1966.
5. Zweng, H. C., Little, H. L., and Peabody, R. R.: Laser photocoagulation and retinal angiography, St. Louis, 1969, The C. V. Mosby Co.

4

PREPARATION OF PATIENT

Preparation of the patient for treatment with argon laser photocoagulation begins with a complete examination of the eye, including the taking of a complete history of visual symptoms, with emphasis on chief complaint and present illness, past ocular history, past general medical history, family history of eye diseases or general diseases with possible eye manifestations, medicines the patient is taking, and any known allergies, including specific inquiry regarding reactions to fluorescein dye injection. Physical examination includes the standard eye examination parameters: distant and near visual acuity, with and without correction. The Amsler grid examination of each eye is most important in all macular problems. External ocular abnormalities are noted; pupil size and reflexes are recorded. Visual field determination is made using the tangent screen before the retina is examined, because of the deleterious effect of funduscopy light on the visual field of sick retinas. Goldmann perimetry is carried out on eyes in which a continuing visual field record is needed, whether the eyes are treated or not. All treated eyes are examined with the Goldmann perimeter. Slit-lamp examination of the anterior segment and anterior vitreous is carried out. Applanation intraocular pressure determination is deferred if an indication for fluorescein angiography is expected, and the pictures taken within a few hours after the tension determination. Retinal photography is compromised at least a little by the effect of topical anesthetics on the corneal epithelium for 2 to 3 hours. Ocular tensions should be recorded before and after pupil dilation, after angiography is completed. Anticipating the need for fluorangiography, we heed Lee Allen's[1] advice for obtaining mydriasis: 1% cyclopentolate hydrochloride (Cyclogyl) and 10% phenylephrine hydrochloride (Neo-Synephrine), in a *viscous* solution, one drop of each every 5 minutes three times. Pupils difficult to dilate sometimes require more applications. Funduscopic examination by indirect and direct ophthalmoscopy is carried out; slit-lamp funduscopy through the corneal diagnostic contact lens is deferred until after intravenous fluorography is done, if that procedure is to be carried out.

Intravenous fluorescein angiography is done unless the suspected pathologic condition is peripheral retinal degeneration; 5 ml of a 10% solution or 3 ml of a

25% solution of fluorescein are injected. Before the procedure is performed, the patient should be advised of the possible side effects of intravenous fluorescein injection. We have carried out over 20,000 intravenous fluorescein examinations, and only one patient has had a serious reaction. The side effects are, from lesser to greater severity, as follows:

1. *Invariable yellowing of the skin,* lasting 1 to 2 hours.
2. *Invariable marked increase in yellow color of the urine,* lasting from 1 to 3 days; in diabetics with renal disease, this effect can last longer.
3. *Nausea,* usually lasting about 2 minutes. The incidence of nausea has decreased in the last several years from approximately 5% to 1% in our experience. If the patient has had previous nausea or vomiting, injecting the dye more slowly, 1 to 2 minutes, usually minimizes or abolishes this symptom.
4. *Vomiting.* About one patient in five who have nausea vomits, an overall incidence of 0.2%.
5. *Hives.* This symptom usually develops within 30 minutes after the dye is injected, but can develop several hours later. Chlorpheniramine maleate (Chlor-Trimeton), 8 mg given by mouth 1 hour before injection of the dye, usually prevents hives. If the hives are very bothersome, an intramuscular injection of 1 ml of 1:1,000 solution of epinephrine (Adrenalin) is helpful if there is no systemic contraindication to its use.
6. *Toxic reactions,* such as fever, muscular aches and pains, or severe headache, can last for several days. If these symptoms are encountered, 100 mg of hydrocortisone succinate (Solu-Cortef) is given intramuscularly and the patient is hospitalized and observed. If further dye injections are required, the patient should be given 100 mg of prednisone orally, 12 hours before, 8 mg Chlor-Trimeton Repetab 1 hour before, and 100 mg of Solu-Cortef intramuscularly 30 minutes before the procedure is carried out. We have had one patient with this symptom complex, who required six fluorescein injections; although there were no serious aftereffects, her discomfort lasted 24 to 36 hours.
7. *Anaphylactoid reaction.* If a patient has had any severe symptoms previously, such as vasomotor collapse and syncope, *intravenous fluorescein is contraindicated.* If such a reaction occurs unexpectedly, an airway must be established, oxygen supplied by means of a face mask, and 1 ml of 1:1,000 epinephrine given. Medical personnel must be prepared to give external cardiac massage and mouth-to-mouth resuscitation until the patient can be moved to a hospital by ambulance. We have seen one such reaction, from which the patient recovered without any residual sequellae.
8. *Death.* Several deaths have occurred throughout the world after intravenous fluorescein injection.[2,3] Many patients who require fluorangiography may have a cardiovascular status distinctly below normal, especially diabetics and elderly patients with senile macular degeneration. Therefore, both physician and photographer must carefully and calmly explain to the

patient what he can expect during the procedure and support him throughout it.

9. *Pregnancy.* Although fetal toxic effects have not been reported from fluorescein injections into the mother, most ophthalmologists do not give the dye to a pregnant woman. If fluorangiography is deemed absolutely necessary, it should be postponed beyond the first trimester, the period of greatest danger to the developing fetus.

Because of the remote danger of severe reaction to fluorescein injection, a physician should remain in the area where the angiogram is taken for at least 30 minutes after the injection is given. He need not remain at the patient's side, but should be able to respond to the photographer's call for assistance within several minutes.

The following should be kept in or near the photography room for use in case of serious reaction to fluorescein injection:

1. Tank of oxygen with a face mask attached
2. Airway
3. Tray containing—
   a. Epinephrine (Adrenalin), 1:1000 solution
   b. Aminophylline solution
   c. Hydrocortisone succinate (Solu-Cortef)
   d. Sterile syringes and needles for intramuscular or intravenous administration of medications
   e. Ammonia inhalant capsules
4. Oral antihistaminic (Chlor-Trimeton or Ornade)
5. Stretcher or gurney with blanket

In our experience, the incidence of serious side effects from intravenous injections of fluorescein is extremely low—low enough that it probably ranks among the safest investigative procedures in medicine. Certainly patients must be advised of possible side effects, so that they can intelligently accept or reject the ophthalmologist's advice to submit to the procedure. The ophthalmologist should assure patients that the recommended examination is a *photographic,* not a *radiologic,* procedure. Some ophthalmologists present the possible side effects to the patients in writing and ask them to acknowledge their understanding of the risks involved by signing a consent form. To date, we have not required such written consent, but a verbal explanation must be given and verbal consent must be obtained.

After the fluoroangiogram is taken, the retinal examination is completed with slit-lamp funduscopy and fluorescein angiography using indirect ophthalmoscopy.

If the ophthalmologist recommends to a patient that his disease be treated with argon laser photocoagulation, an explanation of the nature of the treatment is in order. Several techniques, including a tape recording, written or verbal explanation, or a combination of these, can be used to clarify the procedure to the patient and accompanying family members or friends. (An example of a tape recording explaining argon laser photocoagulation treatment for diabetic retinopathy is given at the end of this chapter.) The discussion of the proposed treatment should be complete enough to satisfy all questions the patient and his family have. The degree of detail will vary with the patient's interest and sophistication. Points to be covered include—

1. *Nature of the disease process.*
2. *Natural history* of the disease process.
3. *Object of treatment—*
   a. Stabilization of vision
   b. Improvement of vision
   c. Prevention of visual loss, short of that expected by the natural course, even though the ophthalmologist expects vision will deteriorate further after treatment.
4. *What photocoagulation does:* changes light energy to heat in order to destroy abnormal structure or tissue or create a retinal scar.
5. *Reassurance* that laser energy is light energy, not ionizing radiation.
6. *Discussion* of possible complications. The patient should be warned that vision may be made worse by treatment. Specifically, he should be warned of the possibility of retinal and vitreal hemorrhage or inadvertent burning of the fovea. The patient should be warned about other complications, depending on the disease entity, as discussed in subsequent chapters (e.g., macular edema after panretinal photocoagulation in proliferative retinal disease).
7. *Expected course of treatment:*
   a. Duration
   b. Number of treatment sessions
   c. Frequency of treatment sessions.
8. *Visual fluctuations* during and after treatment.
9. *Pain during and after the procedure.* Lengthy procedures, as in panretinal photocoagulation, can give eye pain near the end of the treatment session and a headache for several hours after it is over. Enteric-coated sodium salicylate (aspirin), 600 mg, 30 minutes before the procedure usually prevents or ameliorates these symptoms.
10. *Recurrence.* Even if photocoagulation therapy is successful, the patient's problem can recur. Treatment is designed to rid the patient of a specific threat to vision, not to cure the underlying pathologic condition that gave rise to the immediate threat.
11. *Failure.* The patient must be advised that in spite of treatment, vision may decrease; the procedure may be ineffectual.

Above all, the patient must understand that he incurs certain risks with treatment and that no guarantees of success can be given. If he accept the physician's recommendation, the patient signs a permit for surgery, after he has had an opportunity to ask any questions about the recommended treatment. We use the permit reproduced in Fig. 4-1.

PALO ALTO RETINAL MEDICAL GROUP, INC.

– ARGON LASER PHOTOCOAGULATION CONSENT FORM –

PATIENT'S NAME: ______________________________ DATE: ______________

DESCRIPTION OF PROCEDURE TO BE UNDERTAKEN:
ARGON LASER PHOTOCOAGULATION OF THE __________ EYE FOR ______________

____

____

EXPLANATION OF LASER TREATMENT AND RISKS

The laser provides a source of very concentrated light energy. The beam of the argon laser is a bright green color. In medical uses of the laser, the light energy of the laser beam is absorbed by the tissue which is treated, and the light energy is changed into heat energy. The heat energy cauterizes or welds the tissue. In the retina, the laser light beam is used to destroy parts of the retina that are diseased. Small scars are produced in the retina which replace the diseased areas. Because the green light of the argon laser is well absorbed by any red colored substances, it is well absorbed by the abnormal blood vessels which occur in diabetic retinopathy. The argon laser is used to provide benefits in this and in many other retinal diseases.

Usually very little pain is experienced during the laser treatment. If you should experience pain, the strength of the beam or the length of the exposure time can be altered by the physician so that discomfort is minimized.

The eye may be uncomfortable after treatment. Vision is occasionally blurry or blotchy for days to weeks after treatment.

If this technique is applied to your eye, you should be aware of some possible risks of the procedure. As with any operation, complications are possible. Some of the possible complications include:

1. Destruction of visual cells in the center of the retina called fovea, which produces a blind spot in the center of vision.
2. Bleeding from the retina, which may cause reduced vision.

____
Signature of Physician

PATIENT CONSENT

The above explanation has been read by/to me and my questions regarding the treatment and its risks have been answered. I agree to undergo argon laser photocoagulation in my __________ eye.

Although I understand that unforeseen results may occur, I authorize Robert L. Jack, M.D., Hunter L. Little, M.D., H. Christian Zweng, M.D. to perform this procedure. I fully understand that in his best judgment, the potential benefits outweight the risks and give me the best opportunity for maintenance or restoration of sight.

______________________________ ______________________________
Signature of Patient *Signature of Witness*

Fig. 4-1. Argon laser photocoagulation consent form. The physician signs this form and gives it to the patient for him and his family to read before the planned procedure is carried out so he can ask any questions that arise. If the patient agrees to the operation, he signs the form. Although anyone may witness the patient's signing (e.g., nurse or laser room technician), witnessing by a family member is best.

Sedation is required for some patients, especially if the procedure is likely to be lengthy (e.g., as in panretinal photocoagulation in diabetic retinopathy). Diazepam (Valium), 5 mg, administered orally 30 minutes before treatment, usually allays apprehension.

Corneal anesthesia is required with use of the contact lens through which treatment is given. Proparacaine hydrochloride 1% (Ophthaine) is quick, effective, and lasts about 30 minutes.

Retrobular anesthesia is usually not needed. However, it should be considered for patients with (1) extreme photophobia; (2) very low pain threshhold; (3) subretinal neovascular membrane in or close to the fovea; or (4) retinal pigment epithelial disease close to the fovea, especially if close inferiorly because Bell's phenomenon makes a close location just below the macula especially dangerous. If a retrobulbar anesthetic is given, a 1½-inch #23 Atkinson needle should be used to minimize the danger of retrobular hemorrhage. If placed in the muscle cone, 2 ml of either 2% or 4% lidocaine (Xylocaine) gives a satisfactory sensory and motor block.

The patient's head usually should be restrained gently in the slit-lamp rest with an elastic strap around the occiput.

At the end of treatment and after the ophthalmologist has removed the contact lens, he should inspect the corneal epithelium through the slit lamp. If a corneal abrasion has developed, it should be treated in the usual fashion with two eye pads firmly taped on the closed lids.

After treatment is completed, the 1% solution of methyl cellulose used with the contact lens should be irrigated out of the eye. If the procedure has been lengthy (over 15 minutes), the eye is patched, again with two eye pads.

Postoperative instructions vary with the disease process treated. In general, if the retina treated harbors no neovascularization (e.g., vascular proliferative retinopathy or subretinal neovascularization), the patient may continue his activities without modification. If the retina contains neovascularizations, the patient must be instructed to avoid (1) the effect of gravity on the vessels, by not lowering his head below heart level and by sleeping with his head elevated, which he can accomplish by placing a piece of 4-by 4-inch lumber under his mattress across the top of the bed; and (2) the Valsalva effect, which will subject the treated and therefore vulnerable vessels to increased intraluminal pressure, making hemorrhage more likely.

Postoperative analgesia is not necessary for short procedures, but occasionally sodium salicylate, 600 mgm, is needed after longer sessions. Rarely, meperidine (Demerol), 50 mg taken orally, is required.

As with all medical treatments and procedures, there is no substitute for communication with the patient before, during, and after treatment, in terms that he and his family understand. Time and energy spent in patient education are never wasted and are always appreciated by the patient and his family.

TAPED EXPLANATION OF ARGON LASER PHOTOCOAGULATION TREATMENT OF DIABETIC RETINOPATHY

Your doctor has recommended to you that you undergo a treatment called argon laser photocoagulation of your eye for the sake of your vision. Photocoagulation is a process in which a beam of light is focused on your retina, the delicate membrane that lines the inside of the back half of your eye. The retina is about the thickness and consistency of a single sheet of wet Kleenex. It contains cells that change light energy into nerve impulses that travel to the brain, where they are assembled in a mosaic so that you can see images.

Your retina has been damaged by diabetes. Without treatment, you probably will lose vision. However, this is not true in all cases like yours; some cases don't progress. However, visual loss is common enough that your specialist advises treatment rather than allow the natural course of the disease to continue.

The laser beam is an intense light. It is not an X ray. The light energy from the laser is absorbed by pigment and changed to heat. This creates a burn and later a scar. The scar is usually very small because the spot of light used for this purpose is very small. It is hoped that the light beam will burn out the diseased portion of the retina, thus saving your vision from further decline. Sometimes vision improves after this course of treatment; sometimes it remains the same; sometimes it continues to deteriorate.

The technique sometimes involves sealing of leaks from abnormal blood vessels and other structures in the retina. Another technique used destroys the new abnormal blood vessels, which tend to bleed easily, by focusing the beam directly on them. In a third technique, these new blood vessels are treated by an indirect method, which we call panretinal photocoagulation (PRP). In this technique, many exposures of light are focused on the retina to destroy carefully part of the diseased retina. Therefore, areas are very carefully selected that are not in the center of vision but at the side. This technique usually results in a little loss of peripheral vision. Some patients don't notice this, but some do, especially at night.

After you are seated in front of the argon laser phtocoagulator, your chin will be supported by a rest, as will your forehead. A light restraining strap will be placed around the back of your head to keep it well positioned. Drops of anesthetic will be put in your eyes, so you will not feel the diagnostic contact lens that must be placed on your eye for the treatment. The physician will examine your retina first, with a light through the slit lamp, an instrument that permits him to look at the back of your eye through the diagnostic contact lens. He will tell you where to look and will warn you that he is about to treat your eye with the laser beam. When he is ready to treat you, his foot will depress a pedal that triggers shining of the beam for a preselected, short time on your retina. The physician often makes several selections of power of the beam, its size, and exposure time as he goes through the treatment. Depending on the technique used, the number of exposures will range anywhere from a very few up to 500 or more. If at any time during the procedure you feel pain, you should let your physician know. Occasionally some patients are sufficiently sensitive to light or the treatment is so close to the center of their retina that they must receive an injection of anesthetic behind the eyeball. This is not common, however.

After the treatment, the nurse will irrigate your eye and apply an eye patch for several hours. Some patients will experience discomfort in the form of an ache in or around the eye. Usually mild painkillers, such as aspirin or Bufferin, will relieve this discomfort. Some diseases and some treatment techniques allow patients to continue their usual daily routine after treatment, but others require that patients take care of themselves in a certain way. Your physician will discuss this with you. It is highly important that you follow his instructions to the letter.

As with any surgical procedure, photocoagulation may have complications. The greatest danger is bleeding, or hemorrhage, in the retina. The blood vessels of diabetic retinopathy are less healthy than normal and therefore likely to bleed. With the absorption of the argon beam by hemoglobin, the vessel wall is intentionally damaged in certain techniques. This leads to a greater possibility of bleeding. A very small hemorrhage can be absorbed without the patient's knowing it was present. But large hemorrhages can interfere with vision very seriously and take many, many months to clear; occasionally, they never clear. Rarely, the treatment will result in the accumulation of fluid in the center of the retina, the macula, the part of the retina that is used for sharp seeing, such as reading. Usually this blurriness clears in a few weeks or months; rarely, the blurriness remains.

We have already mentioned a small amount of loss of side, or peripheral, vision with one of the techniques that is widely used in treating diabetic retinopathy.

Finally, you must appreciate that, even with treatment, your vision might not improve or remain the same, but may worsen. This might be due to the natural course of the disease, but it can also occur as a result of treatment. Loss of vision from treatment is not common, but it is a definite risk that you must know about and be willing to take.

Argon laser photocoagulation is not a cure for your disease. It is designed to rid the retina of changes that threaten vision now. Even if successful, it does not prevent possible recurrence of retinal changes that might require further treatment. Until the nature of diabetic retinopathy is more clearly understood and means are devised to prevent it, physicians will have to treat it with the best means at hand.

Your ophthalmologist wants you to understand your eye problem and the way he intends to treat it. If you have any questions after listening to this tape, he will be happy to answer them.

REFERENCES

1. Allen, L.: Ocular fundus photography, Am. J. Ophthalmol. **57:**13, 1964.
2. Juillard, G.: Personal communication, 1976.
3. Woolf, M.: Personal communication, 1976.

5

DOCUMENTATION

Documentation of patients receiving argon laser photocoagulation therapy is very important. Only by reviewing case histories, preoperative and posttreatment angiograms, and treatment settings will results obtained with photocoagulation treatment improve. Accordingly, we have developed a set of forms for use in recording treatment data.

The record of laser treatment, which is retained in the patient's chart, is shown in Fig. 5-1. It includes columns indicating number of exposures, spot-size diameter, exposure time, and power setting. If any *one* of the three parameters is changed, the number of exposures is recorded and the count begun again with the new settings. At the end of the treatment session, the total number of exposures is recorded under Treatment on the front summary sheet (described below). The ophthalmologist indicates the sites of treatment on the retinal diagram provided. The technique used is indicated, and any complications are noted. This record contains the basic data taken at every laser treatment session.

A summary sheet entitled Argon Laser Photocoagulation (Fig. 5-2), is placed at the front of the patient's record. It is self-explanatory except for Treatment and Comments. Under the former heading, notation is made only that the patient was treated. Notations regarding quiescence, change of classification or diagnosis, changes in the patient's general health, and so forth, are place under Comments.

The Summary Data Sheet Record (Fig. 5-3) is kept separate from the patient's record, in a file classified according to diagnosis. By referring to each classification file, it is possible to identify all patients treated for any given disease and to quickly review all such patients from the standpoint of treatment parameters. We maintain this file in a set of loose-leaf binders kept in the laser treatment room for ready access at any time during patient treatment.

We have developed a form (Fig. 5-4) for use in computerizing the most important aspects of patients who have been treated or observed. This computer record can be modified as one wishes; in its current form, it is reasonably complete and, if used fully, will permit retrieval of a large amount of information in a very short period of time. *Text continued on p. 75.*

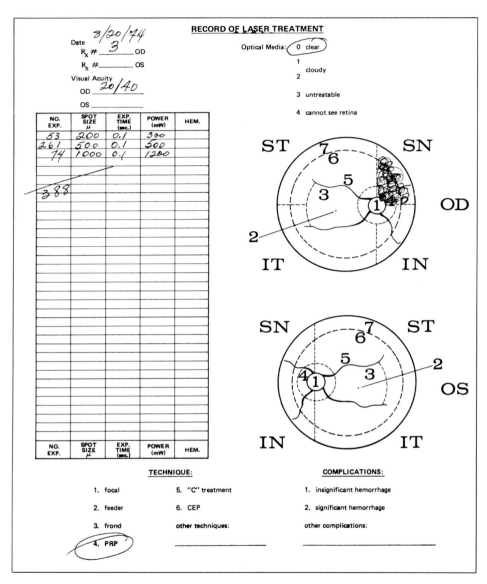

Fig. 5-1. Record of laser treatment. This form is kept in patient's record. Spot-size diameter, exposure time, and power settings are noted. If a hemorrhage occurs, it is noted opposite the settings that were used. Number of exposures for each set of parameters is noted and totaled at end of treatment session. The ophthalmologist indicates on the drawing the area that was treated, clarity of optical media, technique used, and any complications noted.

PALO ALTO RETINAL MEDICAL GROUP, INC.

ARGON LASER PHOTOCOAGULATION

NAME:

GENERAL HEALTH: *mild peripheral neuropathy*
"Borderline" hypertension

AGE: 32   REFERRING DOCTOR:

MEDICATIONS: *Insulin , NPH + reg.*

HISTORY: (ocular & general)
Diabetes Mellitus for 18 yrs. Vision reduced O.D. for 3 mos. ±
No previous photocoagulation Rx.

DX: (& comments)
Diabetic retinopathy , gr. IIB, O.D. ; gr. II B OS.

PHOTO # 1970

DATE	TREATMENT			OD	OS	COMMENTS
			Visual Acuity (corrected)			
8.15.74	Argon laser photocoag. OD	①		20/40	20/20+	Mild vitreous "H" O.D. B4 Rx
8.17.74	" " "	②				
8.20.74	" " "	③				Media now clear O.D.
8.22.74	" " "	④				
9.2.74	" " " OS	①				Valium . 5mgm , B4 Rx
9.5.74	" " "	②				
9.7.74	" " "	③				
9.10.74	" " "	④				
11.2.74	EXAM			20/30	20/25 -1	Vitreous "H" O.D. cleared. Mild bilateral macular edema. Angios taken O.U.
1.16.75	EXAM			20/25	20/25 +1	Macular edema cleared Glial tissue has replaced disc neovascularization. Quiescent O.U.

Fig. 5-2. Argon laser photocoagulation. This sheet is kept on front of patient's eye record, permitting a quick survey of patient's course since treatment began. Not only are treatment sessions recorded, but visits after treatment on which no treatment was given are also recorded.

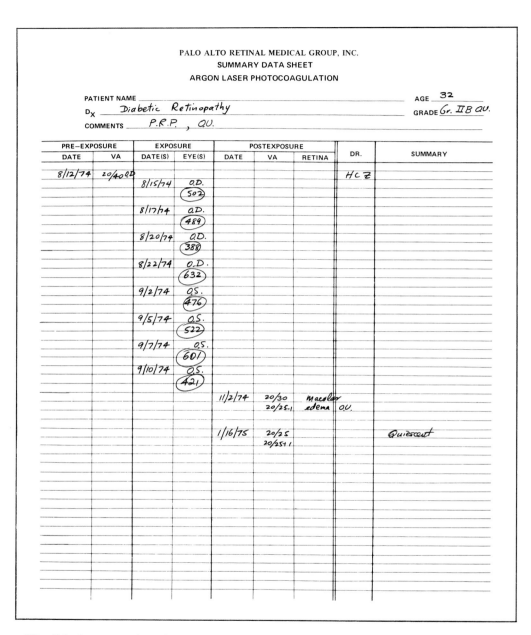

Fig. 5-3. Summary data sheet. This record is kept in loose-leaf folders separate from the patient's record, under diagnosis classifications (e.g., all sheets on patients treated with diabetic disc new vessels are kept together, with subretinal neovascular membranes due to senile maculopathy). This file permits quick review of patients treated, according to diagnosis.

3

NAME _____

Blank = unasked or not done;   U = unknown or undefined;
S = same as previous visit.   (OD = even, OS = odd)

RETINAL RECORD
PALO ALTO RETINAL MEDICAL GROUP
MENLO PARK, CALIFORNIA

SERIAL GENERAL INFORMATION AND EYE EXAM —
GENERAL, SLIT LAMP

		VISIT NUMBER												
		DATE												
GENERAL INFO		**GENERAL PHYSICAL EXAM**												
	3/4	BLOOD PRESSURE (mm Hg)												
	5	BLOOD SUGAR — Glucose fast mg%												
	6	Glucose random mg%												
	7	Glucose 2 hr. P.C. mg%												
	8	normal=0, abnormal=1 Glucose tolerance marginal=2												
		GENERAL MEDICAL INFORMATION												
	10	DIET (number of calories/day)												
	11	URINARY SUGARS — Number of times checked out of 30 days.												

GENERAL MEDICATION: Units (e.g. mgm/cc) should be written following the drug name. Numbers representing the dosage should appear in the flow sheet by total amount administered in AM and by total amount administered in PM. (See codes on page M1.)

		INSULINS (Dose measured in units)	AM	PM	AM	PM	AM	PM	AM	PM	AM	PM	AM	PM
GEN MEDICATIONS	13-15	1)												
	16-18	2)												
	19-21	3)												
		ORAL HYPOGLYCEMIC AGENTS (Dose in mg)												
	22-24	1)												
	25-27	2)												
	28-30	3)												
		OTHER GENERAL MEDICATIONS: List by codes (see page M1). (List dosage and times of administration on page 10.)												
	31	1)												
	32	2)												
	33	3)												

	COMPUTER ENTRY NOS.		OD	OS	OD	OS	OD	OS	OD	OS	OD	OS	OD	OS
EYE EXAM	OD/OS	**EYE EXAM**												
	36/37	**VISUAL ACUITY:** Corrected distance												
	38/39	REFRACTIVE ERROR: Equivalent sphere												
	40/41	VISUAL FIELD: Normal = 0, abnormal = 1,												
	42/43	Central Loss: no = 0, minor = 1, extensive = 2												
	44/45	Concentric Loss: no = 0, if yes % lost												
	46/47	Sectoral Loss: no = 0, if yes % lost												
	48/49	Nerve Fiber Bundle Defect: no=0, if yes % lost												
	50/51	INTRAOCULAR PRESSURE (mm Hg)												
SLIT LAMP		**SLIT LAMP EXAM**												
	56/57	**CONJUNCTIVA:** normal = 0, abnormal = 1												
	58/59	Enter grades. 0 = none, Clumped Cells 1 = slight, 2 = moderate,												
	60/61	3 = severe, 4 = very severe Ischemia												
	64/65	**IRIS:** normal = 0, abnormal = 1												
	66/67	Rubeosis: yes = 1, no = 0												
	70/71	**LENS:** normal = 0, abnormal = 1												
	72/73	Cataract: yes = 1, no = 0												
	74/75	Aphakic: yes = 1, no = 0												
	76/77	Pupillary Membrane: yes=1, no=0												

APRIL, 1974

Continued.

Fig. 5-4. Computer data form. This form is used to record data on patients treated with argon laser photocoagulation, which will be inserted into a computer for ready access, especially for cross-filing information.

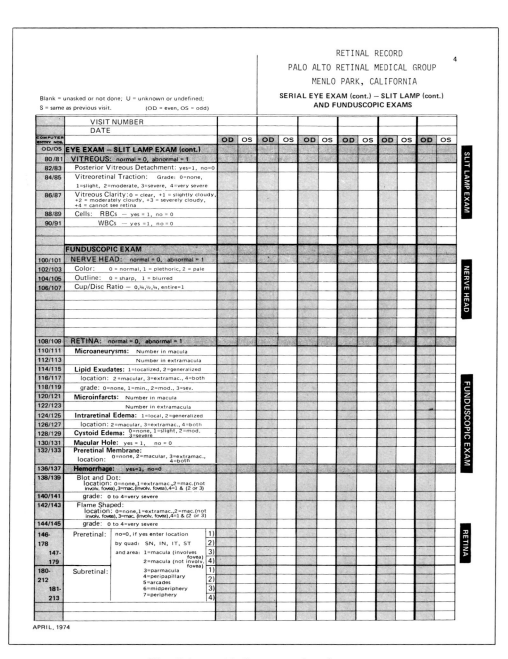

Fig. 5-4, cont'd. Computer data form.

<table>
<tr><td colspan="2">5
NAME _____

Blank = unasked or not done; U = unknown or undefined;
S = same as previous visit.   (OD = even, OS = odd)</td><td colspan="2">RETINAL RECORD
PALO ALTO RETINAL MEDICAL GROUP
MENLO PARK, CALIFORNIA
SERIAL EYE EXAM (cont.) —
FUNDUSCOPIC EXAM (cont.)</td></tr>
</table>

		OD	OS	OD	OS	OD	OS	OD	OS	OD	OS	OD	OS
	VISIT NUMBER												
	DATE												
COMPUTER ENTRY NOS	OD/OS												
	EYE EXAM - FUNDUSCOPIC EXAM (cont.)												
	RETINA (cont.)												
214/215	**Drusen:** 0, 1=few, 2=mod., 3=very many 4=virtually confluent												
216/217	**Pigment Hyperplasia and/or Dispersion**												
	0, +1=slight, +2=mod., +3=severe, +4=very severe												
220/221	**Detachment SR:** yes=1, no=0												
222/223	serous: yes=1, no=0												
224/225	hemorrhagic: yes=1, no=0												
226/227	location: 2=macular, 3=extramac., 4=both												
228/229	foveal involvement: yes=1, no=0												
230/231	size: (disc diameters)												
236/237	**Detachment RPE:** yes (1=single, 2=multiple), no = 0												
238/239	serous: yes=1, no=0												
240/241	hemorrhagic: yes=1, no=0												
242/243	location: 2=macular, 3=extramac., 4=both												
244/245	fibrovascular scar: yes=1, no=0												
246/247	foveal involvement: yes=1, no=0												
248/249	size: (disc diameters)												
254/255	**Inflammation:** yes=1, no=0												
256/257	state: 1=inactive (scar), 2=active												
258/259	If active, enter location & size 1) loc												
260/261	Quad: SN, IN, IT, ST, and size												
262/263	Area: 1, . . . 7 2) loc												
264/265	Size: disc diameters size												
266/267	3) loc												
268/269	size												
270/271	Other locations: yes=1, no=0												
276/277	**ARTERIES:** Normal = 0, abnormal = 1												
278/279	Attenuation: no = 0, 1 = local, 2 = general												
282/283	Corpuscular Flow 1 = local, 2 = general												
284/285	clumping: 0 to 3												
286/287	Occlusion - central: no = 0, old = 1, new = 2												
288/289	Occlusion - branch: no = 0, old = 1, new = 2												
290/291	location: 1 = disc, SN, IN, IT, ST												
292/293	Sheathing: no = 0, yes = 1												
296/297	**VEINS:** normal = 0, abnormal = 1												
298/299	Engorgement: no = 0, 1 = local, 2 = general												
300/301	Tortuosity: no = 0, 1 = local, 2 = general												
302/303	Beading: no = 0, 1 = local, 2 = general												
304/305	Reduplication: no = 0, yes = 1												
306/307	Corpuscular Flow: no = 0, 1 = local, 2 = general												
308/309	clumping: 0 to 3												
310/311	Occlusion - central: no = 0, 1 = old, 2 = new												
312/313	Occlusion - branch: no = 0, 1 = old, 2 = new												
314/315	location: 1 = disc: SN, IN, IT, ST												
316/317	Sheathing: no = 0, yes = 1												

Side labels: RETINA, FUNDUSCOPIC EXAM, ARTERIES, VEINS

APRIL, 1974

Continued.

Fig. 5-4, cont'd. Computer data form.

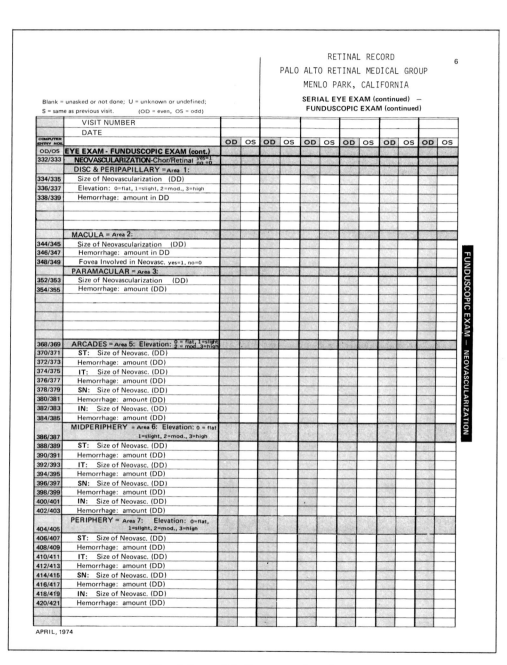

Fig. 5-4, cont'd. Computer data form.

			RETINAL RECORD

PALO ALTO RETINAL MEDICAL GROUP

MENLO PARK, CALIFORNIA

7

NAME _____

Blank = unasked or not done; U = unknown or undefined;
S = same as previous visit.   (OD = even, OS = odd)

**SERIAL EYE EXAM (cont.) - FUNDUSCOPIC
EXAM (cont.) AND FLUORESCEIN ANGIOGRAPHY**

PERIPHERAL RETINA / FUNDUSCOPIC EXAM / FLUORESCEIN ANGIOGRAPHY	COMPUTER ENTRY NOS. OD/OS	VISIT NUMBER / DATE / EYE EXAM - FUNDUSCOPIC EXAM (cont.)	OD	OS	OD	OS	OD	OS	OD	OS	OD	OS	OD	OS
		PERIPHERAL RETINA — NON VASCULAR normal=0, abnormal=1												
	438/439													
	440/441	Lattice work degeneration: yes = 1, no = 0												
	442/443	Cobblestone degeneration: yes = 1, no = 0												
	444/445	Tear: yes = 1, no = 0												
	446/447	Holes: yes = 1, no = 0												
	448/449	Dialysis: yes = 1, no = 0												
	450/451	Retinal detachment: yes = 1, no = 0												
	452/453	no=0, rhegmatogenous detach.:												
	454/455	if yes enter: traction detachment:												
	456/457	1=central 2=peripheral exudative detachment:												
	458/459	3=both retinoschisis:												
	460/461	Buckles: yes = 1, no = 0												
	468/469	**TUMORS:** yes = 1, no = 0												
	474/475	**FLUORESCEIN ANGIOGRAPHY:** normal=0 abnormal=1												

Enter <u>source</u> (retinal or choroidal) below. Then enter **INTENSITY (1, 2, 3) OF LEAK** in flow chart corresponding to <u>location</u> of leak in left column. Enter <u>time of onset</u> of fluorescence (time in seconds from appearance of dye at disc to appearance at lesion) in flow chart below intensity.

	COMPUTER ENTRY NOS.		OD	OS	OD	OS	OD	OS	OD	OS	OD	OS	OD	OS
	476/477	**SOURCE** of leakage: 0=none, 1=retinal, 2=choroidal, 3=both												
		DISC & PERIPAPILLARY = area 1 Inten.												
		Time onset												
		MACULA = area 2 Inten.												
		Time onset												
		2.1 (nearest) leak ≥ ½ DD Inten.												
		from fovea Time onset												
		2.2 (nearest) leak < ½ DD Inten.												
		from fovea Time onset												
		2.3 (nearest) leak involving fovea Inten.												
		Time onset												
		PARAMACULA = area 3 Inten.												
		Time onset												
		IVF LEAKAGE IN OTHER AREAS: yes = 1 no = 0 ARCADES=5, MIDPER=6, PER=7, QUADRANTS: SN, IN, IT, ST.												
	566/567	AREAS OF NONPERFUSION: no=0, mac.=2 xmac.=3, both=4												
	568/569	TRANSMITTED FLUORESCENCE: yes = 1 no = 0												
	570/571	NEGATIVE FLUORESCENCE: yes=1, no=0												
	572	IDIOSYNCRATIC REACTIONS: yes = 1 no = 0												
		(write in reaction)												

APRIL, 1974

Continued.

Fig. 5-4, cont'd. Computer data form.

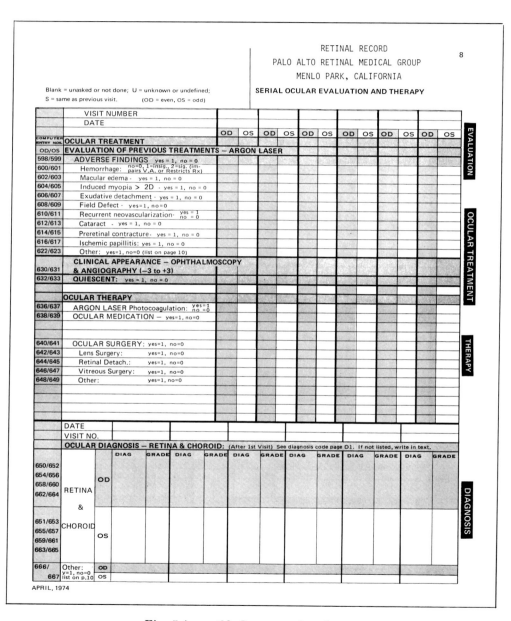

Fig. 5-4, cont'd. Computer data form.

9

NAME _____

Blank = unasked or not done; U = unknown or undefined;
S = same as previous visit.　　(OD = even, OS = odd)

RETINAL RECORD
PALO ALTO RETINAL MEDICAL GROUP
MENLO PARK, CALIFORNIA
SERIAL LAB TESTS AND BLOOD RHEOLOGY

		VISIT NUMBER						
		DATE						
COMPUTER ENTRY NOS.		**LABORATORY TESTS — SCREENING PANEL**						
		Calcium (mg %) 8.5 — 10.5						
		Phosphorous (mg %) 2.5 — 4.5						
	668	Glucose (mg %) 65 — 110 (see p. 3)						
	669	BUN (mg%) 10 — 20						
		Uric acid (mg %) 2.5 — 8.0						
	670	Cholesterol (mg %) 150 — 300						
	671	Total protein (gm %) 6 — 8						
	675	Albumin (gm%) 3.5 — 5.0						
		Total Bilirubin (mg%) 0.15 — 1.0						
		Alkaline phosphatase (mUml) 30 — 85						
		LDH (mUml) 100 — 225						
		SGOT (mUml) 7.5 — 40.0						
	672	TRIGLYCERIDES (TC) (mg%) < 165						
	673	FIBRINOGEN (mg%) 260-500						
	674	**SERUM PROTEIN ELECTROPHORESIS**						
	675	Albumin (gm%) 3.5-5.0						
	676	Alpha 1 Globulin (gm%) 2-4						
	677	Alpha 2 Globulin (gm%) 6-13						
	678	Beta Globulin (gm%) 8-15						
	679	Gamma Globulin (gm%) 10-21						
		COMPLETE BLOOD COUNT (CBC)						
	680	Hgb (gm %)						
		RBC (x 10^6) / mm^3						
	681	PCV (%)						
		WBC (x 10^3) / mm^3						
		URINALYSIS						
	682	Sugar: o, trace=t, 1,2,3,4						
		Casts						
		RBC's						
		WBC's						
	683	Albumin: o, trace=t, 1,2,3,4						
	684	Acetone						
		24 hr. urine protein (gr/24 hr.) 0 — .1						
	685	**BLOOD RHEOLOGY**						
		Rheoscopy (0—5)						
	686	Sedimentation rate: @ 1 hr. (mm) 0—15						
	687	@ 3 hrs.						
	688	Necleopore passage: 5 micron pore						
	689	8 micron pore						
	690	Centrifuge: 1						
	691	2						
	692	Plasma Viscosity						

LABORATORY TESTS (vertical label)

BLOOD RHEOLOGY (vertical label)

APRIL, 1974

Continued.

Fig. 5-4, cont'd. Computer data form.

RETINAL RECORD
10

PALO ALTO RETINAL MEDICAL GROUP

MENLO PARK, CALIFORNIA

PROBLEM-ORIENTED PROGRESS NOTES

Instructions: Notes must be dated and signed. They need not repeat information contained on other pages of this chart. They may include informal comments concerning future plans. Reasons for major therapeutic changes should be fully detailed. Novel observations and significant developments should appear. Problems should be identified by number.

Visit No.	Date	Prob-lem No.	Title of Problem and Progress Note

PROGRESS NOTES

APRIL, 1974

Fig. 5-4, cont'd. Computer data form.

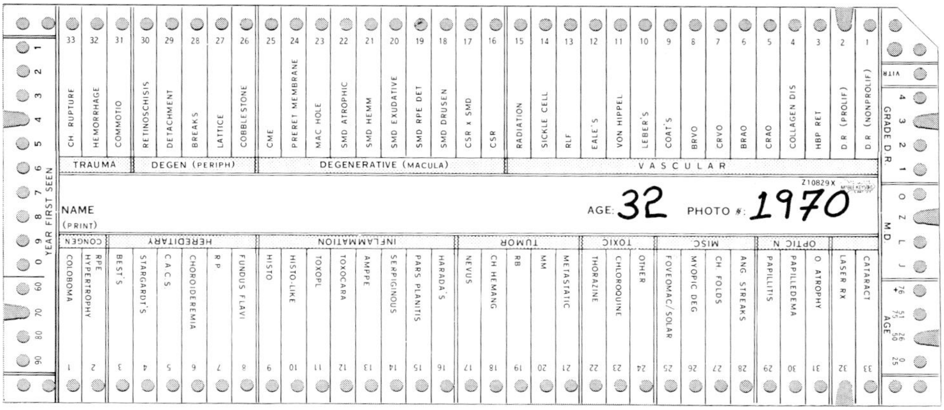

Fig. 5-5. This simple 3¹/₄ by 7¹/₂-inch card is useful in maintaining a diagnostic file, with a minimum of space, work, and expense. As noted in this example, patient is 32 years old, was first seen in 1974, has proliferative diabetic retinopathy on the nerve head (Grade IIB in the authors' classification), and was treated by argon laser photocoagulation.

A much simpler cross-index file, which we have found useful, is shown in Fig. 5-5. When each new patient is seen, a card is prepared listing various conditions diagnosed. When these are punched out, retrieval of the desired cards is very simple, using nothing more complicated than an ice pick, passed through the hole of the parameter that one wishes to sort out. This method of cross-indexing requires a minimum of trained personnel to maintain it and little space to store it.

6

PERIPHERAL RETINAL DEGENERATIVE DISEASES

PERIPHERAL RETINAL BREAKS

The first use made of retinal photocoagulation was creation of a watertight scar around a peripheral retinal break that threatened to develop into a separation of the sensory epithelium. The effectiveness of this treatment is well established,[6,10] but further research has sharpened both the indications and techniques of this treatment form.

The reports of Byer,[1] Straatsma et al.,[9] and Foos,[4] among others, make clear a much higher incidence of peripheral retinal breaks than of sensory retinal separation, leading to the conclusion that by no means does the mere presence of a retinal break constitute an indication for encircling photocoagulation of the break. Undoubtedly, far more breaks have been treated than the natural history indicated needed treatment.

We consider the following to be the indications and contraindications to photocoagulation treatment of peripheral retinal degenerative or traumatic disease:

Indications
1. All breaks that have even a small amount of fluid under the sensory retina; that is, the break must have developed into at least a tiny detachment of the neuroepithelial layer.
2. As a postoperative auxillary to retinal separation surgery. Occasionally after surgery the retinal break will be on the crest of the scleral buckle but not fully on the anterior slope; thus the hole still gapes open, admitting fluid under the sensory retina behind the buckle. Sometimes it is possible to close such a break with photocoagulation.
3. Delimitation of a large retinal separation not yet involving the macula, when surgery must be postponed for any reason. This uncommon indication includes only eyes in which macular vision is still unimpaired, because visual results are usually better when surgery is done before the macular neuroepithelium is also separated. Occasionally, a patient will

76

postpone surgery or be too ill to undergo the planned procedure. Photocoagulation is a temporary measure that may be used in an attempt to protect the macula until definitive surgery can be carried out.

4. Isolation of areas of lattice degeneration containing retinal breaks but without separation of the sensory layer, if either the eye has had an intracapsular lens extraction, has 5 diopters or more of myopia, or the fellow eye has had a retinal separation.

After collapse of the vitreous body, as seen in many older patients, or after an intracapsular lens extraction, the forward-moving vitreous can tear the retina if there is a retinovitreal adhesion, especially where the retina is thinned and weakened, as in retinal tufts and lattice-work degeneration, creating a "fish-mouth" tear or other configuration in which the persistent vitreal tug on the *attached* retinal operculum facilitates passage of liquid vitreous through the tear into the potential space between sensory retina and the retinal pigment epithelial layer. Consequently, the incidence of retinal detachment is higher in aphakic than phakic eyes.[4] However, if the operculum is avulsed form the retina by the tugging force of the anteriorly displaced vitreous, a gaping tear is not created, greatly reducing the danger of retinal separation. Whatever the mechanism, the incidence of separation is definitely higher in aphakic eyes.[5] The well-known higher incidence of retinal separations in an eye contralateral to one that previously sustained a separation[2] bears out the medical aphorism that paired organs tend to suffer the same fate. Similarly, eyes with myopia are known to have a higher incidence of neuroretinal separation.[8] Therefore, a higher index of concern is warranted for eyes with any of the aforementioned characteristics.

Factors unfavorable for use of photocoagulation

1. The separation occupies more than about 1 hour on the clock. A surgical reattachment procedure should be done.

2. The ocular media are too hazy for photocoagulation, due to cornea, lenticular, or vitreal opacities; then transscleral treatment, either cryocoagulation or electrodiathermy, must be given to the break.

3. The separation is already well demarcated by a broad line of pigment. Treatment is unnecessary, because an adhesion between the sensory retina and the pigment epithelium has developed; nature has accomplished the goal of photocoagulation.

4. The pupil cannot be dilated widely enough to permit application of the treatment beam around the break. Transscleral treatment must be given.

5. Flat holes with opercula floating freely over them.

Using these indications and contraindications since May 1969, we have treated 123 eyes with symptomatic retinal breaks, surrounded by at least a small sensory layer elevation, and 11 eyes with retinal breaks without such elevations. All treatment was given with the argon laser slit-lamp photocoagulator, through the three-mirror corneal diagnostic contact lens and with the pupil dilated as widely as possible.

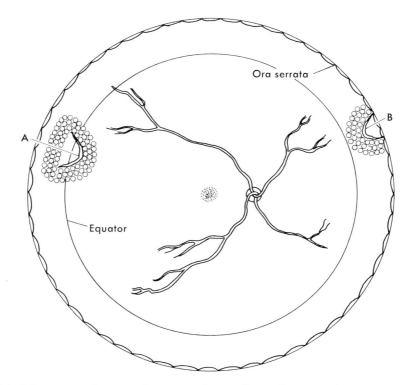

Fig. 6-1. Schematic indicating placement of argon laser photocoagulation lesions around tear in sensory retina at equator *(A)* and at ora serrata *(B)*.

Ideally, a triple row of burns is placed around the break, taking care to coagulate where the sensory and pigment epithelial layers are still in apposition (Fig. 6-1, *A*). No adhesion between these two layers will occur if photocoagulation is given where they are apart. The greatest cause of failure of photocoagulation to delimit a small retinal separation is not coagulating around the *anterior* aspect of the tear. If the break is so far anterior that it is not possible to ring the break, a U-shaped pattern of photocoagulation is used, with the burns placed from ora serrata to ora serrata (Fig. 6-1, *B*). Treatment of tears near or at the ora serrata is facilitated by use of the Eisner scleral depressor with the contact lens[3] (available from Sparta Instrument Co., Fairfield, N.J.) (Fig. 6-2). Usual photocoagulation parameters used are 200- to 500-μm beam diameter, 0.05- to 0.1-sec time exposure, and 300- to 1,000-mW power. All parameters may be varied somewhat, depending on clarity of media, amount of retinal pigment, and obliquity of the beam, to give moderately heavy lesions (Figs. 6-3 to 6-5).

No restrictions are placed on patient activities, except to bar heavy physical exercise, either at work or play (e.g., heavy lifting or tennis) for 2 weeks. All patients are warned about the symptoms of retinal separation:photopsia, showers of black particles before the eye, or both.

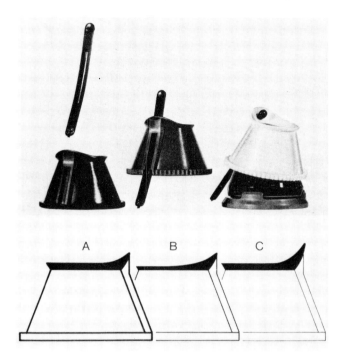

Fig. 6-2. Identation funnel with moveable indenter. This scleral depresser of Eisner is useful with Goldmann 3-mirror contact lens, both to examine the far periphery of retina and to treat it with photocoagulation, especially to surround retinal tear anteriorly with burns. (Courtesy Georg Eisner, Prof. M.D.)

All patients are examined about 2 weeks after treatment, to determine that the photocoagulation lesions adequately surround the break. If they do not, more treatment is given. Patients should be examined annually with indirect ophthalmoscopy with scleral depression or slit-lamp funduscopy through the peripheral mirror of the Goldmann lens.

Since 1969 we have treated 12 eyes with circumferential equatorial prophylactic photocoagulation. This procedure was carried out on two indications:
1. The presence of multiple peripheral retinal breaks, found at the same time or on later examinations, that required photocoagulation based on the previously discussed indications.
2. The presence of lattice degeneration involving at least one quarter of the retinal periphery in an eye with myopia of −5 diopters or more and where the contralateral eye had had a retinal detachment, even if the lattice areas contained no retinal breaks.

All retinal breaks were first treated with a ring of photocoagulations as described above. Circumferential treatment was started at the 2-week postoperative visit. A double row of barely continuous burns was placed at the equator in each quadrant (Fig. 6-6). Treatments were spaced 1 week apart, to minimize the

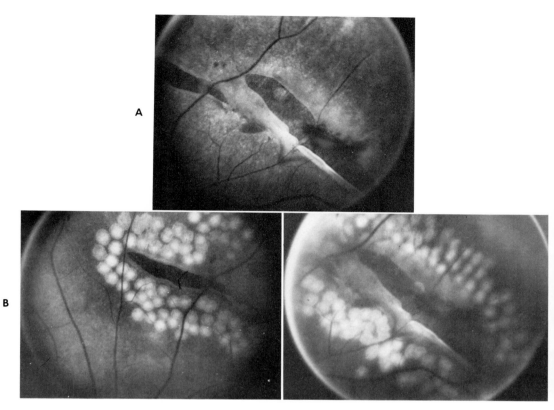

Fig. 6-3. A, Photograph of two traumatic retinal tears in the superotemporal quadrant, left eye, before treatment. **B,** Same eye immediately after argon laser photocoagulation, showing a double to triple row of lesions around the superior tear. **C,** Same eye immediately after argon laser photocoagulation around lower tear.

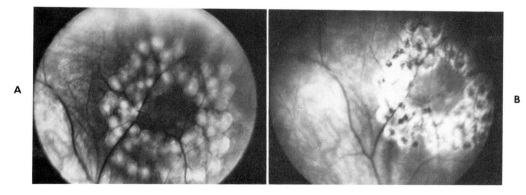

Fig. 6-4. A, Photograph of retinal tear at equator, superotemporal quadrant, right eye, immediately after argon laser photocoagulation, showing double to triple row of lesions. **B,** Same eye 7 weeks after treatment, showing pigmentation that developed in lesions.

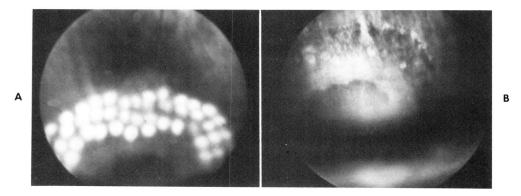

Fig. 6-5. A, Photograph immediately after argon laser photocoagulation around retinal dialysis, left eye. Patient had retinal separation from similar dialysis, right eye. Note double to triple row of photocoagulation lesions from ora serrata to ora serrata. **B,** Same eye 14 days after argon laser photocoagulation, showing pigmented cordon around dialysis.

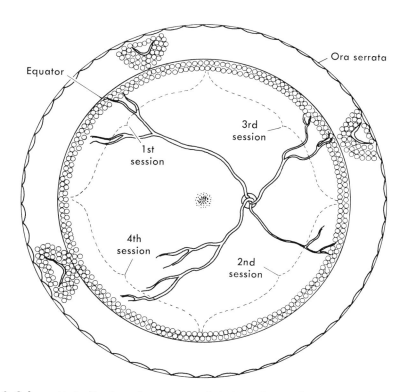

Fig. 6-6. Schematic indicating placement and timing of argon laser circumferential equatorial prophylactic photocoagulation lesions. Treatment sessions are 1 week apart.

Table 6-1. Treatment of retinal breaks

Number of eyes treated	Number of eyes requiring further treatment	Number of eyes with macular complication after photocoagulation treatment
123 with retinal breaks and sensory retinal separation	1	1
11 with retinal breaks without sensory retinal separation	0	0
15 with multiple breaks treated with circumferential equatorial prophylactic photocoagulation	1	0

hazard of maculopathy from treatment. The 15 eyes treated had two to five breaks previously treated. One patient with Marfan's syndrome in whom retinal detachment surgery in the fellow eye had failed developed a neuroretinal separation 2 years after this photocoagulation treatment had been given.

The alternative treatment is the placement of an encircling silicone band at the equator, with circumferential cryotherapy or electrodiathermy at the band site, a procedure more formidable than four weekly outpatient treatments, which do not interfere significantly with the patient's schedule.

Our experience in treating symptomatic retinal breaks from May 1969 to September 1975 is summarized in Table 6-1.

The single eye that required additional nonphotocoagulation therapy (excluding the patient with Marfan's syndrome) was treated with cryocoagulation, because the photocoagulation did not include the anterior lip of the tear and a slight extension of the sensory retinal separation was noted 2 weeks after photocoagulation treatment.

The most common complications of photocoagulation of peripheral retinal breaks are (1) maculopathy, either microcystic macular edema or a preretinal membrane, and (2) vitreous contracture at the edges of the break, resulting in a sensory retinal separation requiring surgery.

The single macular complication in our series was a preretinal membrane, seen about 1 year after photocoagulation treatment, that reduced central vision to 20/50. Although it is questionable that the peripheral treatment caused the maculopathy, this eye is included as a complication of peripheral treatment, an incidence of 0.7%.

RETINOSCHISIS

Retinoschisis rarely presents a threat to central vision by involving the macula. Therefore, treatment is reserved only for those eyes in which the schisis is approaching the macula or gives promise to do so. If the schisis has already reduced central vision or has a hole in its internal layer, it should be treated surgically like a sensory retinal detachment.

The indications we use for photocoagulation are—

1. Retinoschisis that is within 3 disc diameters of the edge of the macula.
2. The presence of holes in both the inner and outer layers of the schisis. If the schisis proceeds through the delimitation, a surgical retinal reattachment procedure must be done.

The technique of argon laser photocoagulation used involves two steps. First, the schisis is delimited by a triple row of lesions placed in intact retina just posterior to the edge of schisis. Because the split in the retina is in the external plexiform layer, photocoagulation must be heavy enough that this layer is included in the final limiting scar. These lesions, therefore, are heavier than needed for limitation of sensory retinal separations from breaks in the retina. Parameters used more peripherally are 500-μm beam diameter, 0.2-sec exposure, and 500-mW power. However, the part of the schisis that is 3 disc diameters or closer to the

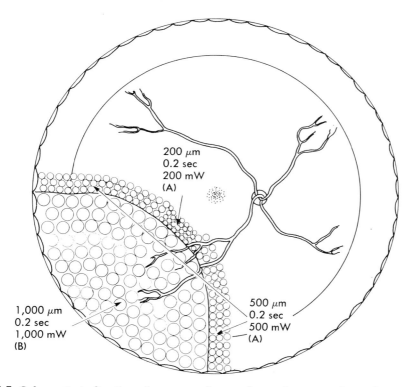

Fig. 6-7. Schematic indicating placement of argon laser photocoagulation lesions in retinoschisis. *A* lesions placed to delimit schisis, *B* to collapse dome of schisis.

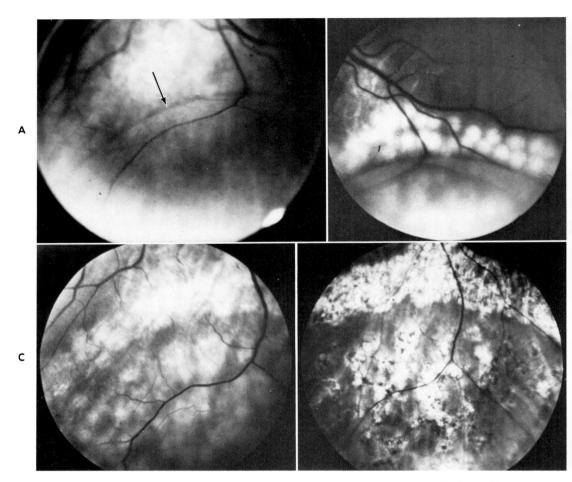

Fig. 6-8. A, Photograph showing inferior retinoschisis, *Arrow,* edge of schisis. **B,** Same eye immediately after argon laser photocoagulation, showing double row of heavy lesions delimiting schisis and lesions placed through dome onto outer leaf of schisis. **C,** Same eye 1 week after treatment, showing reduction of schisis. **D,** Same eye 3 months after treatment, showing complete collapse of schisis. Note continuous trend of pigmented lesions at top of photograph, outlining schisis, and scattered lesions placed through it below.

edge of the macula should not be treated with such parameters, because of possible traction lines across the macula or macular gliosis due to the proximity of relatively heavy photocoagulation. The settings in such a situation are altered to 200-μm beam diameter, 0.2-sec exposure, and 200-mW power (Fig. 6-7, *A*).

Second, the schisis is treated with lesions through the entire dome, with the reaction occuring in the exterior leaf rather than the interior. Settings used are 500 μm, 0.2 sec, and 500 mW or 1,000 μm, 0.2 sec, and 1,000 mW (Fig. 6-7, *B*).

A   B

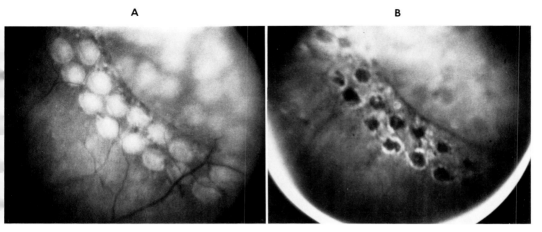

Fig. 6-9. A, Photograph showing retinoschisis in superotemporal quadrant immediately after argon laser photocoagulation. Note double row of heavy lesions and lesions placed through dome onto outer leaf of schisis. **B,** Same eye 5 weeks after treatment, showing band of pigmented scars in front of schisis but with schisis still present despite photocoagulation of dome. Schisis has remained unchanged for 18 months.

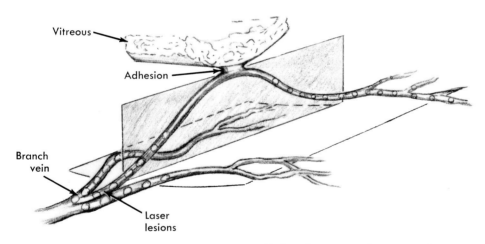

Fig. 6-10. Diagram of peripheral retinal vein pulled up from retina by retracted vitreous to which vein had been adhesed. Photocoagulation lesions must be given to *all* tributaries immediately distal from and proximal to the retracted vein so that it will no longer carry blood.

This technique using xenon arc photocoagulation was originated by Okun and Cibis.[7]

Using these above indications and techniques, we have treated 12 cases of retinoschisis (Figs. 6-8 and 6-9). None has progressed beyond the delimiting scar. In six of the 12, the schisis collapsed with reattachment of the two layers.

RETRACTED VEIN IN RETINAL PERIPHERY

A relatively uncommon finding in the retinal periphery is a normal retinal vein retracted from the plane of the retina by the retracted vitreous to which the vein is adhesed (Fig. 6-10). Unless the retracted vein produces bleeding, no treatment is indicated; however, if bleeding does occur, argon laser photocoagulation is useful in stopping the flow of blood through the vessel. Initial photocoagulation is applied to the various tributary veins, both *distal from and proximal to* the retracted vein. If only the tributaries distal from the retracted vein are closed, blood will reflux up the retracted segment from proximal tributaries. Settings used are 200-μm spot-size diameter, 0.1-sec time exposure, and 300-mW power. These lesions are used to stimulate hyperpigmentation around the vessels that are to be closed with later argon laser photocoagulation. Subsequent treatment is given about 6 weeks after the first session, to give time for the desired hyperpigmentation to develop. The settings of 500 μm, 0.2 sec, and 150 to 200 mW of power are used to go over *all* tributary veins again, as often as needed so that the retracted vein no longer carries blood. As many as six or seven sessions may be required to obtain the desired result. *No attempt* should be made to photocoagulate the retracted vein, because vitreal hemorrhage very likely will occur.

Segmental panretinal photocoagulation should be considered for the area drained by the treated vein to prevent possible retinal neovascularization (see Chapter 14).

SUMMARY

Most eyes with peripheral retinal degenerative disease have excellent central vision. Therefore, only those eyes with vision endangered by their disease (i.e., in danger of a sensory retinal separation or of macular involvement by schisis) should be treated prophylactically, with methods that are effective, produce minimal complications, and cause minor inconvenience to the patient. Our experience indicates that the techniques here described satisfactorily fulfill these criteria.

REFERENCES

1. Byer, N. E.: Clinical study of lattice degeneration of the retina, Mod. Probl. Ophthalmol. **15:**58-67, 1975.
2. Duke-Elder, S., and Dobree, J. H.: System of ophthalmology. X. Diseases of the retina, St. Louis, 1967, The C. V. Mosby Co., p. 795.
3. Eisner, G.: Biomicroscopy of the peripheral fundus, New York, 1973, Springer-Verlag New York Inc.
4. Foos, R. Y.: Tears of the peripheral retina: pathogenesis, incidence, and classification in autopsy eyes, Mod. Probl. Ophthalmol. **15:**68-81, 1975.
5. Hawkins, W. R.: Aphakic retinal detachment, Ophthalmic Surg. **6**(2):66-73, 1975.
6. Meyer-Schwickerath, G.: Light coagulation, St. Louis, 1960, The C. V. Mosby Co.
7. Okun, E., and Cibis, P. A.: The role of photocoagulation in the management of retinoschisis, Arch. Ophthalmol. **72:**309, 1964.
8. Schepens, C. L., and Marden, D.: Data on the natural history of retinal detachment: further characterization of certain unilateral nontraumatic cases, Am. J. Ophthalmol. **61**(2): 213-226, 1966.
9. Straatsma, B. R., et al.: Lattice degeneration of the retina, Trans. Am. Acad. Ophthalmol. Otolaryngol. **78:**87-113, 1974.
10. Zweng, H. C.: Laser photocoagulation in rhegmatogenous retinal separation. In Pruett, R. C., and Regan, C. J., editors: Retina Congress, New York, 1974, Appleton-Century-Crofts.

7

CLASSIFICATION AND INDICATIONS FOR PHOTOCOAGULATION OF MACULAR DISEASES

Clarification of nomenclature and of macular disease syndromes is essential before discussing photocoagulation of macular diseases. Classification of macular diseases can be based on the pathologic findings as visualized during ophthalmologic examination and on histopathologic examination of specimens submitted to the laboratory.[1-3] Differentiation of the terms retinal detachment, retinal edema, and retinal cysts, as applied to the posterior pole of the eye, is required.[4]

Retinal detachment is the separation of the retina from underlying structures, by accumulation of subretinal serous or hemorrhagic fluid or by inflammatory, reactive hyperplastic, or neoplastic cells. The separation can be between the retinal epithelium and Bruch's membrane (retinal pigment epithelial detachment) or between the retinal pigment epithelium and the sensory retina (detachment of the sensory retina), or both separations can exist in the same macula. The detached sensory retina is usually semitransparent, normal in thickness, and without edema; however, with prolonged elevation of the sensory retina, it undergoes edematous changes and cystic degeneration.

Retinal edema is the accumulation of fluid within the retina. This fluid can be intracellular, as manifested in central retinal artery occlusion, where cell death is associated with cell swelling. The fluid can be extracellular from capillary effusion within the retina, as seen in retinal vein thrombosis, diabetic retinopathy, hypertensive retinopathy, and cystoid macular edema in aphakia and chronic uveitis. In both kinds of edema, the retinal thickness is increased and the retinal transparency is decreased.

Retinal cysts are saclike distensions within one of the plexiform layers of the sensory retina and therefore are an exaggerated form of extracellular retinal edema. There is progressive distension within the plexiform layers and oblitera-tion of the adjacent tissues. Rupture of the inner wall of the cyst creates a lamellar retinal hole. Inasmuch as the hole involves only the inner layer of the sensory retina, a rhegmatogenous retinal detachment with accumulation of fluid between the sensory retina and the retinal pigment epithelium cannot occur unless the hole extends through all layers of the sensory retina. Except in macular holes from trauma and in high myopia, macular holes are and usually remain lamellar and therefore do not require treatment with photocoagulation. Occasionally the word cyst is used to describe a retinal pigment epithelial detach-ment (macular cyst). We suggest that cyst be limited to the definition given in this paragraph and retinal pigment epithelial (RPE) detachments be called just that.

The following is a descriptive classification of macular lesions:[2,3]
1. Detachment of sensory retina
   a. Serous
   b. Hemorrhagic
2. Detachment of retinal pigment epithelium
   a. Serous
   b. Hemorrhagic
3. Edema
   a. Intracellular: retinal artery occlusion
   b. Extracellular: cystoid macular edema
      1. Vein occlusion
      2. Diabetes
      3. Hypertension
      4. Aphakia
      5. Chronic uveitis

In addition to a descriptive classification, an etiologic classification of macular diseases is essential:[2]
1. Degenerative
   a. Central serous retinopathy (CSR)
   b. Diffuse retinal pigment epitheliopathy (DRPE)
   c. Senile macular degeneration
   d. Vascular hypertension
   e. Arteriosclerosis
   f. Preretinal membrane contracture
2. Inflammatory
   a. Histoplasmic choroiditis
   b. Histoplasmiclike choroiditis
   c. Toxoplasmosis retinochoroiditis
   d. *Toxocara canis* ocular infestation
   e. Solar retinitis (foveomacular retinitis)
   f. Acute multifocal posterior placoid pigment epitheliopathy (AMPPPE)

    g. Chronic uveitis (including microcystic macular edema after cataract extraction)

3. Metabolic
   a. Diabetes mellitus
   b. Angioid streaks (pseudoxanthoma elasticum and Paget's disease)
   c. High myopia
   d. Heredomacular degenerations (vitelliform, Stargardt's disease, flavimaculatus, and such)
   e. Tapetoretinal degenerations (retinitis pigmentosa)
   f. Cerebromacular degeneration (Tay-Sachs and Niemann-Pick diseases)
   g. Clotting abnormalities (e.g., from estrogen or progesterone medications)
4. Neoplastic
   a. Nevus
   b. Melanoma
   c. Choroidal hemangioma
   d. Metastasis
5. Traumatic: rupture of choroid and Bruch's membrane
6. Toxic maculopathies
7. Congenital anomalies (pit of optic nerve, drusen of the nervehead)

The organization of such a classification is subject to criticism and is certain to change as future knowledge is gained in the understanding of the pathologic physiology of macular diseases. Broad headings of degenerative disorders, inflammatory diseases, metabolic derangements, neoplastic growths, traumatic sequelae, toxic effects, and congenital anomalies are listed. It is debatable whether diabetic retinopathy and its vascular changes should be included under metabolic or under degenerative diseases. Likewise, the various heredomacular diseases, including vitelliform macular degeneration, Stargardt's macular degeneration, flavimaculatus, and retinitis pigmentosa, are included under metabolic disorders, a classification future research may alter. Nonetheless, when viewing the macula, the ophthalmologist is urged to make an accurate description of the macular syndrome in question and to attempt to categorize the syndrome into one of the above-mentioned etiologic groups. Grouping aids in the evaluation of the natural course expected and indications for and expected response to treatment.

The following are criteria for the selection of macular lesions amenable to treatment with photocoagulation:[2]

1. Presence of fluid (serous or hemorrhagic), with localized leakage demonstrated on fluorescein angiography
   a. Intraretinal
   b. Beneath sensory retina
   c. Beneath pigment epithelium
2. Neovascularization
   a. Retinal
   b. Choroidal

Treatment of foveal leakage is usually contraindicated. In all cases, it should be determined whether the natural course of the disease or the scar produced by photocoagulation will produce the greater visual impairment.

Macular diseases that fulfill the above criteria and in which argon laser photocoagulation should be considered are:

1. Central serous retinopathy (CSR)
2. Diffuse retinal pigment epitheliopathy (DRPE)
3. Exudative senile macular degeneration
   a. Serous
   b. Hemorrhagic
4. Histoplasmic choroiditis with subretinal neovascular membrane (SNVM)
5. Angioid streaks with subretinal neovascular membrane (SNVM)
6. Diabetic maculopathy with subretinal neovascular membrane (SNVM)
7. Maculopathy secondary to high myopia with subretinal neovascular membrane (SNVM)
8. Cystoid macular edema (seldom) secondary to aphakia
   a. Aphakia
   b. Branch retinal vein occlusion
   c. Central retinal vein occlusion
9. Congenital pit of optic nerve, with serous detachment of macular sensory retina and drusen of the nervehead with subretinal neovascular membrane (SNVM)
10. Traumatic rupture of choroid and Bruch's membrane with subretinal neovascular membrane (SNVM)

On fluorescein angiography, central serous retinopathy, degenerative retinal pigment epitheliopathy, and serous senile maculopathy show leaks under the retinal pigment epitheliopathy and through a break in the retinal pigment epitheliopathy under the sensory retina. Hemorrhagic senile maculopathy, presumed histoplasmic choroiditis, active angioid streak maculopathy, and Fuchs' spot in high myopia demonstrate subretinal neovascular membranes (SNVM). The maculopathy of diabetes mellitus, chronic branch retinal vein occlusion after cataract extraction, produces serous fluid within the sensory retina. Because the source of fluid under the sensory retina seen with congenital pits of the optic nerve is unknown, it is the only disease entity possibly amenable to argon laser photocoagulation that does not fulfill the above criteria.

Not all cases of the diseases here listed are candidates for argon laser photocoagulation, but all should be seriously considered for such treatment. Each will be discussed separately in subsequent chapters.

Most patients who have macular disease are not candidates for photocoagulation. Included in the nontreatable macular diseases are nonexudative (dry) and cicatricial senile macular degenerations, preretinal membrane contracture, acute multifocal posterior plaquoid pigment epitheliopathy, heredomacular dystrophies, macular holes except holes through the full thickness of the retina as sometimes seen in high myopia and after trauma, and toxic maculopathies.

The prospect of improving or at least retaining some useful central vision is the goal in treating macular diseases with photocoagulation. If treatment destroys foveal vision, that goal will not be achieved, except in a few desperate cases where retention of extrafoveal macular vision appears more likely with treatment than by trusting to the natural course of the disease. As in all medicine, the risk-to-benefit ratio must be carefully weighed and explained to the patient before the decision to treat with photocoagulation is made.

REFERENCES

1. Gass, J. D. M.: Pathogenesis of disciform detachment of the neuroepithelium. I. General concepts and classification, Am. J. Ophthalmol. **63:**573, 1967.
2. Little, H. L.: Macular diseases: classification and treatment with argon laser slit lamp photocoagulation. In Francois, J., editor: Symposium on light-coagulation, Ghent, June 15-16, 1972, The Hague, 1973, W. B. Junk.
3. Maumenee, A. E.: Clinical manifestations, Trans. Am. Acad. Ophthalmol. Otolaryngol. **69:**605, 1965.
4. Zweng, H. C., Little, H. L., and Peabody, R. R.: Laser photocoagulation and retinal angiography, St. Louis, 1969, The C. V. Mosby Co.

8
INVOLUTIONAL MACULOPATHIES

Involutional maculopathies include all primary diseases of the macula that do not have a known traumatic, toxic, inflammatory, or neoplastic etiology. In this classification we place central serous retinopathy (CSR); diffuse retinal pigment epitheliopathy (DRPE); atrophic (SMDA), serous (SMDS), hemorrhagic (SMDH), and cicatricial (SMDC) senile maculopathy; and the several definite heredomacular degenerative maculopathies Best's vitelliform and Stargardt's disease. These diseases can have from relatively mild (CSR) to decidedly severe (SMDH) effect on patients' central vision. At times these disease entities overlap or evolve from one to another. Clear-cut differentiation is therefore sometimes difficult, even for the most experienced retinologist.

The diagnostic terms now used are descriptive, underscoring the need for research leading to a fuller knowledge of the basic mechanisms and causes at work. Only then can diagnoses be made from etiologic factors. All investigators reporting on various aspects of maculopathies must make every effort to be very clear about which disease category is under discussion. Imprecise knowledge as to the cause of maculopathies leads to confusion in prognosis and treatment. Further, very careful diagnostic criteria must be set up to clarify the natural course of each of these maculopathies and to evaluate various treatment modalities in view of the natural history.

The importance of the involutional maculopathies is emphasized by Kahn and Moorhead in their study on blindness.[1] These authors define blindness as best corrected distance in the better eye of 20/200 or a visual field limited to 20° or less at the widest point. They found that "the four largest cross-classification categories with each accounting for about 10% of all additions to blindness registers are: senile retinal degeneration, glaucoma, diabetic retinopathy and senile cataracts." With excellent surgical techniques available to remove cataractous lenses and with improved detection and treatment of glaucoma, involutional maculopathies stand with diabetic retinopathy as the two causes of blindness most in need of improved therapies.

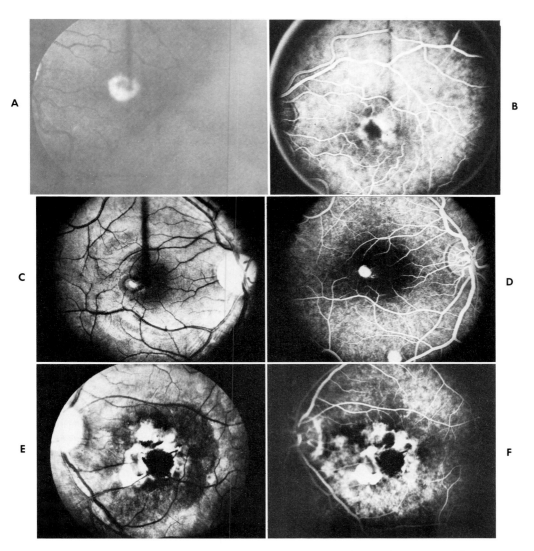

Fig. 8-1. Best's vitelliform maculopathy. **A,** Photograph of left eye of a 45-year-old woman with vision of 20/20. Central area is yellowish in color with a fluid level in it. **B,** Fluoroangiogram of same eye, demonstrating no leakage of dye in macula. **C,** Best's vitelliform maculopathy. Photograph of right eye of a 14-year-old white girl with vision of 20/15. Typical "egg yolk" appearance of macular lesion due to fatty deposits. **D,** Fluoroangiogram of same eye. **E,** Photograph of left eye of same 14-year-old patient. "Egg yolk" appearance has changed to a macular scar. **F,** Fluoroangiogram of left eye in same patient.

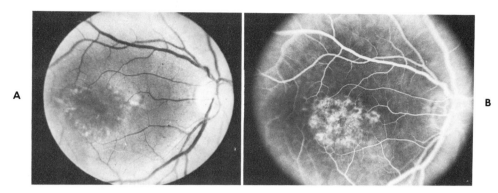

Fig. 8-2. Stargardt's maculopathy. **A,** Photograph of posterior pole of right eye, showing atrophic-appearing macula with irregular pigmentation at RPE level. Yellowish flecks are seen in and around macula. VA, 20/200. **B,** Fluoroangiogram of same eye, showing staining of yellowish irregular flecks with dye. Staining gradually fades with time.

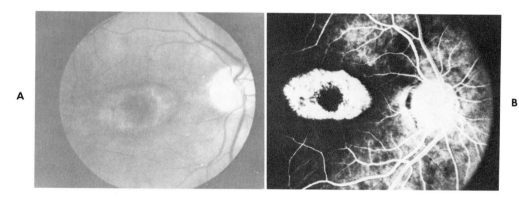

Fig. 8-3. Chloroquine maculopathy. **A,** Photograph of right eye, showing bull's-eye pattern of a depigmentation in macula of 45-year-old white woman. VA, 20/40. **B,** Fluorangiogram of same eye, showing marked transmitted fluorescence from underlying choroid in area of macular depigmentation. Fluorescence does not change over time.

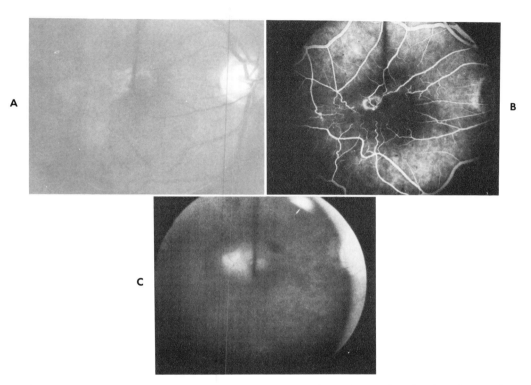

Fig. 8-4. A, Photograph of right eye showing preretinal membrane that developed several months after an incident of amaurosis fugax, from which patient recovered 20/20 vision. In succeeding months, vision slowly decreased to 20/50. Membrane is a fine irregular grayish yellow structure immediately above macula, puckering the surface of the retina! **B,** Fluoroangiogram showing staining of membrane in early venous phase, with traction on paramacular vessels evident. **C,** Late exposure in same angiogram sequence, showing leakage of dye from capillaries under traction by membrane.

Fig. 8-5. A, Fundus photograph of right eye of 67-year-old woman, showing macular lamellar hole *(large arrow)* caused by retraction of vitreous body. Operculum *(small arrow)* is seen on back of retracted vitreous. **B,** Fluoroangiogram showing transmitted fluorescence from underlying choroid exactly occupying area of lamellar hole.

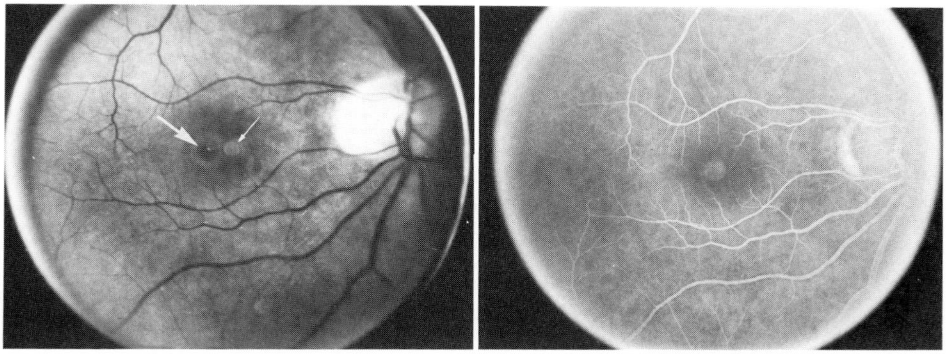

Because this book concerns itself with treatment with argon laser photocoagulation, no further mention will be made of Best's vitelliform maculopathy (Fig. 8-1) or Stargardt's disease (Fig. 8-2), chloroquine maculopathy (Fig. 8-3), preretinal membrane (Fig. 8-4), and lamellar macular holes (Fig. 8-5), because argon laser photocoagulation is not useful in the treatment of these maculopathies.

REFERENCE

1. Kahn, H. A., and Moorhead, H. B.: Statistics on blindness in the model reporting area: 1969-1970. U.S. Department of Health, Education, and Welfare (National Institutes of Health), publication no. 73, 1970, p. 427.

9

CENTRAL SEROUS RETINOPATHY

Central serous retinopathy is a lively topic among ophthalmologists interested in retinal disease, and controversy surrounds its diagnosis, etiology, course, treatment, and even its name. Twenty-five years ago, the term central angiospastic retinopathy[2] was favored, because many of the patients were described as "hard-driving and tense, with compulsive personalities"[5] or as undergoing some crisis in their personal or public lives.[6] However tense some of these patients seemed, they did not give definite evidence of angiospasm, as measured by elevated blood pressures, narrowing of retinal arterioles, or a higher incidence of vascular accidents than expected. In recent years the terms central serous retinopathy and choroidopathy have been favored, depending on the user's belief that the initial pathologic site is in the retina or choroid. The best and most recent evidence indicates that first there is a loss of adhesion between the retinal pigment epithelium (RPE) and Bruch's membrane, giving an RPE detachment, because serum passes readily through Bruch's membrane from the choriocapillaris, with a later rupture of the zona occludens between cuboidal cells of the RPE,[1,3,7] allowing the serum to seep under the sensory retina. Perhaps, therefore, retinopathy is the better term. The reason for loss of adhesion between the RPE and Bruch's membrane is unknown.

Central serous retinopathy (CSR), then, is a disease of the macula in which serum leaks through an underlying serous retinal pigment epithelial detachment, lifting the sensory retina from the RPE on which it normally lies. Such detachments of both retinal pigment epithelial and sensory retinal layers are similar to those seen in exudative senile macular degeneration. Differentiating these two entities is sometimes difficult, but very important, as will be discussed.

The patient's chief complaint is usually abrupt loss of vision or distortion in the form of micropsia or metamorphopsia. Occasionally he will also note a "gray film" in the affected eye, with reduced light and color sensitivity.

A detailed history should include specifically—

1. Nature and duration of visual symptoms.
2. Whether the complaints are increasing or decreasing.

3. Extent to which symptoms are interfering with the patient's life style.
4. Whether the patient has had any similar episodes and, if so, their duration and treatment.
5. Any medication being taken for the current episode.

Examination of the patient should include—

1. Best corrected distance and near vision in each eye.
2. Amsler grid examination.
3. Central visual field: 1-mm white target at 1 meter or 3-mm white target, if necessary.
4. Color-vision testing with Ishihara plates.
5. Ophthalmoscopic examination with direct and indirect systems and, after photography, with slit-lamp funduscopy through a diagnostic corneal lens.
6. Retinal fluorescein angiography with stereoscopic views, if available. Photographic exposures should be taken of the macula and paramacular areas during the arterial and venous phases and 10 to 15 minutes after the injection of the dye.
7. In some cases fluorescein angiography should be done at the slit lamp to help clarify the existence of a leak. At times, the presence or absence of a leak, as opposed to transmitted fluorescence or staining, is difficult to ascertain from an angiogram; rarely, the leak is not seen on the angiogram because it is out of the posterior pole but can be seen by fluorangioscopy.

No doubt some of the confusion about central serous retinopathy is due to imprecise diagnostic criteria. We have developed a set of objective criteria for diagnosing CSR, to exclude other causes of serous detachments of the sensory epithelium of the macula and to permit meaningful comparisons with similar cases, treated or untreated, reported by other investigators:

1. Serous detachment of the sensory retina in the macula, seen on slit-lamp ophthalmoscopy. Although all such retinas should be visualized by indirect and direct ophthalmoscopy, slit-lamp funduscopy gives the most critical view for determining whether there is fluid under the sensory retina. The fluid is clear, as contrasted with the usually turbid or cloudy fluid seen in exudative senile macular degeneration.
2. An active leak, as demonstrated on fluorescein angiography.
3. Absence of drusen and of extensive changes in the retinal pigment epithelial layer.
4. Absence of retinal or subretinal hemorrhage or lipoidal deposits is a prerequisite for the diagnosis of central serous retinopathy.

This disease is perhaps part of a spectrum of maculopathies, with central serous retinopathy at the mild end and hemorrhagic senile macular degeneration at the severe end (see Chapter 7).

The detachment of the sensory retina can vary from very low to high, with yellow deposits on the posterior surface of the elevated layer often seen. If the detachment is low, often the presence of the fluid can be detected through the slit

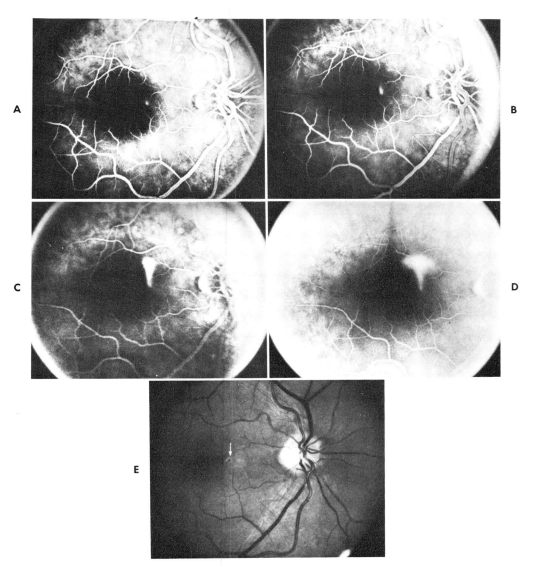

Fig. 9-1. A, Fluoroangiogram in arteriovenous phase of right retina of 35-year-old white man with serous detachment of macular sensory retina. A leakage point is seen near nasal edge of macula. Note irregular fluorescence above and below nerve head. VA, 20/40. **B,** Later fluoroangiogram of same retina, showing dye diffusing from initial leaking point. Note fluorescence from other areas does not change shape. **C,** "Plume" of fluorescence from leaking point seen in **A** is now well established as dye rises to top of sensory retinal detachment. **D,** Fluorescent "plume" has now reached top of sensory retinal detachment, and dye has started to flow down sides of detachment. **E,** Photograph of same retina 4 months after argon laser photocoagulation treatment. Note small area of hyperpigmentation at treatment site *(arrow)* surrounded by aura of hypopigmentation. VA, 20/25.

lamp only by noting the shadow just next to the retinal vessels, cast by them on the retinal pigment epithelium.

The appearance of the retinal fluoroangiogram is variable, as the disease is variable. Leakage of dye may be obvious or subtle. A leak is diagnosed when a fluorescent dot or area seen during the arterial or venous phase spreads, blurring its edges in the delayed films and forming a pool of fluorescein under the sensory retina.

In typical cases, the angiogram shows a small area of fluorescence in the arterial or early venous phase, with fairly rapid spreading of the fluorescent pattern, in the form of a "smokestack" or "plume," until the space under the detached sensory retina is filled with the dye. The plume is dye leaking through a tiny break in the RPE detachment. When leakage is brisk it forms the characteristic plume pattern because the incoming fluid has a lower specific gravity than does the fluid already under the sensory retina. The lighter fluid rises to the top of the detach-

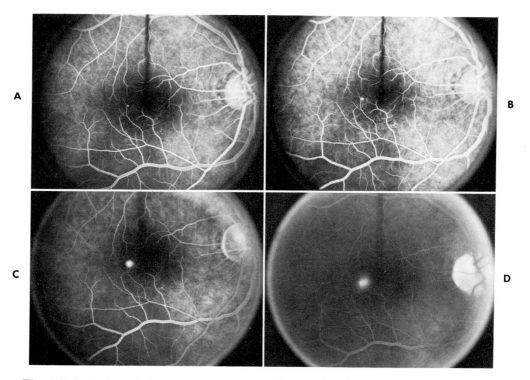

Fig. 9-2. A, Early retinal fluoroangiogram of a 46-year-old white man with serous detachment of macular sensory retina, with dotlike leak noted temporal from fovea. **B,** Leak has increased in midarteriovenous phase of fluoroangiogram. **C,** Further blurring of fluorescent dot seen as angiogram progresses. **D,** Delayed fluoroangiogram showing diffusion of dye under sensory retina.

ment sensory retina and then flows down its sides (Fig. 9-1). The initial dot of fluorescence is produced by the increased concentration of dye trapped under a small, sometimes tiny, RPE detachment (Fig. 9-2).

Sometimes the leak is not as brisk or as obvious as just described. Great care must be taken to follow all fluorescent dots through the entire series of photographs; 5- by 7-inch enlargements of crucial frames are useful. In the late frames, areas of leakage are recognized by diffusion of the dye under the sensory retina (Fig. 9-3). If the funduscopic appearance is typical of a serous detachment of the sensory retina, but no leak is found on the angiogram, two possibilities should be considered: either the leak has sealed but not enough time had passed for absorption of the subretinal fluid, or the leak is beyond the area photographed. In such instances fluorescein angioscopy should be done to examine the retina beyond the posterior pole, especially in or just above the superior temporal vascular arcade, either at the slit lamp or with the indirect ophthalmoscope, using the cobalt blue filter on the instrument. Peripheral choroidal and retinal tumors, which can cause serous detachments of the macula, must be suspected. Congenital optic nerve pits can also cause serous detachments of the sensory retina in the macula (Fig. 9-4).

We have treated four eyes with serous detachment of the sensory retina with congenital pits of the optic nerve head. We have treated the pits directly to no avail. However, with treatment to the arc of retina at the temporal edge of the nerve head and areas of RPE leakage within the serous detachment, we have collapsed the detachment but without improvement of visual acuity (Fig. 9-4).

Special care must be taken to detect any subretinal neovascular membrane that might be causing the serous elevation of the macula or can be mistaken for it. Such cases must be treated much differently than central serous retinopathy, as discussed in Chapters 11 and 12.

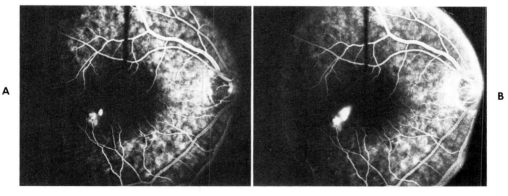

Fig. 9-3. Fluoroangiogram (**A,** earlier; **B,** later) of right retina with serous detachment of macular sensory retina, showing two leaks, one brisk and one more indolent.

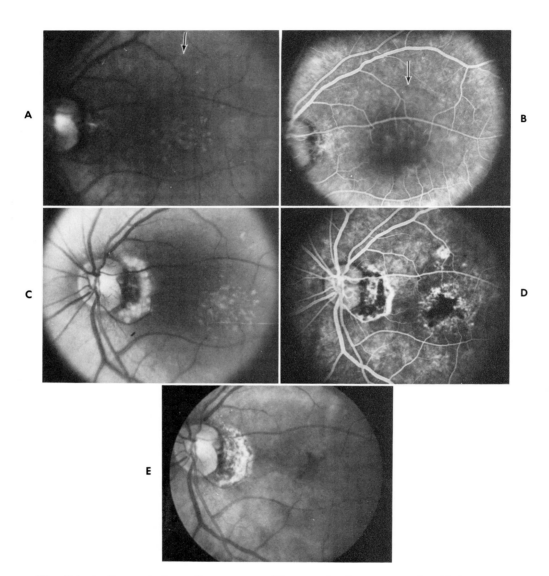

Fig. 9-4. A, Congenital pit of optic nerve. Photograph of posterior pole of left eye with serous detachment of sensory retina (*arrow,* superior edge). Yellow flecks centrally are lipoproteinaceous deposits on posterior surface of detached sensory retina. VA, 20/200. **B,** Fluoroangiogram showing outline of sensory retinal detachment (*arrow,* superior edge). **C,** Photograph immediately after argon laser photocoagulation just off temporal edge of nerve head. Settings used: 200 μm, 0.1 sec, 200 mW. **D,** Fluoroangiogram 1 month after treatment. Sensory retinal detachment has collapsed. VA, 20/80. Area of negative fluorescence at temporal edge of nerve head due to pigmentation from treatment. **E,** Photograph taken on same day as **D,** showing sensory retinal detachment has collapsed.

Transmitted fluorescence from the underlying choroid through areas of pigment atrophy in the RPE often is seen immediately adjacent to areas of hyperpigmentation, also representing reaction in the RPE to the disease.

Based on the above diagnostic criteria, we have used argon laser photocoagulation to treat 112 eyes in 105 patients with classic CSR, as described. Our technique is as follows:

Anesthetic. Topical anesthetic only is used; retrobulbar block is not necessary. Occasionally, diazepam (Valium) 5 to 10 mg orally 30 minutes before treatment is indicated for a tense patient.

Settings. Beam diameter, 100 to 200 μm; exposure time, 0.05 to 0.1 sec; power, 150 to 200 mW. It is usually best to begin with the smaller beam diameter, shorter time exposure, and lower power (100 μm, 0.05 sec, 150 mW), and then increase the power by 50 mW until a medium coagulation—more beige than white in color—is obtained.

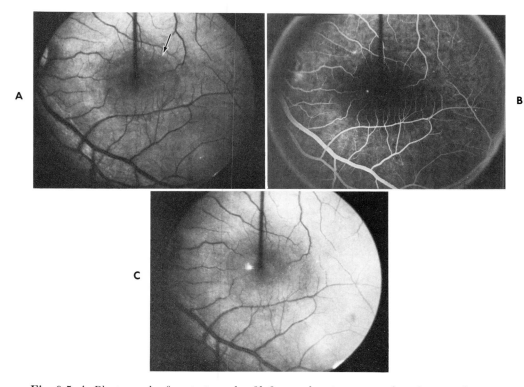

Fig. 9-5. A, Photograph of posterior pole of left eye, showing serous detachment of sensory retina *(arrow)* in 46-year-old white man. VA, 20/30. **B,** Fluoroangiogram of left eye of 44-year-old white man with central serous retinopathy, showing leakage of dye from point about 400 μm nasal from fovea. **C,** Photograph of same eye immediately after argon laser photocoagulation treatment, showing burn directly on point of leakage.

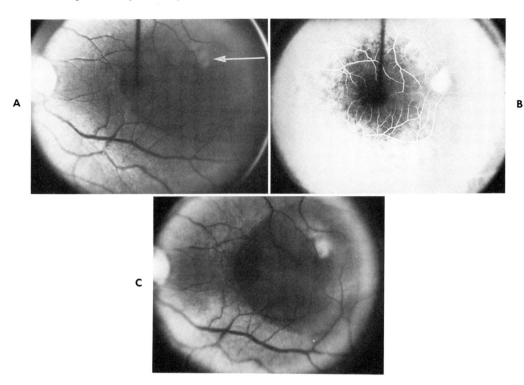

Fig. 9-6. A, Photograph of left retina of 48-year-old white man with serous detachment of sensory retina, with underlying retinal pigment epithelial detachment *(arrow).* **B,** Fluoroangiogram of same eye, showing dye filling RPE detachment and beginning to leak out under sensory retina. **C,** Photograph of same retina immediately after argon laser photocoagulation treatment. Entire RPE detachment has been coagulated.

Area treated. The point of leakage, as determined by fluorescein angiography, is treated (Figs. 9-5 to 9-7). Occasionally, fluorescein angioscopy is done, with the patient seated at the photocoagulator slit lamp, to ascertain the exact point of leakage.

Number of exposures. Usually one to five "medium" coagulations are required.

Follow-ups. Four weeks after treatment.

In our group of 105 patients treated, there were approximately nine times as many males as there were females; all patients were white. There was no essential difference in laterality; seven males (6.2%) were treated bilaterally. The age of patients at the time of treatment ranged from 22 to 58 years (average, 41.6, median, 43) (Fig. 9-8). The time from onset of disease to treatment ranged from 2 days to 5 years (average, 6 months). The number of exposures per eye ranged from 1 to 158 (average, 29) and the number of treatment sessions varied from one

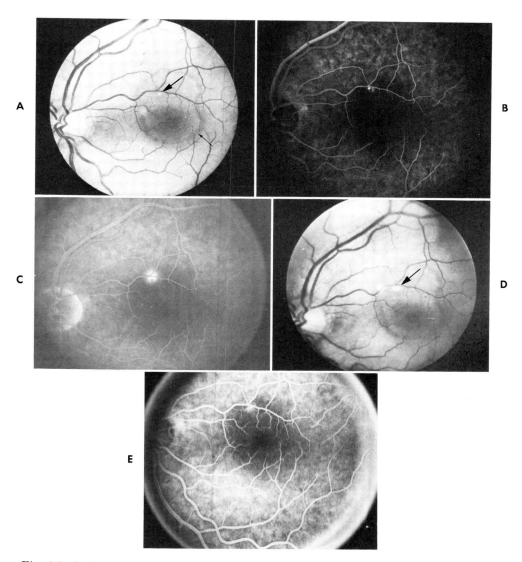

Fig. 9-7. A, Fundus photograph of left eye of 47-year-old woman, showing serous detachment *(small arrow)* of macular sensory retina before treatment. *Large arrow,* RPE detachment. **B,** Fluoroangiogram (venous phase) showing RPE detachment densely filled with fluorescein. Small RPE window defect is seen immediately temporal from RPE detachment. **C,** Fluoroangiogram (late phase) showing fluorescein leaking from under RPE detachment to under sensory retina. **D,** Fundus photograph immediately after argon laser photocoagulation of RPE detachment *(arrow).* **E,** Fluoroangiogram (venous phase) 6 weeks after treatment, showing window defect but no leakage of fluorescein.

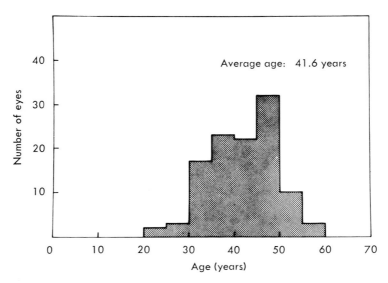

Fig. 9-8. Histogram showing age distribution grouped in half-decades of 112 eyes with central serous retinopathy treated with argon laser photocoagulation.

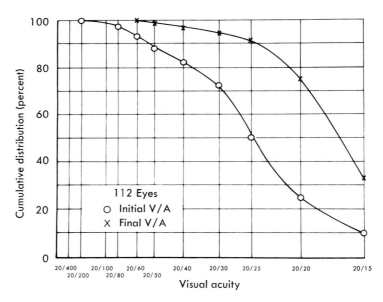

Fig. 9-9. Cumulative distribution expressed as percent of visual acuities of eyes with central serous retinopathy, before treatment with argon laser photocoagulation and at end of follow-up.

NOTE: Throughout this volume, cumulative distribution charts appear as shown in Fig. 9-9. Analysis of these charts can yield much information. Visual acuities are ranged on the abscissa, and the accumulated percentages of eyes in the series on the ordinate. By traversing from right to left, the reader can determine the percent of eyes in the total series that saw at a given vision level or better. For example, in Fig. 9-9, 91% of eyes saw 20/25 or better after treatment, compared with 50% before treatment.

to five (average, 1.3). Patients were usually seen 3 to 4 weeks after treatment, for reevaluation of all parameters examined initially. They were returned to the referring ophthalmologists when the sensory epithelial detachment cleared and no leakage was seen on fluorescein angiography. Follow-up time by us depended, therefore, on the patients' course; the range was 1 to 54 months (average, 10 months).

All patients had symptoms of either visual loss or distortion to a degree that was bothersome enough that they elected to have treatment, even though they were advised that their disease was usually self-limiting.

Fig. 9-9 shows the percent cumulative distribution of visual acuities of all 112 eyes before treatment and at the end of follow-up.

Males appeared to do better than females visually (Figs. 9-10 and 9-11). In both groups 50% of eyes had visual acuity of 20/25 or better before treatment. At the end of follow-up, 92% of eyes in males had 20/25 V/A or better, contrasted with 80% in females; however, the small number of females (10) makes the difference of questionable significance.

Fig. 9-12 shows the results in individual eyes, relating acuity before treatment to that at the end of follow-up in each eye treated. No significant visual loss (2 lines or more) occurred in any eye in this series. Sixty-one eyes (54%) improved (2 lines or more), and 51 (46%) were essentially unchanged; however, 27 of the 51 eyes (53%) had v/a of 20/20 or better before treatment and thus could not improve 2 lines or more on the Snellen chart. Excluding these 27 eyes, it was pos-

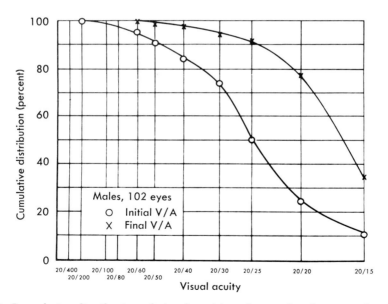

Fig. 9-10. Cumulative distribution of visual acuities of eyes of males treated with argon laser photocoagulation, before treatment and at end of follow-up.

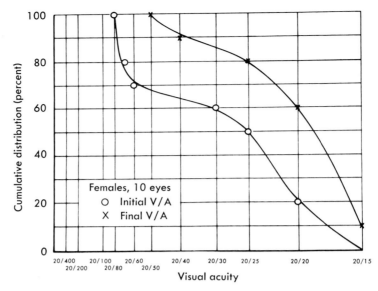

Fig. 9-11. Cumulative distribution of visual acuities of eyes of females treated with argon laser photocoagulation, before treatment and at end of follow-up.

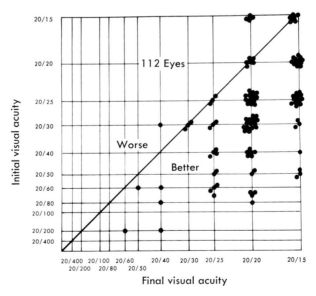

Fig. 9-12. Scatter diagram relating pretreatment visual acuity of each eye with central serous retinopathy treated with argon laser photocoagulation with visual acuity at end of follow-up. Total series, 112 eyes.

sible that 85 eyes could improve visually 2 lines or more; 61 (72%) did, and 24 (28%) were unchanged.

It is of interest that 55 eyes (almost 50%) were treated for their second or later episode of central serous retinopathy (the largest number of episodes was seven), and 55 eyes were treated for their first (in two of the 112 eyes, it was impossible to determine if the episode treated was the first). This finding underscores the recurrent nature of the disease.

We presumed that eyes with recurrent disease would fare less well than those treated on their first episode, but data from this series did not bear out that expectation. Pre- and posttreatment visual acuities of patients treated for their first episode and those treated for a second or later episode are shown in Figs. 9-13 and 9-14; Fig. 9-15 compares the final acuities in the two groups directly. The small difference between the two curves is not significant; eyes treated for recurrent episodes fared as well visually as eyes treated on their first episode.

Seven eyes (6.25%) in this series developed recurrence of sensory retinal detachment after successful treatment of the first episode (Table 9-1). Five eyes (9.1%) were from the group of 55 treated for a second or later episode, and two eyes (3.6%) had been treated for the first, indicating again the recurrent nature of central serous retinopathy. Careful comparison of the original pretreatment angiogram with one taken at the time of recurrence showed that three of the

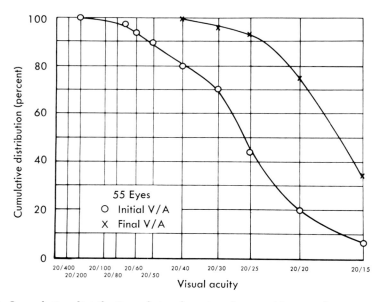

Fig. 9-13. Cumulative distribution of visual acuity of eyes with central serous retinopathy treated with argon laser photocoagulation, before treatment and at end of follow-up. Series of 55 eyes treated on first episode of central serous retinopathy.

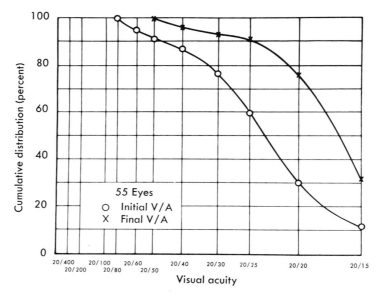

Fig. 9-14. Cumulative distribution of visual acuity of eyes with central serous retinopathy treated with argon laser photocoagulation, before treatment and at end of follow-up. Series of 55 eyes treated on second or later episode.

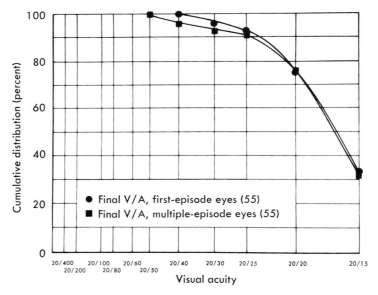

Fig. 9-15. Cumulative distribution of visual acuities of eyes treated with argon laser photocoagulation. Direct comparison of eyes treated on first episode of central serous retinopathy versus eyes treated on second or later episode. No significant difference.

Table 9-1. Recurrent cases of central serous retinopathy

	Same lesion	New lesion	Same and new lesions	Total	Incidence
Eyes treated on second or later episodes	2	2	1	5	5/55 = 9.1%
Eyes treated on first episode	1		1	2	2/55 = 3.6%

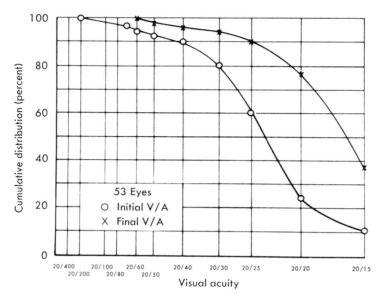

Fig. 9-16. Cumulative distribution of visual acuity of eyes treated with argon laser photocoagulation, before treatment and at end of follow up. Age of patients in this series, ≤ 41 years.

seven retinas leaked from the same point, two leaked from a new site, and two from both the old and a new point simultaneously. Therefore, the angiogram of the entire posterior pole should be examined carefully in eyes with recurrent CSR, rather than assume that recurrence is a reactivation of the previously treated leak.

We expected older patients to do less well visually at the end of follow-up than younger ones, but visual outcome did not vary significantly in the two groups, divided at the average age of 41 years (Figs. 9-16 to 9-18).

Another factor that we considered might affect visual prognosis is length of time from onset to treatment. We thought that perhaps the earlier a case is treated, the more complete the visual recovery will be. Some patients are quite vague in pinpointing the exact time of onset of disease. Appreciating the possibil-

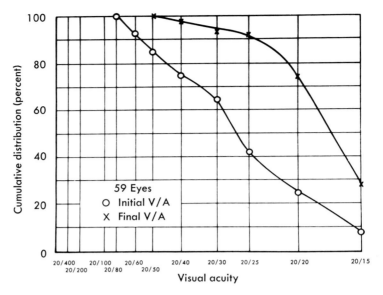

Fig. 9-17. Cumulative distribution of visual acuity of eyes with central serous retinopathy treated with argon laser photocoagulation, before treatment and at end of follow-up. Age, ≥ 42 years.

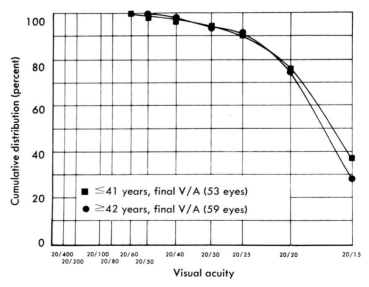

Fig. 9-18. Cumulative distribution of visual acuity of eyes with central serous retinopathy treated with argon laser photocoagulation, at end of follow-up. Direct comparison of 53 eyes ≤ 41 years with 59 eyes ≥ 42 years. No significant difference.

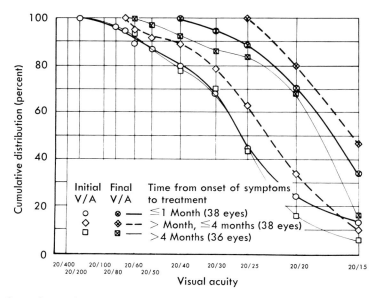

Fig. 9-19. Cumulative distribution of visual acuity of eyes with central serous retinopathy treated with argon laser photocoagulation, before treatment and at end of follow-up. Comparison of visual results in three groups divided according to duration of symptoms before treatment.

ity of patient error, we nevertheless divided all treated eyes into three subgroups of almost equal size: those who had had symptoms for less than 1 month (Group A), longer than 1 month but less than 4 months (Group B), and longer than 4 months (Group C); data are shown in Fig. 9-19. Best results were obtained in Group B, in which all eyes had visual acuity of 20/25 or better at the end of follow-up, suggesting that treatment during that symptom interval gives optimal visual results.

There are three potential complications of argon laser photocoagulation treatment: coagulation of the fovea, choroidal hemorrhage, and development of a subretinal neovascular membrane (SRNM). None has occurred in our experience. With the settings suggested, a choroidal hemorrhage is extremely unlikely. However, coagulation of the fovea must be guarded against by photocoagulating no closer than 300 μm from the fovea and by having the patient focus on the slit-lamp fixation light with his other eye, to avoid eye movement that inadvertently might place the fovea in the treating beam. Leaks on a line directly below the fovea are especially worrisome due to Bell's phenomenon induced by photophobia during treatment. Shorter exposure times (e.g., 0.05 sec or less) are useful in such circumstances. Development of a subretinal neovascular membrane is a very serious complication. The ophthalmologist must be alert to detect a small SRNM on the original angiogram. Treating a SRNM with the "light" or "moderate" lesions used in CSR may hasten the growth of the SRNM. Persistent leaks after treatment should be treated with heavy lesions, if proximity to the fovea permits.

Central serous retinopathy is usually a self-limited disease. As reported by Klein et al.,[4] the visual prognosis without treatment is good. Therefore, indications for treatment must be drawn carefully. Patients often react to their symptoms seemingly out of proportion to the degree of visual loss or distortion present. It is possible that the common observation is true: these patients are tense and hard-driving and thus present themselves for examination more often than do more phlegmatic, less observant people with the same amount of visual difficulty. The former desire an explanation of the change in their visual status very early in the course of the disease; the latter are not as worried or curious, so the disease can pass without medical advice ever being sought. Therefore, the degree to which visual symptoms interfere with the patient's life style should weigh heavily in the joint patient-physician decision of whether to treat with argon laser photocoagulation. In a controlled study Watzke, Barton, and Leaverton demonstrated

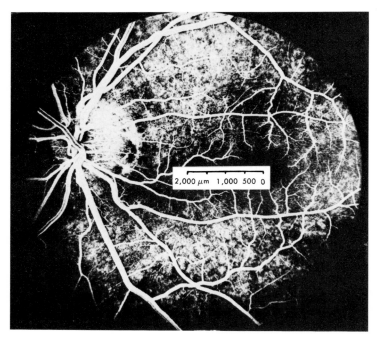

Fig. 9-20. Fluoroangiogram of an emmetropic eye, with a scale indicating distances from the retina. This print is a four-times enlargement of the negative taken with a Zeiss fundus camera, which in turn is a 2.5-times enlargement of the retina. Therefore, the magnification from the retina to the photograph is a factor of 10, and 1 cm on the photograph is equal to 1 mm on the retina.

that treatment significantly shortened the duration of ocular symptoms in eyes treated with ruby laser photocoagulation, compared with eyes given no treatment. They found "there was a significant difference between the two groups. Treated patients had a duration of disease of 2.5 to 7.5 weeks, with a median duration of 5 weeks from treatment to cure. Contrast this with the untreated group who showed a recovery time of 11 to 26 weeks, with a median of 23 weeks. This was statistically significant at the 1% level (P < 0.01) by the two-sample t-test."[8] Therefore, argon laser photocoagulation should be offered as an option to patients whose symptoms seriously interfere with their daily activities.

The leak must be at least 300 μm from the fovea, as measured on fluorescein angiogram. Photocoagulation of a leak closer than 300 μm is possible, but there is greater risk of foveal damage.

Distances on the retina may be estimated by accounting for the magnification that is inherent in the photograph under observation. There is a 2.5 times magnification in the Zeiss fundus camera from the retina of an emmetropic eye to the film plane. Thus, a contact print made from the negative would be a 2.5 times enlargement of the retina: 300 μm on the retina would be 750 μm, or 3/4 mm, on the print. If enlargements are made, the magnification from the negative to the enlargement should be multiplied by 2.5 in order to obtain the magnification from the retina. Fig. 9-20 shows a fluoroangiogram with a scale corrected for the retina. The figure is an enlargement four times the size of the negative and therefore is 10 times larger than the retina. Thus, 1 cm on the photograph is 1 mm on the retina.

Microcystic macular edema in the detached sensory epithelium is rare but constitutes a strong indication for treatment. Such cases have had a prolonged detachment of the sensory retina, and there is greater danger of permanent visual reduction.

In conclusion, our experience indicates that argon laser photocoagulation, with indications and settings as recommended, is safe and effective in treating central serous retinopathy. Done by an experienced clinician, such treatment probably shortens the duration of visual morbidity. However, classic central serous retinopathy is self-limiting, with a generally good visual prognosis without treatment.

REFERENCES

1. Feeney, L.: Intercellular junctions; sites of permeability barriers and cellular communication, Invest. Ophthalmol. **13**:811-814, 1974.
2. Gifford, S. R., and Marquardt, G.: Central angiospastic retinopathy, Arch. Ophthalmol. **21**:211-228, 1939.
3. Hogan, M. J., Alvarado, J. A., and Weddell, J. E.: Histology of the human eye, Philadelphia, 1971, W. B. Saunders Co., p. 410.
4. Klein, M. L., Van Buskirk, E. M., Friedman, E., et al.: Experience with nontreatment of central serous choroidopathy, Arch. Ophthalmol. **91**:247, 1974.
5. Klien, B. A.: Macular lesions of vascular origin. II. Functional vascular conditions leading to damage of the macula lutea, Am. J. Ophthalmol. **36**:1-13, 1953.
6. Lipowski, Z. J.: Psychosomatic aspects of central serous retinopathy, Psychosomatics **12**:398-401, 1971.

7. Shakib, M.: Fluorescein angiography and retinal pigment epithelium, Am. J. Ophthalmol. **74**:206, 1972.

8. Watzke, R. C., Barton, T. C., and Leaverton, P. E.: Ruby laser photocoagulation therapy of central serous retinopathy, Trans. Am. Acad. Ophthalmol. Otolaryngol. **78**:205-211, 1974.

ADDITIONAL READINGS

Gass, J. D. M.: Pathogenesis of disciform detachment of the neuroepithelium. II. Idiopathic central serous choroidopathy, Am. J. Ophthalmol. **63**:587-615, 1967.

Gass, J. D. M.: Photocoagulation of macular lesions, Trans. Am. Acad. Ophthalmol. Otolaryngol. **75**:580-608, 1971.

L'Esperance, F. A., Jr.: Argon and ruby laser photocoagulation of disciform macular disease, Trans. Am. Acad. Ophthalmol. Otolaryngol. **75**:609-625, 1971.

Maumenee, A. E.: Macular diseases: pathogenesis, Trans. Am. Acad. Ophthalmol. Otolaryngol. **69**:691-699, 1965.

Peabody, R. R., Zweng, H. C., and Little, H. L.: Treatment of persistent central serous retinopathy, Arch. Ophthalmol. **79**:166-169, 1968.

Spalter, H. F.: Photocoagulation of central serous retinopathy, Arch. Ophthalmol. **79**:247-263, 1968.

Wessing, A.: Central serous retinopathy and related lesions, Mod. Probl. Ophthalmol. **9**:148-151, 1971.

Wise, G. N., et al.: Photocoagulation of vascular lesions of the macula, Am. J. Ophthalmol. **66**:452-459, 1968.

10

DIFFUSE RETINAL PIGMENT EPITHELIOPATHY

We have observed a group of eyes with maculopathy bearing considerable resemblance to central serous retinopathy (CSR). However, there are differences that set this group apart; thus, in our opinion, they merit a separate classification. Ophthalmologists have noted cases like these in reports on CSR,[1,2] commenting that some eyes do not develop a course similar to the typical case. Because evidence of widespread retinal pigment epitheliopathy disturbance is a common finding in these eyes, we suggest this disease be called diffuse retinal pigment epitheliopathy (DRPE).

Eyes studied differed from those with CSR in several aspects ophthalmoscopically. Diffuse and extensive hyper- and hypopigmentation were present in the retinal pigment epithelium (RPE) layer. Macular sensory retinal detachment was low in all of these eyes, lower than it tended to be in CSR. Fluoroangiograms displayed much more blocked and transmitted fluorescence than is seen in the typical case of CSR, reflecting greater disturbance of RPE pigmentation (Figs. 10-1 to 10-4). In none of the angiograms of these eyes was leakage brisk enough to produce a plume pattern, as is often seen in CSR. Occasionally, it was impossible to find a leak on fluoroangiography or angioscopy, despite the presence of a small amount of persistent subretinal fluid (Fig. 10-5).

Thirty-three eyes were categorized as having DRPE. Table 10-1 compares this group with 112 eyes with central serous retinopathy, described in Chapter 9.

The population characteristics of the two groups did not vary significantly. The same striking sex difference was present in both; age groups were similar, although patients with DRPE were 3.4 years older on the average than were patients with CSR (Fig. 10-6); all patients were white.

Indications for treatment of DRPE are the same as for CSR:

1. Serious interference in the patient's activities, from symptoms, such as metamorphopsia and blurred vision, generated by sensory epithelial elevation in the macula

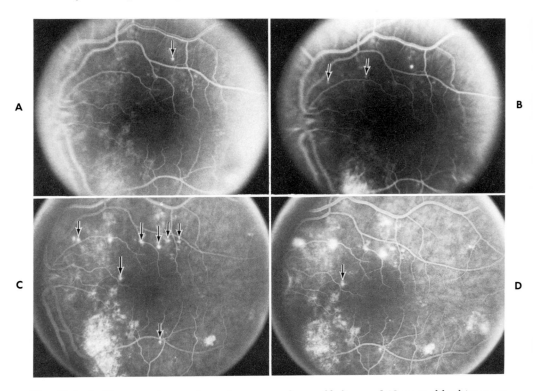

Fig. 10-1. A, Fluoroangiogram in early venous phase of left eye of 43-year-old white man. VA, 20/15. A low serous detachment present only along superotemporal arcade. Vision in right eye 20/200, due to serous detachment of macula present for 5 years (see Fig. 10-2). Only one "bright" leak seen *(arrow).* **B,** Later in venous phase, fluoroangiogram suggests two more leaks *(arrows).* Note transmitted fluorescence along inferotemporal vessels. **C,** Later exposure in same angiographic sequence shows seven more possible leaks *(arrows).* **D,** Later exposure of same angiographic sequence, showing blurring of fluorescence around many suspect dotlike areas of fluorescence but not around one noted in **C,** which therefore probably is not a leak *(arrow).*

    2. Leakage no closer to the fovea than 300 μm, as measured on the fluoroangiogram

    Treatment techniques are the same as described for CSR (see Chapter 9).

    The greater chronicity of the disease process in the group with DRPE is suggested by the longer follow-up time (both range and average) made necessary by persistence or recurrence of visual symptoms associated with macular sensory epithelial detachment. Moreover, experiences with treatment of the two groups make evident the increased chronicity of DRPE, as shown in Table 10-2.

    The greater number of treatment sessions (2.2 versus 1.3) and the greater

Text continued on p. 123.

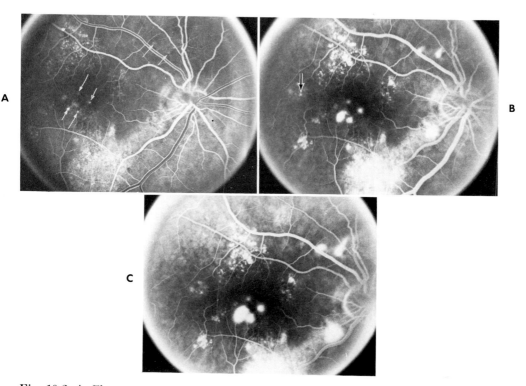

Fig. 10-2. A, Fluoroangiogram, early venous phase, of right retina of patient in Fig. 10-1. VA, 20/200. Blurred vision intermittent for 5 years. No photocoagulation treatment given. Note transmitted fluorescence along inferotemporal vessels, similar to that seen in other eye (Fig. 10-1, C. *Arrows* indicate seven probable leaks). **B,** Later exposure in same angiographic sequence, showing blurring of fluorescein pattern in seven sites noted in **A.** Another possible leak *(arrow)* has developed. **C,** Later exposure in same angiographic sequence, showing further blurring of fluorescence, indicating active leakage of serum into multiple RPE detachments and under sensory retina.

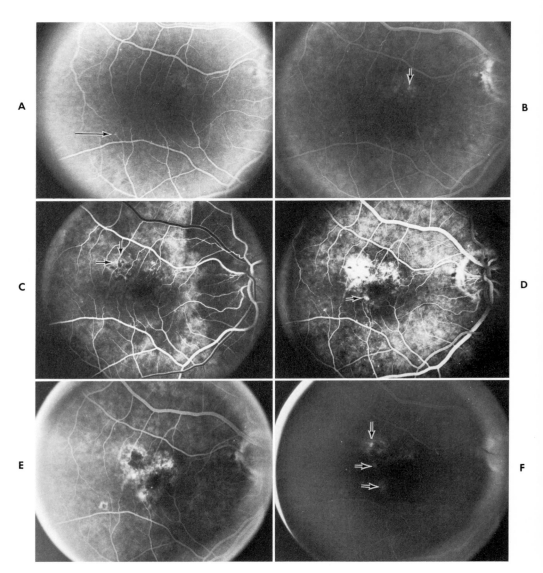

Fig. 10-3. For legend see opposite page.

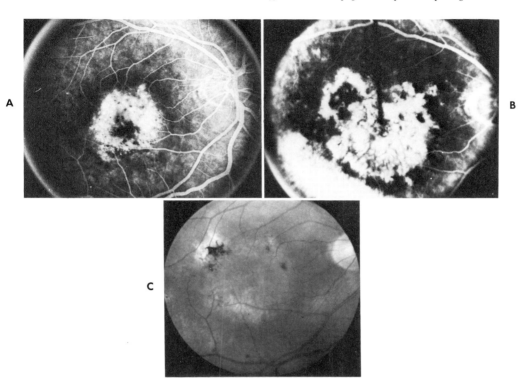

Fig. 10-4. A, Fluoroangiogram in midvenous phase in right eye of 39-year-old white man with vision of 20/25. Low serous sensory retinal detachment in posterior pole. Left eye normal. Mother had well-documented hemorrhagic senile macular degeneration in both eyes. **B,** Fluoroangiogram of same eye 8 years later, showing considerable extension of process. VA, 20/50. Low sensory retinal detachment persists. **C,** Photogram taken same day as **B,** showing hypopigmentation, and hyperpigmentation also evident in posterior pole.

Fig. 10-3. A, Fluoroangiogram in early venous phase of right eye of 52-year-old white man with 2-month history of blurred vision. A low sensory retinal detachment seen. VA, 20/25-2. Patient's mother had well-documented hemorrhagic senile macular degeneration. Exposure shows transmitted fluorescence in superonasal quadrant and a tiny area of fluorescence (*arrow*) at inferonasal edge of macula. **B,** Later exposure in same angiographic sequence, showing development of another tiny leak (*arrow*). No treatment given. **C,** Early venous phase of fluoroangiogram of same eye 3 months later. VA now 20/50. Process has extended temporally. Serous detachment of macular sensory retina still low. Two leaks present (*arrows*). **D,** Later venous phase of same angiographic sequence, showing blurring of fluorescence in superotemporal quadrant. Leakage now evident near edge of perifoveal capillary net (*arrow*) and at edge of nerve head at 11 o'clock. Argon laser photocoagulation given to all suspected leaks in macula and paramacular areas. **E,** Fluoroangiogram, venous phase, 3 weeks after **C** and **D.** VA, 20/25. Low sensory retinal detachment still present. Hyperpigmentation from treatment seen as negative fluorescence. **F,** Late exposure of same angiographic sequence, showing persistent leaks (*arrows*).

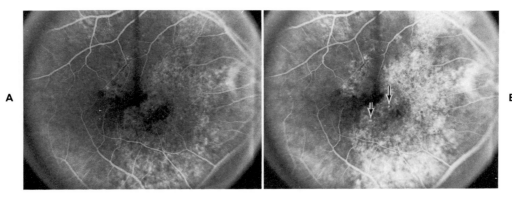

Fig. 10-5. A, Fluoroangiogram of right eye of 46-year-old white man with 7-year history of intermittent blurred vision. Serous detachment of sensory retina very low. No treatment given. VA, 20/30-2, with metamorphopsia. Exposure shows extensive transmitted choroidal fluorescence alternating with areas of blocked fluorescence due to hyperpigmentation at RPE level. **B,** Several dots of fluorescence become brighter *(arrows)* in this exposure of same angiogram, but no definite leaks found.

Table 10-1. Comparison of eyes with CSR and with DRPE

	CSR	DRPE
Number of eyes	112	33
Male patients	102 (91%)	31 (94%)
Female patients	10 (9%)	2 (6%)
Age of patients:		
Range	22 to 58 years	27 to 63 years
Average	41.6 years	45 years
Time from onset to treatment:		
Range	2 days to 5 years	2 days to 15 years
Average	6 months	27 months
Follow-up:		
Range	1 to 54 months	1 to 70 months
Average	10 months	27 months

Table 10-2. Treatment summary of 112 eyes with CSR and 33 eyes with DRPE

	CSR	DRPE
Number of treatment sessions per eye:		
Range	1 to 5	1 to 5
Average	1.3	2.2
Number of exposures per eye:		
Range	1 to 158	2 to 500
Average	29	89
Bilaterality	8/104 (7.7%)	6/27 (22%)
Recurrence rate	$\cong$ 50%	$\cong$ 100%
Quiescent at end of follow-up	100%	68%

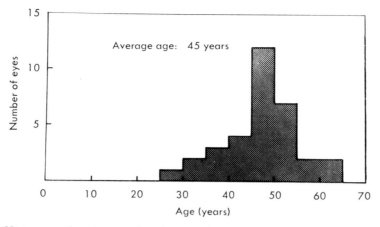

Fig. 10-6. Histogram showing age distribution of patients with DRPE. Compare with Fig. 9-7.

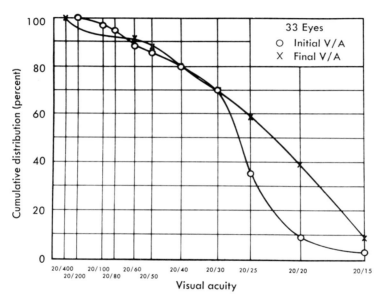

Fig. 10-7. Cumulative distribution of visual acuity of eyes before treatment and at end of follow-up. Compare with Fig. 9-8.

number of argon laser exposures, both range (1 to 158 versus 2 to 500) and average (29 versus 89), indicate the greater difficulty experienced in treating eyes with DRPE than with typical CSR. The 100% recurrence rate of DRPE and the fact that only 68% of eyes with DRPE were quiescent at the end of follow-up furnish evidence of the chronicity of this disease. There was a higher incidence of bilateral treatment given for symptomatic sensory retinal detachments among

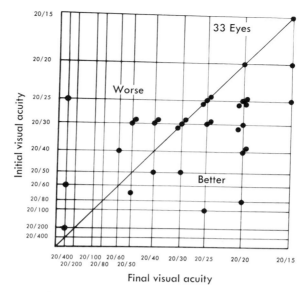

Fig. 10-8. Scattergram showing visual acuity of eyes at beginning of study, related to vision at end of follow-up time (see text).

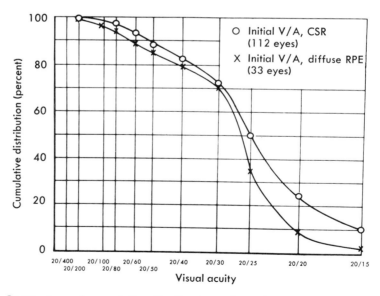

Fig. 10-9. Comparison of cumulative distributions of visual acuities in eyes before treatment for central serous retinopathy and for diffuse retinal pigment epitheliopathy. Curves are very similar.

those with DRPE: 6 of 27 patients (22%), compared with 8 of 104 (7.7%) with CSR. The chi-square test shows a statistical significance of $P < 0.05$.

Visual prognosis is better for CSR than for DRPE. Acuities before treatment and at end of follow-up are shown in Fig. 10-7; visual change in each eye with DRPE is demonstrated in Fig. 10-8. In none of the eyes with CSR treated with argon laser photocoagulation did vision deteriorate significantly (2 lines or more on the Snellen chart) over the follow-up time, but vision in five of the 33 eyes with DRPE (15.2%) did deteriorate. A direct comparison of visual acuities in the two groups is shown in Figs. 10-9 and 10-10. Although initial acuities were virtually identical, the final vision in eyes with DRPE was significantly worse than in eyes with CSR: 105 of 112 eyes with CSR had final vision of 20/30 or better, as compared with 23 of 33 eyes in the group with DRPE. This is significant to $P < 0.001$. At the end of the follow-up period, all eyes treated for CSR had visual acuity of 20/60 or better. In the group with DRPE, vision in three eyes (9%) was worse than 20/60: all had acuity of 20/400 at the end of the follow-up period, whereas before treatment they had had 20/25, 20/60, and 20/200 respectively.

Comparison was made in final visual acuities between eyes treated 4 months or less after onset of symptoms, compared with eyes for which the symptom onset–treatment interval was greater than 4 months. Initial visual acuity curves are very similar (Fig. 10-11), which permits valid comparison of final acuities. A difference does exist, but its statistical significance is low, $P < 0.1$.

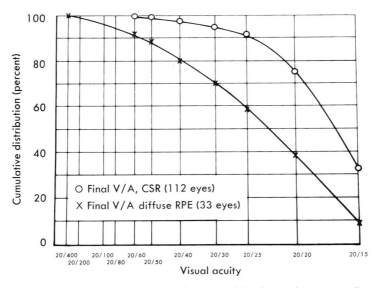

Fig. 10-10. Comparison of cumulative distributions of final visual acuities after treatment for central serous retinopathy and for diffuse retinal pigment epitheliopathy. Former group fared statistically better visually.

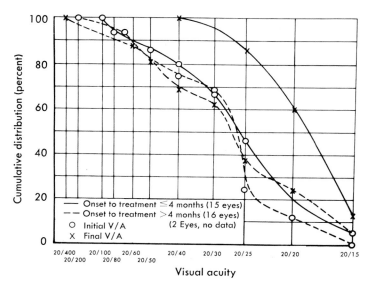

Fig. 10-11. Cumulative distributions of initial and final visual acuities in eyes with DRPE treated within 4 months of onset compared with those treated longer than 4 months after onset. Although visual results were better in former group, difference was of low statistical significance.

In summary, we believe that eyes with heretofore called chronic CSR can be grouped in a separate category. Compared with eyes with typical CSR, eyes with DRPE exhibit the following characteristics: (1) RPE disease is more widespread, (2) there is greater chronicity of course of disease, and (3) visual prognosis is worse.

REFERENCES

1. Watzke, R. C., Burton, T. C., and Leaverton, P. E.: Ruby laser photocoagulation therapy of central serous retinopathy. I. A controlled clinical study; II. Factors affecting prognosis, Trans. Am. Acad. Ophthalmol. Otolaryngol. **78:**205, 1974.

2. Klein, M. L., Van Buskirk, E. M., Friedman, E., et al.: Experience with nontreatment of central serous choroidopathy, Arch. Ophthalmol. **91:**247, 1974.

11
SENILE MACULAR DEGENERATION

Senile macular degeneration (SMD) afflicts many who are still in their economically productive years. Thus, loss of macular vision usually means economic blindness (20/70 or worse VA), because reading capability is lost. When it occurs in persons who have retired from active economic pursuits but are still leading a vigorous and involved life, impairment of reading vision is also a grievous loss. Therefore, careful study of these patients is warranted to accurately diagnose and classify their macular disease to determine the natural history of the several stages of this maculopathy and to evaluate therapies that may give promise of arresting the disease process.

In years past, the nomenclature has been confusing because many terms were used to describe what investigators have come to agree are different stages of the same disease process:[6] senile macular degeneration, senile drusen, Kuhnt-Junius macular degeneration,[8] Doyne's honeycomb choroiditis,[3] and Hutchinson-Tay's central guttate choroidopathy.[7] Due largely to the work of Maumenee[9] and Gass,[4,5] a classification has emerged that is based on ophthalmoscopic appearance, histopathologic examination, and fluoroangiographic interpretation reflecting stages of SMD. Although this work has united the seemingly diverse aspects of SMD into a unified whole, ophthalmology cannot provide an etiologic classification at this time.

Although there is no conclusive evidence, enough instances of familial occurrence have been reported[2,11] to implicate heredity as a factor in SMD. However, even with proof of familial incidence, the proximate mechanisms of atrophy of photoreceptors and the development of localized elevations of RPE and subretinal neovascular membranes remain to be clarified. Inasmuch as hypoxia is a well-established cause of retinal neovascularization, there may be a vascular/nutritional basis for elaboration of a "vasoproliferative factor" that stimulates the growth of subretinal neovascular membranes.

We classify senile macular degeneration as follows:

Stage I: Nonexudative

Stage II: Serous detachment RPE

Stage III: Serous detachment RPE combined with overlying sensory retinal detachment

Stage IV: Exudative hemorrhagic detachment of RPE with or without detachment of sensory retina (vascular)

Stage V: Cicatricial

NONEXUDATIVE SMD (Stage I)

Ophthalmoscopically, multiple drusen, some confluent, are seen along with hyper- and hypopigmentation of the retinal pigment epithelium (RPE). The process can involve part of the macula or the entire posterior pole. The macula has a mottled, or moth-eaten, appearance. Drusen may be found in the retinal pe-

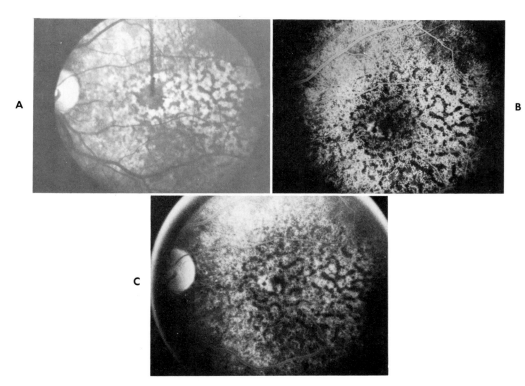

Fig. 11-1. A, Photograph of posterior pole of left eye, showing multiple drusen and RPE hyperpigmentation in 25-year-old woman. VA, 20/20. VA in right eye, 30/30. **B,** Fluoroangiogram same day, showing staining of drusen and multiple ribbonlike areas of negative fluorescence where RPE hyperpigmentation blocks fluorescein transmitted from underlying choroid. **C,** Later exposure in same fluorangiographic sequence, showing that staining areas have not enlarged, indicating they are either drusen that have taken up the dye or window defects in RPE pigmentation allowing fluorescein to be transmitted from underlying choroid. True leakage spreads out in time.

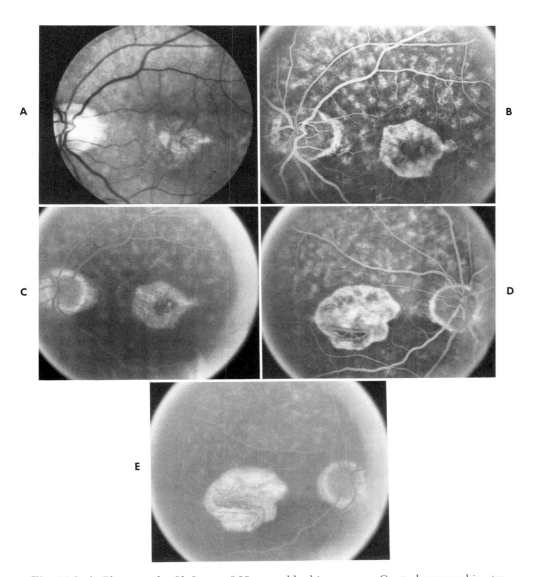

Fig. 11-2. A, Photograph of left eye of 68-year-old white woman. Central geographic atrophy of RPE and multiple drusen seen. Large choroidal vessels and bare sclera seen in area of depigmentation, but no choriocapillaris. VA, 20/400. **B,** Fluoroangiogram of same eye. Drusen have taken up the dye, and sclera is stained. **C,** Later exposure in same angiogram, showing fluorescence fading from drusen. Sclera staining is less vivid but still present. No leakage seen, demonstrating that no diffusion of dye occurred. **D,** Fluoroangiogram of right eye of same patient, showing similar central geographic atrophy of RPE and drusen staining. VA, 20/400. **E,** Late fluoroangiogram showing large choroidal vessels dark against background of scleral staining.

riphery as well. Cholesterol crystals are sometimes seen in the macula. Fluorescein retinal angiogram shows early fluorescence from the underlying choroid, through "window" defects in the RPE, and staining of the drusen. Neither of these areas of fluorescence enlarges with time, as does true leakage (Fig. 11-1). Included in this category are eyes with geographic or areolar pigment atrophy (Fig. 11-2). Vision can vary from 20/20 to 20/400.

Nonexudative senile macular degeneration in most instances is probably caused by the same disease processes leading to exudative senile macular degeneration. The occurrence of nonexudative macular degeneration in one eye and exudative disease in the second eye and the natural history of drusen in nonexudative choroidal macular degeneration support the conclusion that one is dealing with the same disease process in both. Furthermore, serous detachments of the retinal pigment epithelium *sometimes* resolve, leaving a flat dry macula with circumscribed atrophy of the RPE.

Gass[6] observed 49 patients with macular drusen and reported their rate of visual loss. Over an average follow-up time of 4.9 years, nine of the 49 (18%) developed loss of central vision in one eye, and in five (10%) of the nine, loss of vision in the second eye to less than 20/200 occurred within 1 year after onset of symptoms in the second eye. Gass also reported on the visual results in 91 eyes with macular drusen, followed for 4 years, the fellow eye of which had already lost central vision to senile disciform maculopathy: "Thirty-one of the 91 patients (35%) developed loss of central vision in the second eye secondary to disciform detachment and degeneration of the macula." Visual loss from macular drusen can develop as a result of continued atrophy of photoreceptors or development of disciform detachments of the macula.

Cleasby[1] reported on 20 eyes with drusen only, which he had treated with argon laser photocoagulation: "All patients were treated under topical anesthesia with the argon laser (Coherent Radiation Model 800) with a 50 or 100 micron size application at 0.1 seconds. The power setting used was that which was just sufficient to give a minimally visible reaction and ranged from 125 to 500 mW. The average number of applications was 249, with a range of 86 to 406. The usual treatment pattern was a broad ring of closely spaced applications around the fovea, somewhat narrowed in the papillomacular zone, making sure to cover any drusen present. Of the 20 eyes with treated non-exudative senile maculopathy (NSM), only one patient has developed exudative senile maculopathy (ESM) in a follow-up period of six months to two years. The only complication during treatment was a minute hemorrhage in one patient. This was stopped by more intense photocoagulation. For evaluation of visual results, a loss of two or more lines on the Snellen chart or Jaeger card was rated 'worse' and a gain of two or more lines was rated 'better.' Of the 20 eyes photocoagulated, three were better, 12 the same and five worse. Thus, 75% maintained their vision. The only profound loss was the patient who developed ESM three months after treatment and deteriorated from 20/20 and J1 to 20/200 and J14 (vision in his other eye, seen initially with ESM, was 3/200 and JO)."

We have no experience in treating nonexudative senile macular degeneration with photocoagulation. Furthermore, we are concerned that treatment of drusen with photocoagulation might cause the tiny neovascularizations, demonstrated in some drusen in histologic studies by Sark,[12] to grow and precipitate the hemorrhagic stage of senile maculopathy. We report Cleasby's experience as a possible future treatment approach that requires a controlled series with long follow-up before its value is known.

EXUDATIVE: SEROUS
RPE detachments (Stage II)

Leakage of serum through Bruch's membrane elevates a "blister" of RPE (Fig. 11-3). The cause of loss of the normal adhesion between the RPE and Bruch's membrane is unknown. Such separations may be in the fovea, macula, paramacula, or perimacula. They appear as yellowish or pinkish-gray oval or elliptiform elevations, sometimes with scalloped boundaries, always with smooth edges. On fluorescein angiograms, RPE separations typically fill with dye early, demonstrating the normal permeability of Bruch's membrane to serum. RPE detachments often have surface pigmentation, arranged in a roughly cruciate distribution ("hot cross bun" pigmentation) (Figs. 11-4 and 11-5). Vision can range from 20/20 (even if the separation involves the fovea) to 20/100.

Management concepts

Outside the macula. RPE detachments not involving the macula should be observed but not treated actively, because they do not interfere with vision. On the initial examination, 35-mm color photography and retinal fluorescein angiography should be carried out. The patient should be seen at intervals of 3 to 6 months. He should be instructed to test macular vision daily with Amsler grid ob-

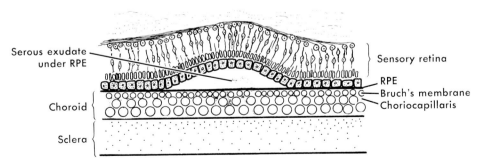

Fig. 11-3. Illustration of serous detachment of the retinal pigment epithelium from underlying Bruch's membrane. Stage II senile macular degeneration.

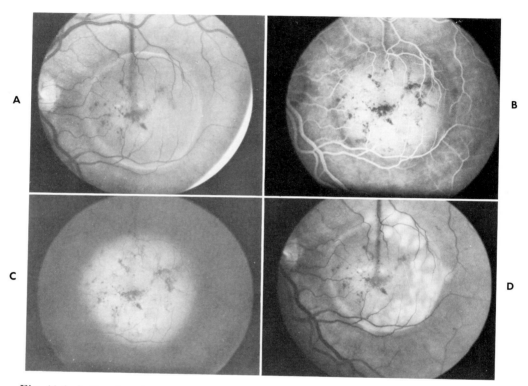

Fig. 11-4. A, Fundus photograph of large retinal pigment epithelial detachment 4 to 5 mm in diameter. Edges are sharp. "Hot cross bun" pigmentation present on surface of detachment. VA, 20/30−2. **B,** Fluoroangiogram of same retina, showing early filling of entire detachment with dye. **C,** Late fluoroangiogram of same eye. Edges of detachment are sharp and regular. **D,** Photograph showing a double row of argon laser photocoagulation immediately after treatment of temporal third of RPE detachment.

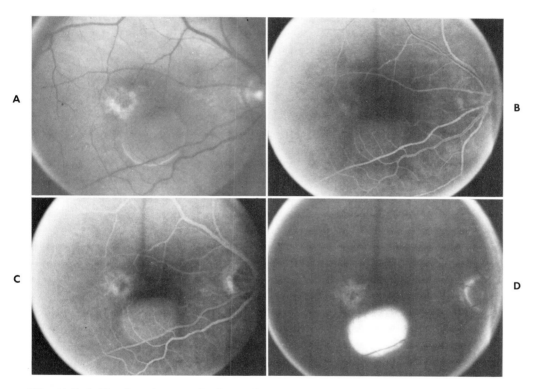

Fig. 11-5. A, Fundus photograph of retinal pigment epithelial detachment about 2 mm in diameter, occupying inferior portion of macula and extending into paramacula. VA, 20/40. Hypopigmentation is noted in superotemporal portion of macula, indicating previous RPE disturbance. **B,** Fluorangiogram same day as **A.** RPE detachment nearly completely filled in early venous phase. **C,** Later exposure in same angiographic sequence, demonstrating full filling of RPE detachment. **D,** Delayed exposure in same angiographic sequence, showing intense fluorescence in RPE detachment. *Continued.*

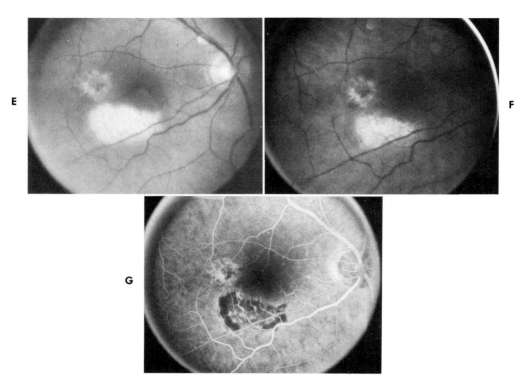

Fig. 11-5, cont'd. E, Photograph immediately after RPE detachment treated with argon laser photocoagulation. Entire detachment photocoagulated, except for portion within 300 μm of fovea. **F,** Photograph 2 weeks after treatment, showing resolving photocoagulation lesions with collapse of RPE detachment. **G,** Fluoroangiogram same day as **F,** showing choroidal fluorescence blocked due to hyperpigmentation of treatment. RPE detachment has collapsed.

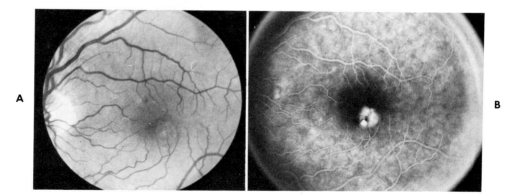

Fig. 11-6. A, Photograph showing asymptomatic RPE detachment in macula. VA, 20/15. **B,** Fluoroangiogram same day. RPE separation abuts fovea but does not involve it. Pigmentation seen on surface of detachment.

servations and advised to return for reexamination promptly if he notes a change in the Amsler grid pattern that is consistent for 3 days. At the regular 3- to 6-month examination, visual parameters should be carefully retested and fluorescein angiography carried out if there is any question of enlargement of the detachment.

Within the macula. Detachments not involving the fovea should be observed only as described above (Fig. 11-6). Since the larger detachments of the RPE are predisposed to the development of subretinal neovascular membrane, treatment is indicated if the detachment has enlarged on angiography or visual symptoms have developed, such as decreased acuity or metamorphopsia.

Detachments involving the fovea should be treated, but only if one third of the detachment is 300 μm or more from the fovea; treatment within 300 μm of the fovea can endanger it.

If the macula in the fellow eye has been destroyed by hemorrhagic senile maculopathy, there is a stronger indication for treatment.

Very careful observation must be made to detect any subretinal neovascular membrane. The treatment technique is different, and the prognosis for vision is much worse in that stage, as discussed later in the section on exudative hemorrhagic senile macular degeneration.

Technique of argon laser photocoagulation. Lesions should be moderately heavy in intensity. Recommended parameters are 200-μm spot size diameter, 0.1- to 0.2-sec time exposure, and 200- to 300-mW power.

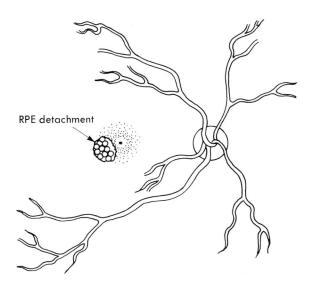

Fig. 11-7. Diagram showing extrafoveal macular RPE detachment. Treatment lesions cover all of detachment 300 μm or more from fovea.

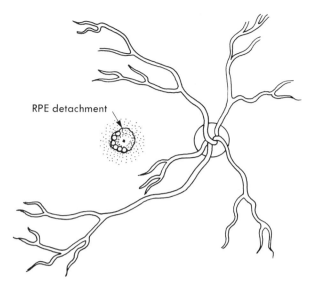

Fig. 11-8. Diagram showing single row of photocoagulation placed in temporal periphery of small RPE detachment. Pattern may be placed nasally if greater area of detachment is nasal. Lesions should be no closer than 300 μm to fovea. At least one third of detachment should be treated.

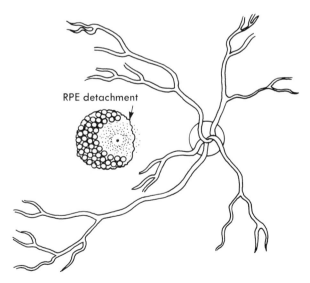

Fig. 11-9. Diagram showing C pattern of photocoagulation of large RPE detachment almost centered on fovea. Double row of lesions shown in temporal portion of detachment, with none closer than 300 μm to fovea.

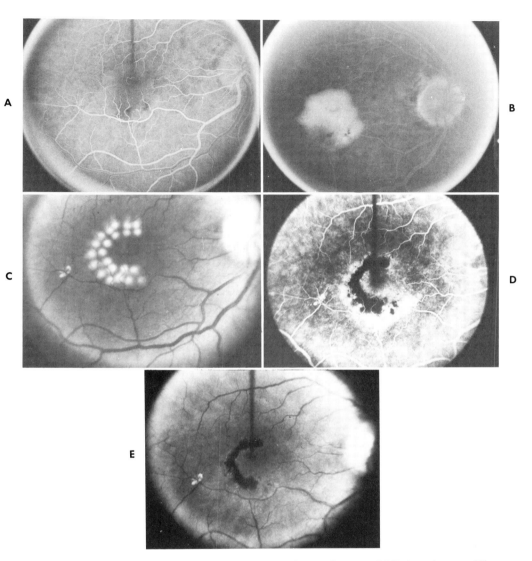

Fig. 11-10. A, Fluoroangiogram in early venous phase, showing RPE detachment filling with dye. VA, 20/40. **B,** Same fluoroangiogram, late exposure, showing sharp, scalloped edges of RPE detachment. **C,** Photograph immediately after argon laser photocoagulation. C-pattern technique used. **D,** Postoperative angiogram 3 months after treatment. RPE detachment has collapsed. Hyperpigmentation due to treatment blocks choroidal fluorescence, and area of pigment atrophy around hyperpigmentation transmits choroidal fluorescence. VA, 20/20−2. **E,** Photograph 3 months after treatment, showing hyperpigmentation in treatment site.

Three patterns of placement of the lesions may be used. If the whole RPE detachment is 300 μm or more from the fovea, the entire elevation should be photocoagulated (Fig. 11-7). If part of the detachment is within 300 μm of the fovea, treat as much of it as is outside that distance (Fig. 11-5).

If the detachment encroaches on the fovea but is relatively small (i.e., 500-μm diameter), treat at least one third of the elevation 300 μm or more from the fovea (Fig. 11-8).

If the detachment encroaches on the macula but is greater than 500 μm in diameter, the C pattern of photocoagulation suggested by Wessing[14,15] is used. A double row of lesions is placed in a semicircle at the temporal edge of the detachment (Figs. 11-4, 11-9, and 11-10).

We treated 17 eyes with RPE detachments with ALP using the above criteria and observed them for 6 to 55 months (average, 28 months). Seven patients (41%) were male, 10 (59%) were female; they ranged in age from 32 to 71 years (average, 59). Four (23%) of the 17 improved visually (two lines or more on the Snellen Chart); seven (42%) remained the same; six (35%) worsened. This small treated group not matched with control untreated eyes does not give enough data to permit a definitive statement about efficacy of treatment. Furthermore, we are unaware of any report on the visual fate of untreated RPE detachments with which we could compare our group. One aspect of our experience deserves emphasis: four eyes (23%) developed subretinal neovascular membranes during follow-up, 4, 6, 12, and 35 months after treatment respectively. These RPE detachments were ½ disc diameter or larger. Eyes with RPE detachments are susceptible to progression from avascular to vascular degeneration, as discussed in the next section.

RPE separation with overlying sensory retinal detachment (Stage III)

When a break develops in the separated RPE, leakage of serum under the sensory epithelial layer elevates it (Fig. 11-11). The break occurs in the zonula occludens, which normally binds the RPE cells together in a watertight seal. The sensory retinal detachment is seen on funduscopy as a gray-yellow elevated area with diffuse edges, as opposed to the sharp edges seen in RPE detachments. The underlying fluid is often turbid or murky. On fluorescein angiography, the underlying RPE detachment fills with dye early, but the overlying sensory retinal detachment usually fills more slowly and the edges are blurred. Often the full extent of the latter detachment is obvious only in delayed films (Figs. 11-12 to 11-14). Any sensory retinal exudative detachment must be suspected of either harboring a subretinal neovascular membrane or of having an environment in which one can grow later (Fig. 11-24).

Indications for argon laser photocoagulation. Treatment is indicated on diagnosis, because of vision reduction and the likelihood of progression to hemorrhagic senile maculopathy. Teeters and Bird[13] observed 18 maculas with avascular exudative senile maculopathy for 4 to 19 months, during which time 12

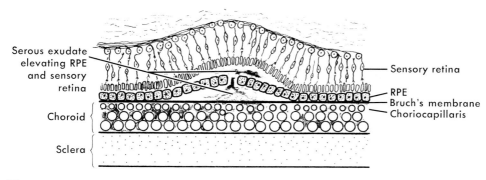

Serous exudate elevating RPE and sensory retina

Choroid

Sclera

Sensory retina

RPE
Bruch's membrane
Choriocapillaris

Fig. 11-11. Diagram of serous detachment of retinal pigment epithelium, with secondary serous detachment of overlying sensory retina occurring through break in RPE. Stage III senile macular degeneration.

(67%) developed subretinal neovascular membranes (hemorrhagic SMD). Since the leakage site frequently involves the fovea or even the entire macula, only those eyes with localized leakage points not involving the fovea are amenable for laser photocoagulation. Thus, fluorescein angiography is essential in determining which eyes should be treated.

Technique of argon laser photocoagulation. Only the underlying RPE detachment should be treated.

The serous fluid under the elevated sensory retina is usually turbid; therefore, higher power density and longer time exposures are required than for simple RPE detachments. Initial parameters are 100- to 200-μm spot size, 0.1 sec, and 200-mW power; the power is then increased by 50-mW increments until 400 mW is reached. If lesions are not obtained at that level, exposure time should be increased to 0.2 sec, with the power reduced to 200 mW. Power is increased as before, to obtain "dirty" white lesions on the RPE detachment (Figs. 11-12 to 11-14).

Postoperative examination, including retinal fluoroangiography, should be carried out every 2 weeks until the sensory and RPE detachments have flattened.

We have treated 59 eyes with combined RPE and sensory retinal detachments (Stage III), with argon laser photocoagulation (Coherent Radiation Models 800 and 900), and have followed these eyes for from 6 to 54 months. Patients ranged in age from 45 to 82 years (average, 65). Of these patients, 54% were female and 46% were male; all were white.

Results were evaluated by comparing visual acuity before treatment with that on the last follow-up visit. Because this study was not controlled and randomly assigned, visual results were compared with those in 18 untreated eyes reported on by Teeters and Bird.[13]

The 59 eyes with avascular sensory retinal detachments treated in this series were subdivided into two groups. Group 1, comprising 35 eyes followed for 6 to 19

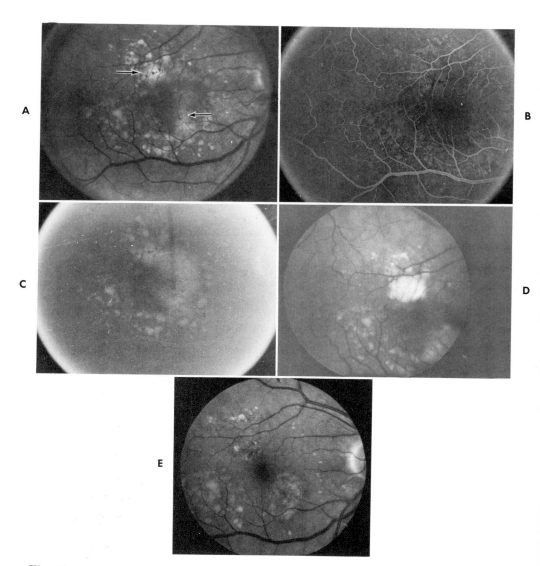

Fig. 11-12. A, Retinal photograph showing sensory retinal detachment overlying two RPE detachments *(arrows).* VA, 20/30. Hyperpigmentation is especially marked over RPE detachment at superior edge of macula. **B,** Fluoroangiogram same day. In early venous phase, RPE detachments are accumulating dye; sensory retinal detachment is not. Multiple drusen show staining with dye. **C,** Late exposure of same angiographic sequence, showing sensory retinal detachment filled with dye. Edges fuzzy. Fluorescence from drusen unchanged from early exposures, indicating staining with, not leakage of, dye. **D,** Photograph immediately after argon laser photocoagulation. Upper RPE detachment treated more heavily. **E,** Photograph 3 months after photocoagulation, with resolution of both RPE detachments and overlying sensory retinal separation. VA, 20/20−1.

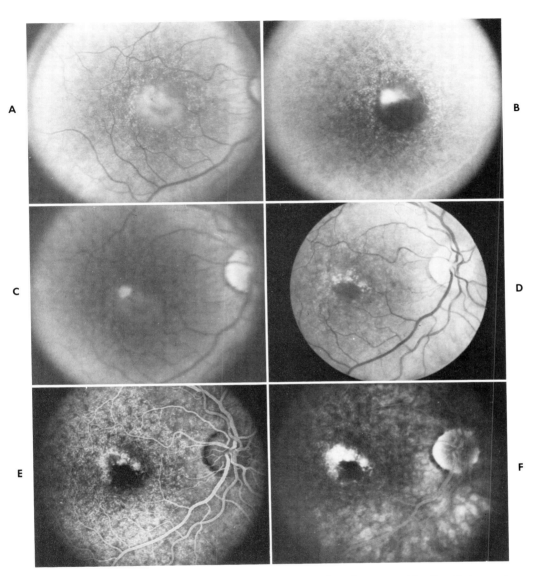

Fig. 11-13. A, Photograph of retina with sensory retinal detachment visible. Small pigment fleck seen on underlying RPE detachment. Many drusen in posterior pole. Other eye, similar appearance. VA, 20/30. **B,** Fluoroangiogram in venous phase, showing intense hyperfluorescence in RPE detachment, with serum containing dye leaking out under sensory retinal detachment. Drusen bodies show staining with fluorescein. **C,** Photograph immediately after argon laser photocoagulation. Only RPE separation treated. **D,** Photograph 3 months after treatment. VA, 20/20 − 1. Sensory retina flat. **E,** Fluoroangiogram, venous phase, same day as **D,** showing transmitted fluorescence from choroid through area of hypopigmentation from argon laser photocoagulation treatment. **F,** Late exposure in same fluoroangiogram. No RPE detachment seen, nor dye leakage under sensory retina.

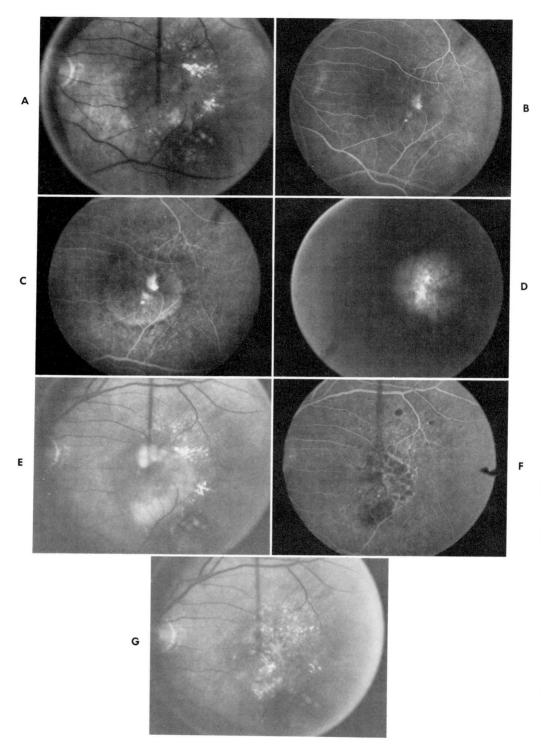

Fig. 11-14. For legend see opposite page.

months, was selected to match the Teeters and Bird group of 18 avascular eyes followed for 4 to 19 months; group 2 was composed of 24 eyes followed for 20 to 54 months. Fig. 11-15 shows that the initial visual acuity curves of the three groups were reasonably similar; Fig. 11-16 illustrates the final visual acuity curves of the same three groups. Both treated groups show improvement over the

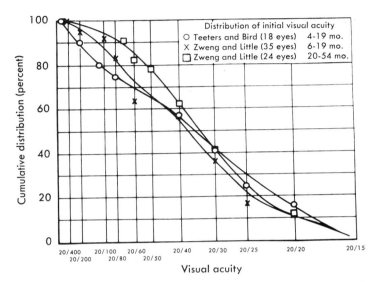

Fig. 11-15. Avascular exudative senile maculopathy (Stage III). Cumulative distribution of visual acuity curves of eyes at start of study. Comparison of 18 untreated eyes reported by Teeters and Bird with 59 treated eyes, broken into two groups according to length of follow-up time. Curves not significantly different.

Fig. 11-14. A, Photograph of posterior pole of left eye, showing serous elevation of sensory retina. At temporal edge, lipid deposits are seen. Presence of lipids often indicates presence of subretinal neovascular membrane (SRNM), although none was found in this case. Benign nevus present inferotemporally from macula. Drusen seen on nevus and above macula. VA, 20/30−2. **B** and **C,** Fluoroangiograms showing dye leaking from RPE detachment under sensory retinal detachment, gradually outlining it. One other tiny RPE detachment present under sensory retinal detachment, but not leaking serum under it. In late film, **D,** edges of sensory retinal elevation fuzzy. **E,** Photograph immediately after argon laser photocoagulation. Treatment more extensive than now recommended. Current concept is to treat RPE detachment only. **F,** Fluoroangiogram 3 months after treatment, demonstrating flattening of both sensory retina and RPE detachment. Hyperpigmentation seen in treated area. RPE detachment not leaking was not treated and is still present. **G,** Photograph same day as **F,** showing collapse of sensory retinal detachment, with absorption of much of lipid deposited temporal from macula.

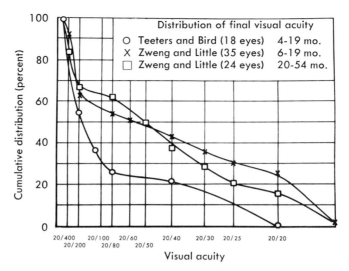

Fig. 11-16. Avascular exudative senile maculopathy (Stage III). Cumulative distribution of visual acuity curves of eyes at end of study. Curves of two treated groups show significantly better visual results than untreated group (see text).

Table 11-1. Exudative senile macular degeneration: avascular (Stage III)

	Follow-up (months)	Final vision	
		≥20/80*	≥20/40†
18 Untreated eyes (Teeters and Bird)	4 to 19	5 (27%)	4 (22%)
59 Treated eyes (Zweng and Little)	6 to 54	34 (59%)	24 (42%)

*Significant at P < 0.03 level.
†Significant at P < 0.05 level.

Teeters and Bird untreated eyes. Of interest is that the final visual acuity curves of both treated groups are similar, in spite of the longer follow-up of group 2. Two especially significant points of vision data that can be compared are acuities of 20/80, because some macula is still functioning at that level, and 20/40, because reading usually is possible without magnification. In the Teeters and Bird group, four of 18 eyes (27%) had 20/80 vision or better; in the two treated groups, 24 of 59 eyes (59%) had 20/80 or better. This is statistically significant at a P < 0.03 level. Four of 18 untreated eyes (22%) had acuity of 20/40, as compared with 24 of 59 treated eyes (43%). This is significant at the P < 0.05 level, and is even more significant in view of the longer follow-up time of our patients (Table 11-1).

Of special interest is comparison of rate of progression from avascular to vascular maculopathy. Although there were 59 eyes in our series, accurate data regarding progression in the 6- to 19-month interval was available only for 49. The rate of progression in the Teeters and Bird group was 67%; in 49 treated

Table 11-2. Progression of senile macular degeneration: avascular to vascular

Follow-up (months)	Avascular (Stage III)	Vascular (Stage IV)	Percent
Teeters and Bird 4 to 19	18	12	67
Zweng and Little 6 to 19	49	13	27

Significant at P < 0.0005 level.

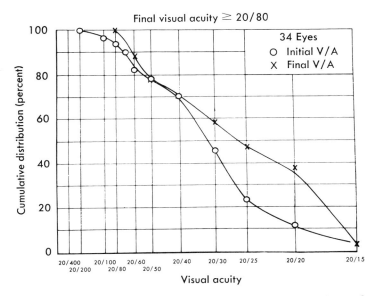

Fig. 11-17. Avascular exudative senile maculopathy (Stage III). Cumulative distribution of visual acuities of 34 eyes treated with argon laser photocoagulation; final VA, 20/80 or better. Only two eyes had VA worse than 20/80 *before* treatment.

eyes, followed for the same length of time, it was 27%. This is statistically significant at the P < 0.0005 level (Table 11-2).

Further analysis showed that eyes with visual acuity of 20/80 or better at the end of follow-up had 20/80 before treatment with only two exceptions; thus patients with initial vision of less than 20/80 are not likely to recover macular function after photocoagulation (Fig. 11-17).

EXUDATIVE: HEMORRHAGIC (VASCULAR)
RPE detachment with overlying sensory epithelial detachment, with subretinal neovascular membrane (Stage IV)

Funduscopic findings differ from those in Stage III in that usually there is hemorrhage, which can be either dark maroon in color if under the RPE or brighter red if under the sensory retina (Fig. 11-18). Lipoidal deposits are often

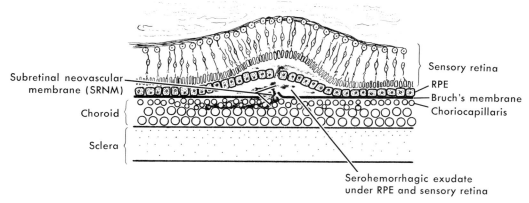

Sensory retina

Subretinal neovascular—
membrane (SRNM)

RPE
Bruch's membrane
Choroid
Choriocapillaris

Sclera

Serohemorrhagic exudate
under RPE and sensory retina

Fig. 11-18. Hemorrhagic exudative senile maculopathy (Stage IV). Diagram representing ingrown neovascular membrane, from choroid through break in Bruch's membrane under retinal pigment epithelium (RPE), with hemorrhage under both RPE and detached overlying sensory retina.

present at the edge of the elevated sensory retina. The subretinal neovascular membrane (SRNM) can sometimes be seen as a dirty-gray irregular circle or oval under the RPE. The characteristic appearance of the membrane on fluorescein angiogram is an irregular area of fluorescence that becomes more dense with time, with the density greater at the edge of the area than centrally ("bicyclewheel"), with a lacy, open appearance in early photographs (Figs. 11-19 and 11-20).

Indications for argon laser photocoagulation. The natural visual course of stage IV senile macular degeneration is generally downhill; thus treatment with argon laser photocoagulation should be considered carefully on diagnosis. However, the entire net must be destroyed or the patient's condition is probably worsened by treatment, because incompletely treated SRNM can recur with great exuberance (Fig. 11-21). Photocoagulation must be heavy in order to eradicate the SRNM; thus the distance from the edge of the membrane to the fovea is a critical factor, because the fovea is endangered by photocoagulation if treatment is given too close to it. We recommend that treatment be undertaken if the SRNM is no closer than 400 μm to the fovea. Only if the physician is experienced and the patient is aware of the risk incurred with treatment should SRNMs that come up to 200 μm of the fovea be photocoagulated. The grim prognosis given by the natural history of this disease is the sole justification for heavy photocoagulation this close to the fovea.

Technique of argon laser photocoagulation. It is advisable that the patient be given a retrobulbar anesthetic.

A barrier of photocoagulation is placed initially, as recommended by Patz,[10] to mark the edge of the SRNM nearest the fovea. The edge is determined by

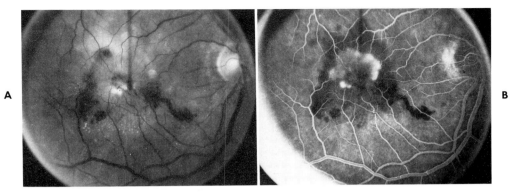

Fig. 11-19. A, Fundus photograph of right retina with hemorrhagic exudative maculopathy. Blurred vision for 2 months. VA, 20/200. Sensory retina elevated across macula and paramacula by serosanguinous exudate. Flecks of lipid seen at inferior edge of elevation. **B,** Early venous phase of fluoroangiogram on same day. Subretinal neovascular membrane (SRNM) seen as irregular circle of fluorescence underlying almost entire macula. Surrounding area of decreased fluorescence due to subretinal hemorrhage blocking choroidal fluorescence. Because SRNM underlies fovea, argon laser photocoagulation is contraindicated.

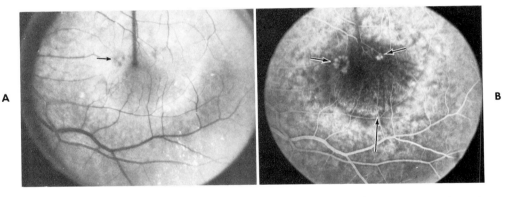

Fig. 11-20. A, Photograph of left eye, showing serous elevation of sensory retina in entire macula, with several flecks of blood *(arrow)* above macula and lipid deposits inferiorly. VA, 20/40. **B,** Fluoroangiogram same date, showing three subretinal neovascular membranes in macula. Largest membrane *(long arrow)* underlies entire macula; two smaller membranes *(short arrows)* are within the larger.

carefully relating the position of the SRNM in the fluoroangiogram to the macular landmarks as viewed by slit-lamp funduscopy. Occasionally, fluorescein angioscopy at the time of treatment is necessary to locate the frond precisely. The settings used to make the visual barrier are 50-μm spot size diameter, 0.05-sec exposure, 150- to 200-mW power, or just enough to give barely discernible lesions (Fig. 11-22).

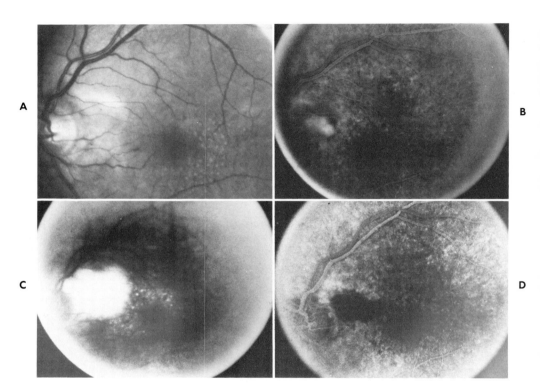

Fig. 11-21. A, Photograph of posterior pole of left eye with exudative detachment of sensory retina just off optic nerve head superotemporally. Drusen seen temporally from macula. VA, 20/60. **B,** Fluoroangiogram same day in late venous phase, showing pooling of dye from subretinal neovascular membrane (SRNM). Some staining of drusen seen, and tiny areas of negative fluorescence due to flecks of hyperpigmentation at RPE level. **C,** Late exposure of same fluoroangiogram, showing considerable leakage of dye from SRNM. **D,** Fluorangiogram 2 weeks after heavy argon laser photocoagulation, showing negative fluorescence in area, with no apparent residual SRNM. VA, 20/25+2. **E,** Photograph 2 weeks after treatment, showing scarring from treatment. Exudative sensory retinal detachment has cleared. VA, 20/25. **F,** Fluoroangiogram 3 months after first treatment, showing growth of SRNM (*arrow*) now threatening fovea. VA, 20/25. **G,** Photograph immediately after heavy argon laser photocoagulation of SRNM. This was last treatment given. **H,** Fluoroangiogram 4 months after **F** and **G.** SRNM has now extended far temporally from macula. VA, 20/400. **I,** Photograph same day as **H,** showing white scarring from treatment and sensory retinal exudative detachment overlying persistent SRNM temporal from treated area.

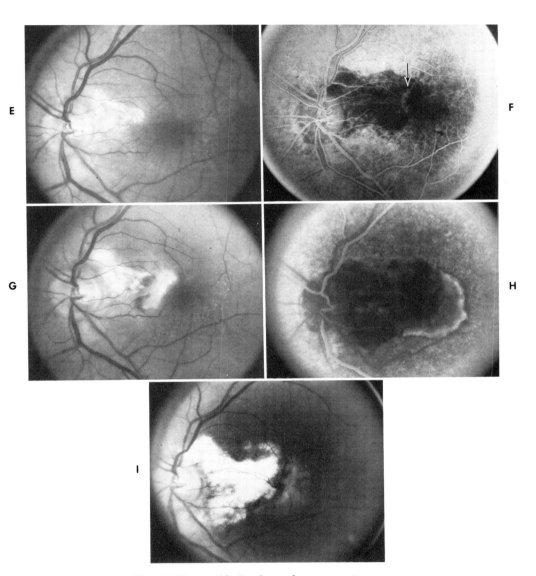

Fig. 11-21, cont'd. For legend see opposite page.

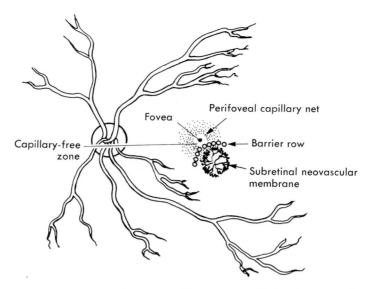

Fig. 11-22. Diagram illustrating placement of barrier row of light photocoagulation lesions just beyond edge of subretinal neovascular membrane nearest fovea, indicating closest that treatment lesions should come to fovea. Lesions made with 50-μm, 0.05-sec, 150- to 200-mW power settings.

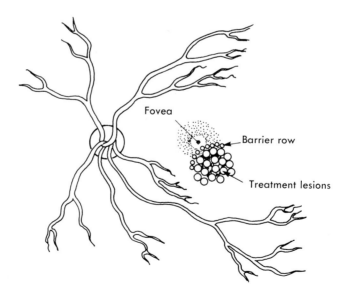

Fig. 11-23. Diagram showing placement of heavy lesions on subretinal neovascular membrane, extending to barrier row of lesions previously given. Treatment lesions made with 200-μm, 0.2- to 0.5-sec, 400- to 600-mW power settings. Lesions beyond macula may be made by 500 μm, 0.5 sec, 600 to 800 mW to give very heavy coagulations.

Treatment lesions should be chalk white. Settings that usually give the required heavy burns are 200 μm, 0.2 sec, and 400 to 500 mW in the macula; 500 μm, 0.5 sec, 800 mW outside the macula (Figs. 11-23 to 11-25).

The ophthalmologist must make clear to the patient that, in order to avert the danger of bleeding from the treated lesion, he must avoid the effect of gravity (by not lowering his head below heart level) and the Valsalva effect (by avoiding lifting, straining, coughing, and sneezing), both of which increase intraluminal pressure in the vessels damaged by photocoagulation.

Very close observation of the patient after treatment is of greatest importance. The lesion should be reexamined with retinal fluorescein angiography approximately every 2 weeks until the active and dangerous SRNM is replaced by a scar.

If further treatment is indicated, the same technique is used.

We have used argon laser photocoagulation to treat 84 patients with the hemorrhagic stage of senile macular degeneration (SMD). Thirty-one were male (37%), and 53 were female (63%); they ranged in age from 48 to 86 years (average, 69). Follow-up time of this group of patients varied from 6 to 48 months (average, 15.3 months). (Fig. 11-26). Because this study was not carried out in a randomized fashion, a comparison was made with the visual acuities of a group of 63 untreated eyes with hemorrhagic SMD reported by Teeters and Bird.[13] Their observations make plain the discouraging visual prognosis for patients with hemorrhagic SMD. Teeters and Bird followed their untreated group for from 6 to 24 months; therefore, we compared 53 of the 84 treated eyes, also followed for 6 to 24 months (Figs. 11-27 and 11-28), with the untreated series. The number of eyes with 20/80 vision before and after the study shows the difference between the two groups (9 of 63 untreated eyes, as opposed to 14 of 53 treated) to be of low significance ($P < 0.01$). Further analysis of the treated patients indicates that two groups of eyes fared better than did the others. In the first group the widest diameter of the subretinal neovascular membrane (SRNM) before treatment, as measured on fluoroangiogram, was no greater than 800 μm, or approximately half the diameter of the optic nerve head (Fig. 11-29). In the second group the distance from the fovea to the nearest edge of the SRNM was greater than 400 μm (Fig. 11-30). In both groups final visual acuity curves were distinctly better than for the untreated eyes reported by Teeters and Bird. The smaller the SRNM, the easier it is destroyed by photocoagulation. The greater the distance from fovea to SRNM, the heavier the treatment can be, the most important factor in destroying the SRNM.

In retrospect, we have identified three negative factors that contributed to our experience:

1. Some eyes were treated too lightly with photocoagulation when treatment was carried out before the significance or even existence of subretinal neovascular membranes was appreciated.
2. Many eyes were not followed as closely (i.e., every 2 weeks) as we now recommend after treatment. *Text continued on p. 156.*

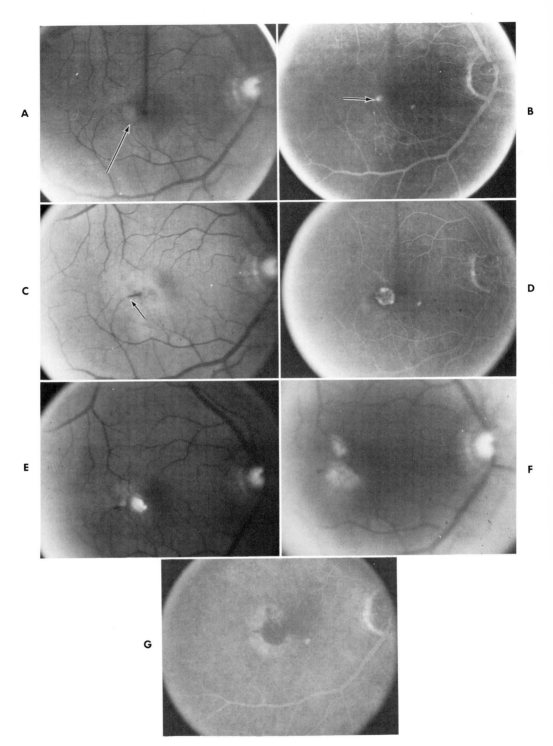

Fig. 11-24. For legend see opposite page.

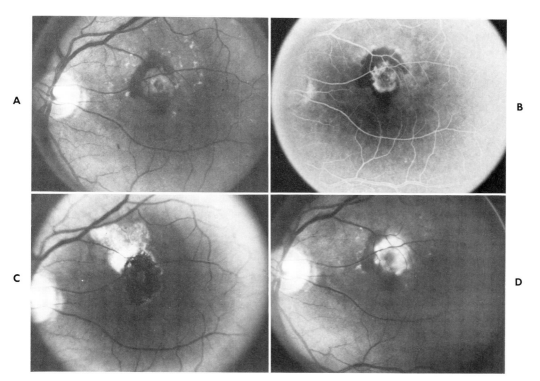

Fig. 11-25. A, Photograph showing serous elevation of sensory retina involving entire macula and extending to superotemporal vascular arcade. Halo of hemorrhage surrounds central lesions, with flecks of lipid seen farther out in separation. VA, 20/200. **B,** Fluoroangiogram same day, showing SRNM underlying central portion of sensory retinal elevation. **C,** Photograph immediately after argon laser photocoagulation of SRNM. Lesions heavy. **D,** Photograph 3 months after treatment. Intervening treatments given for recurrence of SRNM where it extended superiorly; no extensions developed closer to fovea. Hyperpigmentation seen centrally with bare sclera above it. VA, 20/80.

Fig. 11-24. A, Photograph of posterior pole of right eye with small sensory retinal serous elevation *(arrow)*. VA, 20/20. Macula of other eye destroyed by hemorrhagic senile maculopathy. **B,** Fluoroangiogram same day. Tiny area of intense fluorescence indicates RPE detachment *(arrow)*. Dye leaking out of RPE detachment under sensory retinal detachment. **C,** Photograph of same eye 5 weeks later, showing increase in sensory retinal detachment, with small linear hemorrhage *(arrow)*. VA, 20/30. **D,** Fluoroangiogram same day as **C.** SRNM now present. **E,** Photograph immediately after first argon laser photocoagulation of SRNM. VA, 20/60. **F,** Photograph after second argon laser photocoagulation, given 1 week after the first, which did not completely destroy SRNM. **G,** Fluoroangiogram 2 weeks after second treatment. No evidence of SRNM. Dark central area of negative fluorescence due to pigmentation generated by treatment. Fluorescence transmitted from choroid is seen around treated area due to pigment atrophy in RPE. VA, 20/50+2. Two months later, VA improved to 20/20−2.

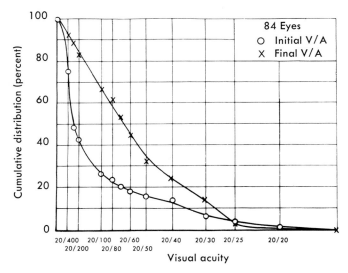

Fig. 11-26. Vascular senile maculopathy (Stage IV). Cumulative distribution of visual acuity curves of eyes before argon laser photocoagulation and at end of follow-up, 6 to 48 months (average, 15.3 months).

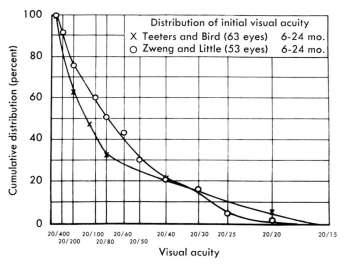

Fig. 11-27. Vascular senile maculopathy (Stage IV). Cumulative distribution of visual acuity curves of eyes entering study. Comparison of 63 untreated eyes with 53 treated eyes reported by Teeters and Bird. Both groups followed 6 to 24 months. Curves not significantly different.

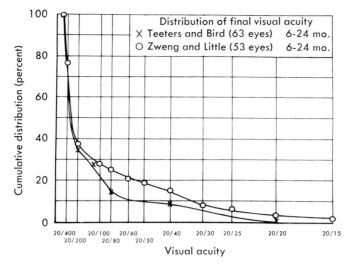

Fig. 11-28. Vascular senile maculopathy (Stage IV). Cumulative distribution of visual acuity curves of eyes at end of study. Comparison of 63 untreated eyes with 53 treated eyes. Both groups followed 6 to 24 months. Curves not significantly different.

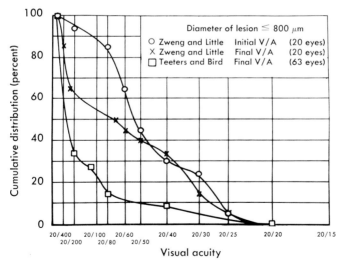

Fig. 11-29. Vascular exudative senile maculopathy (Stage IV). Cumulative distribution visual acuity curves of eyes before argon laser photocoagulation and at end of follow-up, 6 to 24 months. In all treated eyes, subretinal neovascular membrane measured ≤800 μm at its widest extent on fluorangiogram.

3. Very few eyes were treated with the patient under retrobulbar anesthesia. Any ocular movement during the 0.2-sec treatment interval results in less than full treatment to the part of the SRNM photocoagulated during the early part of the exposure, and undertreating any part of the SRNM virtually ensures its full recurrence.

Even with heavy photocoagulation and close follow-up, central vision is sometimes lost, as demonstrated in Fig. 11-31. The right macula had been destroyed

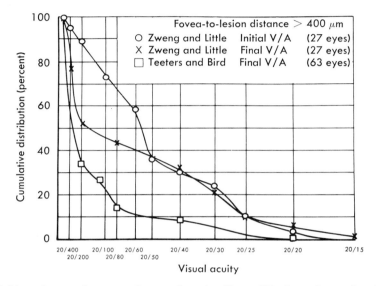

Fig. 11-30. Vascular exudative senile maculopathy (Stage IV). Cumulative distribution visual acuity curves of eyes before argon laser photocoagulation and at end of follow-up, 6 to 24 months. In all treated eyes, distance of nearest edge of subretinal neovascular membrane to fovea was ≥ 400 μm.

Fig. 11-31. A, Fluoroangiogram of left eye of 53-year-old white woman whose right macula had been destroyed by hemorrhagic senile maculopathy 18 months previously. Subretinal neovascular membrane noted in inferonasal quadrant of macula. VA, 20/40, due to serous elevation of sensory retina over fovea. **B,** Photograph immediately after heavy argon laser photocoagulation. **C,** Photograph 2 weeks after treatment. Acute coagulation has not completely resolved, as shown by white spot in center of treated area. VA, 20/25. **D,** Fluoroangiogram same day as **C,** apparently demonstrating that subretinal neovascular membrane had been destroyed. **E,** Fluoroangiogram 2 weeks after **D,** demonstrating recurrence of subretinal neovascular membrane. VA, 20/40. Membrane deemed too close to fovea to permit further photocoagulation. **F,** Fluoroangiogram 3 weeks after **E.** Membrane has extended across entire macula. VA, 20/200. **G,** Fluoroangiogram 3 weeks after **F.** Membrane has now grown past temporal edge of macula.

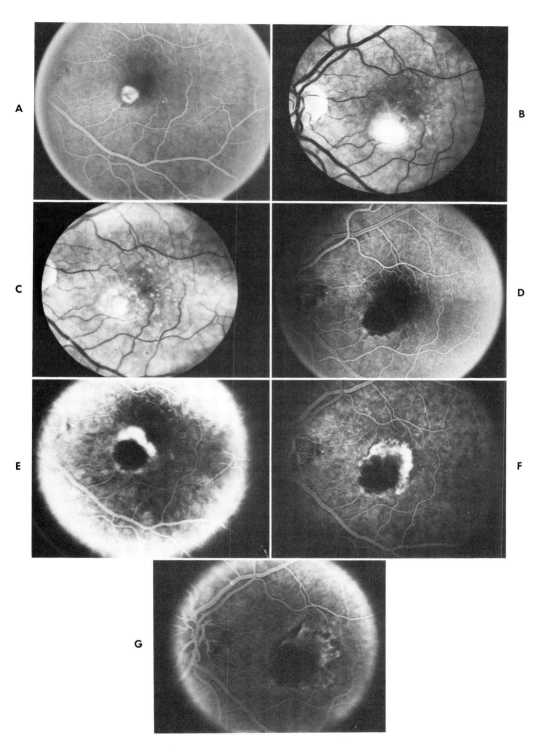

Fig. 11-31. For legend see opposite page.

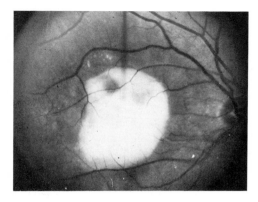

Fig. 11-32. Cicatricial senile maculopathy (Grade V). Kuhnt-Junius macular degeneration. Photograph showing mound of glial and fibrous tissue replacing macula. Sensory retina flat on scar tissue.

18 months previously by hemorrhagic SMD. A peripapillary subretinal membrane developed in the left eye. Despite careful and heavy treatment and weekly observation, the membrane proceeded across the macula, destroying it. Such cases make clear the difficulties and frustrations involved in treating this form of senile maculopathy. However, we have observed complete destruction of a SRNM by argon laser photocoagulation often enough to suggest that a randomized study be carried out, with treated eyes being compared with untreated controls. We are now carrying out such a study, in order to clarify the role of photocoagulation in hemorrhagic SMD.

CICATRICIAL (Stage V)

In the cicatricial stage of senile maculopathy, the normal macular architecture is replaced by a glial and fibrous tissue scar. The sensory retina may be flat on the scar or still elevated by serous or serohemorrhagic exudate (Figs. 11-32 and 11-33). If elevated, lipid is seen commonly in the retina, at the edge of the elevation. Staining of scar tissue is seen on fluorescein angiography, as is leakage of dye if the sensory retina is elevated. Vision is 20/200 to finger counting peripherally.

There is no useful application of argon laser photocoagulation in the cicatricial stage of SMD.

OTHER CAUSES OF SUBRETINAL NEOVASCULARIZATION

Although hemorrhagic senile maculopathy is probably the commonest disease in which subretinal neovascular membranes (SRNM) are seen, it is by no means the only one. Other conditions in which SRNM may occur include:

1. Histoplasmic choroiditis

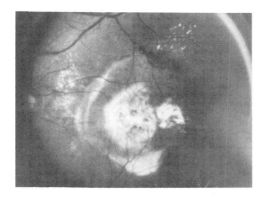

Fig. 11-33. Cicatricial senile maculopathy (Grade V). Photograph showing sensory retina detached over scar replacing macula. Lipid seen at nasal and superotemporal edges of elevated retina.

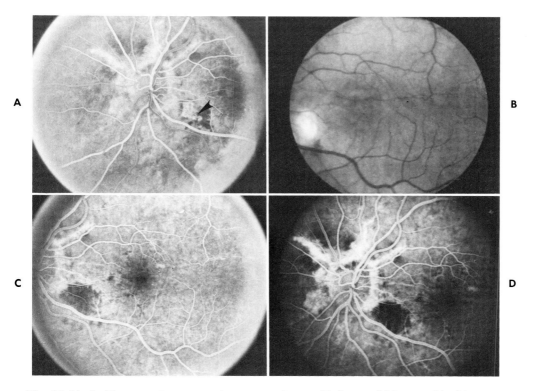

Fig. 11-34. A, Fluoroangiogram, early venous phase, of left eye of 34-year-old white man with pseudoxanthoma elasticum. His only sibling, a brother 6 years older, lost macular vision in both eyes from angioid streaks of retina. Angiogram shows transmitted choroidal fluorescence through breaks in Bruch's membrane radiating out from nerve head. One area of subretinal neovascularization present *(arrow).* Adjacent area of negative fluorescence due to hemorrhage. VA, 20/15, with metamorphopsia. **B,** Photograph immediately after treatment, showing heavy photocoagulation therapy to SRNM. **C,** Fluoroangiogram 1 week after treatment, showing absence of SRNM. VA, 20/15. A little fluorescence seen around vascular twig at temporal edge of lesion. **D,** Fluoroangiogram 6 weeks after argon laser photocoagulation, showing negative fluorescence in lesion, due to pigmentation induced by treatment. VA, 20/15. Metamorphopsia cleared.

2. Senile choroidal macular degeneration
3. Angioid streaks
4. Traumatic ruptures of Bruch's membrane
5. Chorioretinal scars (rarely, toxoplasmosis)
6. Postphotocoagulation chorioretinal scar
7. Myopic degeneration (Fuch's spot)
8. Overlying choroidal nevi (rarely)
9. End-stage Best's vitelliform macular degeneration
10. Optic nerve drusen

Another relatively widespread disease, at least in the midwestern United States, that demonstrates SRNM is presumed *histoplasmic choroiditis*. The role of argon laser photocoagulation in the treatment of this disease is discussed in Chapter 11. Other diseases in which SRNM may occur are *angioid streaks* (Fig. 11-34), as usually seen in *pseudoxanthoma elasticum, high myopia* with development of a *Fuch's spot* in the posterior pole (Fig. 11-35), and old *traumatic choroidal ruptures* (Fig. 11-36); they are also seen in association with *drusen of the nerve head* (Fig. 11-37).

The principles previously discussed in this chapter apply in the photocoagulation treatment of SRNMs, in whichever disease entity they are found. If all neovascularizations are responses to hypoxic stimuli, successful photocoagulation treatment aids the patient in surviving visually only the episode being treated. Successful photocoagulation *does not* insure against recurrent episodes. Therefore, the patient's visual state must be kept under surveillance by both the ophthalmologist and the *patient*. A macular review by the ophthalmologist, including fluoroangiograms, every 4 to 6 months in quiescent cases is useful but no substitute for repeated observations by the patient. Therefore, we recommend

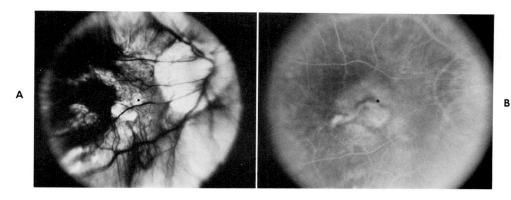

A

B

Fig. 11-35. A, Fundus photograph of right eye of a 51-year-old white woman with Fuch's spot in posterior pole. VA, 20/400. Marked peripapillary atrophy present, showing choroidal vessels. Hemorrhage is seen in macula. **B,** Fluoroangiogram of same eye shows subretinal neovascularization in macula.

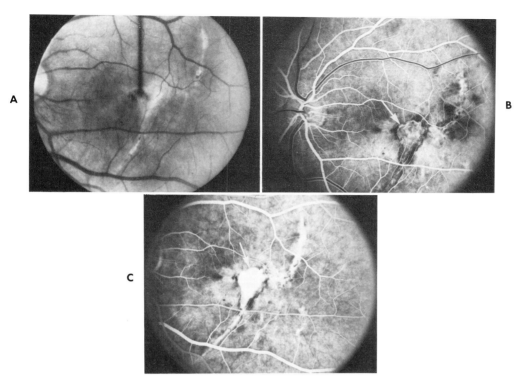

Fig. 11-36. A, Fundus photograph of left eye of 47-year-old man 13 months after eye had been struck a direct blow by a tennis ball. Vision, 20/30−1. Two typical curvilinear choroidal ruptures seen, with small hemorrhage and serous elevation of macula. **B,** Fluorangiogram in early venous phase, showing subretinal neovascularization *(arrow)* arising from choroidal rupture. **C,** Midvenous phase of same angiogram, showing full filling of subretinal neovascular membrane *(arrow)*.

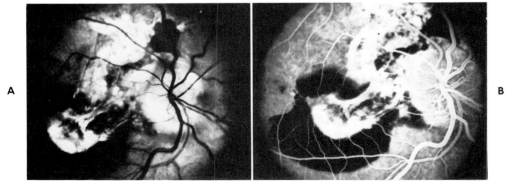

Fig. 11-37. A, Fundus photograph of right eye of 15-year-old white male with drusen of nerve head. Hemorrhage is present in macula and above nerve head. Fibrovascular tissue is present in macula and and superotemporal vascular arcade. **B,** Fluoroangiogram of same eye. A subretinal neovascular membrane is seen in macula.

that the patient use the *Amsler grid* daily. If he notes a definite change in the grid's appearance to the eye(s) under surveillance (i.e., new or enlarged scotomas or metamorphopsia), which persists for several days, the patient should report his findings to the ophthalmologist promptly. In this way, investigation can be carried out early in the course of an episode, when photocoagulation treatment might be helpful, rather than late (when the fovea is involved), when photocoagulation is usually contraindicated.

REFERENCES

1. Cleasby, G.: Idiopathic focal subretinal neovascularization. In Blach, R. K., editor: Macular workshop, Bath, England, May 1975, London, Moorfields Eye Hospital.
2. Deutman, A. F., and Jansen, L. M. A. A.: Dominantly inherited drusen of Bruch's membrane, Br. J. Ophthalmol. **54:**373, 1970.
3. Doyne, R. W.: Peculiar conditions of choroiditis occurring in several members of the same family, Trans. Ophthalmol. Soc. U.K. **19:**71, 1899.
4. Gass, J. D. M.: Pathogenesis of disciform detachment of the neuroepithelium. III. Senile disciform macular degeneration; IV. Fluorescein angiographic study of senile disciform macular degeneration, Am. J. Ophthalmol. **63:**616, and 645, 1967.
5. Gass, J. D. M.: Stereoscopic atlas of macular diseases, St. Louis, 1970, The C. V. Mosby Co.
6. Gass, J. D. M.: Drusen and disciform macular detachment and degeneration, Trans. Am. Ophthalmol. Soc. **70:**409, 1972.
7. Hutchinson, J., and Tay, W.: Symmetrical central choroidoretinal disease occurring in senile persons, R. London Ophthalmol. Hosp. Rep. **8:**231, 1875.
8. Junius, P., and Kuhnt, H.: Die scheibenfornige Etargung der Netzhautmitte (degeneratio maculae luteae disciformis), Basel, 1926, S. Karger AG.
9. Maumenee, A. E.: Serous and hemorrhagic disciform detachment of the macula, Trans. Pac. Coast Otoophthalmol. Soc. **40:**139, 1959.
10. Patz, A.: Personal communication, 1973.
11. Pearce, W. G.: Doyne's honeycomb retinal degeneration; clinical and genetic features, Br. J. Ophthalmol. **52:**73, 1968.
12. Sark, S.: Normal aging changes in the macular region. In Blach, R. K., editor: Macular workshop, Bath, England, May 1975, London, Moorfields Eye Hospital.
13. Teeters, V. W., and Bird, A. C.: The development of neovascularization of senile disciform macular degeneration, Am. J. Ophthalmol. **76:**1, 1973.
14. Wessing, A., and Meyer-Schwickerath, G.: Lichtchirurgische Behandlung und soustige chirurgische Massnahmen bei Maculaaffectionen, Ber. Dtsch. Ophthalmol. Ges. **73:**585, 1975.
15. Wessing, A., and Spitznas, M.: Exudative senile maculopathy. In L'Esperance, F. A., editor: Current diagnosis and management of chorioretinal disease, St. Louis, 1977, The C. V. Mosby Co.

12
HISTOPLASMIC MACULOPATHY

BACKGROUND

Histoplasma capsulatum is a fungus that has infected approximately 30 million people in the United States.[13,23] The initial infection is seldom diagnosed, because it usually occurs as a minor illness with fever and malaise; however, it can occur as an overwhelming pulmonary infection, particularly in patients with chronic lung disease. The only known natural host for *H. capsulatum* is the bat, which harbors the organism in its stomach. *H. capsulatum* in humans is endemic to the Ohio, Missouri, and Mississippi River valleys. The epidemiology of infections caused by this organism is poorly understood.

CLINICAL PICTURE

Histoplasmic choroiditis is a distinct uveitis syndrome, initially described by Krause and Hopkins[8] in 1951 and popularized by Woods and Wahlen[31] in 1960 and later by Van Metre and Maumenee in 1964.[27] Clinical findings consist of multiple central and peripheral small atrophic choroidal lesions, atrophic peripapillary scars, and serous or hemorrhagic detachment of the retinal pigment epithelium or of both the retinal pigment epithelium and the sensory retina within the macula. Hyvarinen, Lerer, and Knox[7] first documented with fluorescein angiography the presence of a neovascular membrane beneath the retinal pigment epithelium. The subretinal neovascular membrane, usually associated with greenish discoloration of the overlying retinal pigment epithelium and surrounded by a signet ring pattern of hyperplastic retinal pigment epithelium, frequently hemorrhages into the fovea and destroys central vision. These clinical findings are seldom observed before the patient is in his third decade and occur in otherwise healthy individuals with clear ocular media.

The neovascular membrane from the choroid extends through Bruch's membrane into the subretinal space. Hemorrhage may occur beneath the retinal pigment epithelium, between it and the sensory retina, or in the sensory retina.

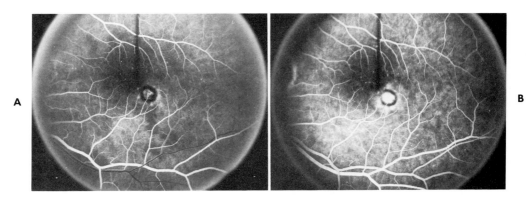

Fig. 12-1. A, Moderate fluorescence of choroidal lesion seen on early venous phase of angiogram. **B,** Same lesion as in **A.** Prolonged fluorescence with blurred margins indicates leakage from lesion.

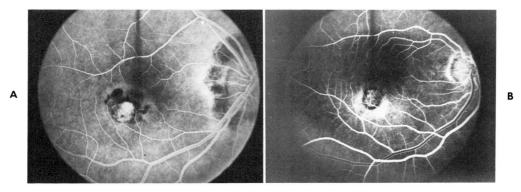

Fig. 12-2. A, Pretreatment angiographic study showing dark subretinal pigment epithelial lesion, with hemorrhage outlined by choroidal fluorescence. VA, 20/30. **B,** Network of choroidal neovascular channels seen on arterial phase of angiogram.

Fluorescein angiography is useful in ascertaining the activity of the lesions. Both active lesions and inactive lesions may fluoresce during the choroidal phase; however, only active lesions manifest a prolonged fluorescence with subsequent blurred margins (Fig. 12-1). In macular lesions the extent of hemorrhage under the retinal pigment epithelium can be determined by the pattern of negative fluorescence in the choroidal phase; that is, the choroidal fluorescence is obliterated locally by the hemorrhage (Fig. 12-2, *A*). Furthermore, the subretinal neovascular membrane in the disciform lesion may be localized by leakage of the dye; this can best be detected by high magnification with the biomicroscope and on stereoscopic angiograms.

The following findings are associated with a subretinal neovascular membrane:

1. Fine network of neovascular channels seen on arterial phase of the fluorescein angiogram (Fig. 12-2, *B*)
2. Cartwheel appearance of the neovascular membrane, with heavier staining at the peripheral margin
3. Scalloped margins of the neovascular membrane
4. Foci of intense fluorescence, frequently termed "hot spots," seen on both early and late phases of the angiogram
5. Hemorrhage around the margin of the neovascular membrane, seen ophthalmoscopically or with angiography as an opaque area that obliterates the background choroidal fluorescence
6. Lipid or proteinaceous exudate, frequently seen in senile macular degeneration, but seldom seen in histoplasmic choroiditis

PRESUMPTIVE EVIDENCE

Van Metre and Maumenee[27] noted a 93% incidence of positive histoplasmin skin tests in patients with fundi as described, in contrast to a 25% incidence of positive histoplasmin skin tests in patients with other types of ocular lesions. Furthermore, chest x-ray examinations of this group showed a 90% incidence of fibrocalcific changes, in contrast to a 54% incidence in the control group. Because serologic tests can revert to normal with time, as noted by the 16% incidence of positive tests versus 3% in the control, these authors recommended the skin test as an accurate means to detect a former exposure to the *Histoplasma* organism. Presumptive evidence strongly supports the possibility that *H. capsulatum* causes the distinct uveitis syndrome.

EXPERIMENTAL EVIDENCE

Although *H. capsulatum* has not been proved to be the cause of histoplasmic choroiditis, Walma and Schlaegel,[28] using presumptive evidence, have estimated that 23% of the cases of granulomatous uveitis in the United States are caused by that organism. Hoefnagels and Pijpers[5] were able to isolate it from an eye with panophthalmitis, which is not usually seen in presumed histoplasmic choroiditis; the diagnosis was made initially by a positive biopsy of gingivitis of the right lower jaw, but the skin test was negative. Smith and Singer[24] produced the typical picture of human disseminated focal peripheral choroiditis in monkeys by injecting *H. capsulatum* into the vitreous cavity. Wong and Green[30] produced typical histoplasmic choroidal lesions in albino rabbits, using intravenous injections of *H. capsulatum*. Organisms were identified within lesions only when the animals were killed within 2 weeks of the intravenous injection, but were not found after the period of acute infection. Maumenee[15] showed a histopathologic section of an eye from a patient with granulomatous choroiditis, in which organisms resembling *H. capsulatum* were demonstrated by means of the Gomori methenamine silver preparation. The organism could not be identified with other stains that are usually positive with *H. capsulatum*. In summary, experimental and histopathologic material supports the possibility that the clinical entity of histoplasmic choroiditis is caused by *H. capsulatum*.

NATURAL COURSE

Histoplasmic choroiditis probably represents a delayed hypersensitivity to the *Histoplasma* antigen, with subsequent scar formation and choroidal neovascularization growing under the retina through a break in Bruch's membrane. Time must be included as a factor in assessing the different choroidal responses of people exposed to the *Histoplasma* organism. Possibly it takes years to develop the clinical symptoms of histoplasmic choroiditis; this would explain the absence of choroidal lesions in the 134 cases of proved histoplasmosis reviewed by Spaeth.[26] Schlaegel[20] has noted that ocular findings are not seen until about 20 years after the development of a positive skin test. This is not unlikely, inasmuch as patients with histoplasmic choroiditis syndrome have been known to develop new choroidal lesions while under the care of an ophthalmologist. Possibly there is a difference in virulent strains of the organism, accounting for the varied clinical findings in humans.

Krill and co-workers[9] studied the natural course of disease in 45 patients, followed up for from 1 to 20 years, in whom the presumptive diagnosis of histoplasmic choroiditis has been made, which they called multifocal inner choroiditis. The initial lesions appears as a discrete, small, yellow or orange infiltrate in the inner choroid, measuring less than ⅓ disc diameter, situated in the peripapillary, macular, and peripheral regions of the fundus. The choroidal lesions then subside, leaving a focal area of choroidal atrophy associated with hyperplasia of the overlying retinal pigment epithelium. There is a strong propensity for the macular lesions to undergo hemorrhagic change, manifested initially by retinal pigment epithelium elevation, which appears dark gray with a surrounding faint red halo. Subsequently, the hemorrhage may break through the retinal pigment epithelium into the sensory retina and rearely into the vitreous. In most cases, the hemorrhagic changes are preceded by edema or serous detachment of the overlying retinal pigment epithelium and the sensory retina. The subsequent growth of new vessels from the choroid through Bruch's membrane gives rise to hemorrhage. Retinal edema, serous detachment, or hemorrhagic change in the macular region accounts for the visual impairment. The eventual appearance of the macular lesion is a hypertrophic organized hemorrhagic disciform scar. Krill and associates report a 77% incidence of macular involvements, with a 57% incidence of impaired vision of 20/200 or worse; surprisingly, 20% of their patients with macular lesions showed improvement in visual acuity to 20/30 or better; however, there was only a 6% chance of maintaining or recovering 20/15 vision.

Gass[3] first observed the significance of asymptomatic macular scars, noting that one in five became active lesions. Smith, Knox, and Jensen[25] documented the significance of small asymptomatic scars in the macula of the fellow eye in 12 patients who had disciform macular disease. Of the 12 eyes, which initially had 20/20 vision, only four had vision of 20/25 or better, and three had 20/200 or worse after a 4- to 102-month follow-up. Ryan[19] reported the development of activity in a macula that previously had been noted as normal with ophthalmoscope and fluorescein angiography. In observing 1,000 patients with presumed histoplasmic choroiditis, Schlaegel[20] observed that one in five eyes with atrophic macular lesions become active and that one in 50 similar nonmacular lesions become active.

THERAPY

Because of the profound loss of central vision and because of a 52% to 87% chance of bilateral occurrence (24% to 67% incidence involving both maculas), an effective form of therapy is needed.[14, 21] Giles and Falls[4] reported no improvement with administration of systemic amphotericin B. Also finding this agent ineffective, Van Metre and Maumenee[27] and Makley et al.[14] at one time advocated histoplasmin desensitization. Because of the possibility of flare-ups of choroidal lesions associated with injection of the histoplasmin antigen, Schlaegel and co-workers[21] once recommended desensitization as a prophylaxis in individuals who have alrady lost one macula and have no lesion threatening the second macula or in individuals with only peripheral choroidal lesions. O'Connor[17] observed that desensitization does not improve the visual prognosis in patients with histoplasmic choroiditis and that desensitization plays no beneficial role in reducing cellular immunity. The use of systemic steroids has been recommended in the management of macular lesions; some ophthalmologists believe that retrobulbar injections of depot steroids are equally as effective as systemic steroids and less hazardous to the patient. The recommended daily dosage of systemic steroids is 60 mg of prednisone or its equivalent, for 2 weeks, after which it is gradually reduced. Schlaegel[20,21] advocates that the patient check his vision daily with the Amsler grid and that when visual distortion occurs he take 100 mg of prednisone daily for 1 week. If the condition worsens, the dosage of prednisone is increased to 150 mg every other day for 1 week. Thereafter, photocoagulation is performed if no improvement is noted. Schlaegel observed improvement in 81 of 108 patients treated with prednisone. Elliott[1] reported that if steroids help, symptoms improve, usually within 4 days. Twenty to 40 mg of methylprednisolone acetate (Depo-Medrol) or its equivalent should be given by retrobulbar injection every 3 days during periods of activity. Hyndiuk and Reagan[6] have demonstrated in primates that retrobulbar injections of tritium-labeled steroids achieve a higher concentration in the choroid than do systemic steroids.

Photocoagulation therapy

Photocoagulation with xenon arc, ruby laser, or argon laser has been advocated for treatment of histoplasmic choroiditis.* The purpose of photocoagula-

---

*References 2, 10-12, 16, 18, 21, 29, 32.

tion is to destroy the subretinal neovascular membrane (SRNM), in order to preserve macular function. The success of treatment is largely dependent on its ability to eradicate the SRNM without destroying the fovea; therefore, results are influenced by the location of the lesion with respect to the fovea.

Material

Since November 1969, we have used argon laser slit-lamp photocoagulation in the management of histoplasmic choroiditis with macular involvement in 49 eyes. All eyes were followed for from 6 months to 5 years. The purpose of treatment was to destroy choroidal neovascularization, usually associated with serous or hemorrhagic detachment of the retinal pigment epithelium, as shown by fluorescein angiography.

Technique

Careful correlation was made between the subretinal neovascular frond and the retinal anatomic landmarks, by comparing the fluorescein angiogram to colored photographs of the retina and at times by use of fluorescein angioscopy during treatment. Treatment parameters were 200-μm beam diameter, 0.2-to 0.4 sec exposure, and 400 to 500 mW power, applied to the area of the frond to give heavy photocoagulation lesions (see Fig. 11-23). Before the treatment lesions were given, a demarcation line at the edge of the frond nearest the macula was made with a row of faint lesions of 50-μm, 0.05 sec, and 100 to 150 mW, which afforded a visual guide to treatment of the frond nearest the fovea (see Fig. 11-22). Treatment was not given closer than 200 μm to the fovea. Only four patients received retrobulbar anesthetic. Repeat photocoagulation was done within 1 week if residual leakage was demonstrated on fluorescein angiography. Studies were repeated at 2 and 4 weeks and at 3 months, to detect recurrent activity.

Results

A favorable response, noted by resolution of serous and hemorrhagic subretinal fluid, was recorded in 63% of the eyes treated (Table 12-1). Visual acuity improved in only 22.5% of eyes, was unchanged in 24.5%, and worsened in 53%.

While the ideal study is one with a randomized control and a treated group of

Table 12-1. Argon laser photocoagulation of histoplasmic maculopathy (49 eyes > 6-month follow-up)

	Clinical appearance (%)	*Visual acuity* (%)*
Better	63	22.5
Same	8	24.5
Worse	29	53.0

*A 2-line difference on the Snellen chart justifies a change in visual acuity.

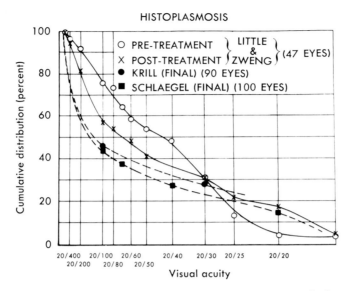

Fig. 12-3. Cumulative distribution of visual acuities of treated eyes and of untreated eyes.

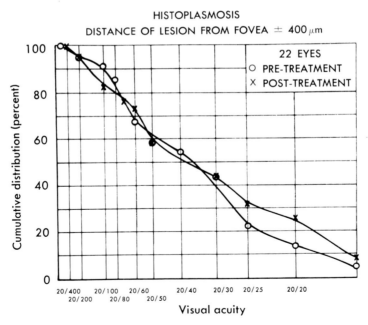

Fig. 12-4. Cumulative distribution of pre- and posttreatment visual acuities in eyes with lesions 400 μm or more from the fovea.

eyes, comparison of any treatment modality with the natural history is useful. We compared this experience with two untreated groups: one with 100 eyes, reported by Schlaegel et al.,[22] and the other with 90 eyes, followed at various intervals of from 1 to 20 years, reported by Krill et al.[9]

Fig. 12-3 shows the pretreatment and posttreatment visual acuities in our series, as compared with the final visual acuities in untreated eyes recorded by Krill and by Schlaegel. Unfortunately, initial acuities are not available in the two studies on the natural history. The cumulative distribution of visual acuities of the treated eyes in our current series was only slightly better than that of the untreated eyes reported by Krill and by Schlaegel.

The most favorable response to treatment occurred in eyes where the margin of the lesion was greater than 400 μm from the fovea (Fig. 12-4); a final visual acuity of 20/50 or better was recorded in 60% of these eyes. Furthermore, when pretreatment visual acuity was 20/80 or better, 70% of the treated eyes maintained visual acuity at that level or better, and 50% had 20/50 or better vision (Fig. 12-5). In Krill's and Schlaegel's untreated series, only 35% of eyes had acuity of 20/50 or better.

In conclusion, photocoagulation seems to be beneficial when the margin of the subretinal neovascular membrane is at least 400 μm from the fovea and when pretreatment visual acuity is 20/80 or better. Once the SRNM extends to the

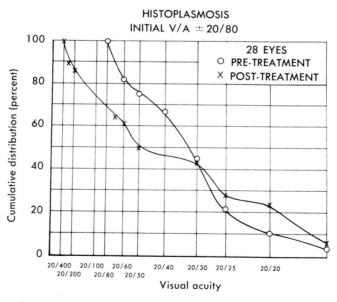

Fig. 12-5. Cumulative distribution of pre- and posttreatment visual acuities in eyes with VA of 20/80 or better pretreatment (i.e., if 75% of eyes had 20/50 or better pretreatment, only 50% had 20/50 or better posttreatment).

perifoveal capillary net, the amount of photocoagulation required to destroy the neovascular membrane usually results in destruction of the fovea as well. In the absence of these criteria, the natural course öf the disease probably does not produce significantly different results than those from argon laser photocoagulation.

Recurrence

Failure to destroy the subretinal pigment epithelial neovascular membrane with the initial photocoagulation treatment occurred in 26% of treated eyes. Most had been treated with minimal coagulation burns (Fig. 12-6, *A* and *B*), and

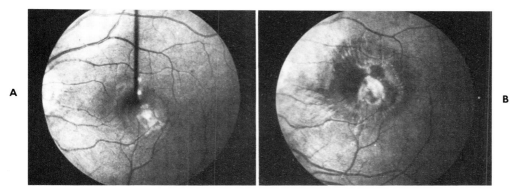

Fig. 12-6. A, Pretreatment appearance of histoplasmic choroiditis, showing serous detachment of sensory retina and localized subretinal lesion. VA, 20/30. **B,** Increased size of subretinal neovascular membrane, with hemorrhage noted 3 months following inadequate argon laser photocoagulation. VA, 20/400.

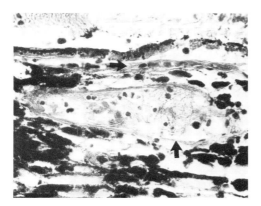

Fig. 12-7. Coagulative necrosis *(arrows)* of all choroidal vessels after argon laser photocoagulation lesion in rhesus monkey.

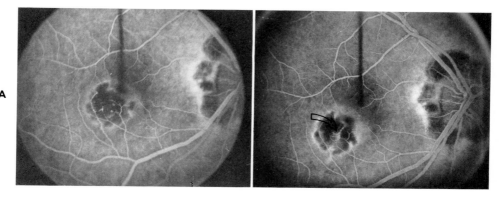

Fig. 12-8. A, Same patient as in Fig. 12-2. Absence of demonstrable leakage in blocked fluorescence 2 days after argon laser photocoagulation. **B,** Recurrent choroidal neovascularization 16 days after photocoagulation.

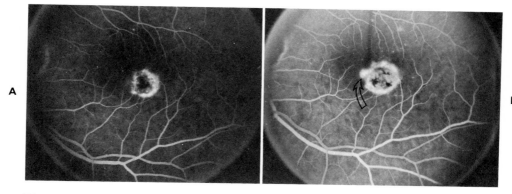

Fig. 12-9. A, Posttreatment angiographic appearance 8 weeks after argon laser photocoagulation. **B,** Recurrent choroidal neovascularization at margin of chorioretinal scar (*arrow*), which occurred 2 years after treatment.

without repeating fluorescein retinal angiography to detect residual vessels in the early postoperative period.

As demonstrated in the rhesus monkey (Fig. 12-7), intense burns produced with high power and prolonged exposure time, using moderate to large spot sizes, cause coagulative necrosis of all the choroidal vessels within the lesion. Intense coagulation burns of this magnitude are necessary to destroy subretinal neovascular membranes.

Recurrent choroidal neovascularizations, as demonstrated on angiography by initial destruction of vessels, occurred in 13% of treated lesions; however, only two of 49 treated eyes (4%) had recurrent choroidal neovascularization from the

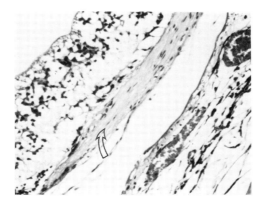

Fig. 12-10. Subretinal fibrous membrane *(arrow)* between Bruch's membrane and sensory retina.

previously treated lesion 1 year after treatment, in contrast to the 20% occurrence of new lesions within the same follow-up period.

In one eye, recurrence of choroidal neovascularization developed within 3 weeks of treatment (Fig. 12-8, *A* and *B*), suggesting that the vessels had not been totally destroyed. In this 5-year study, the longest period between destruction of neovascularization and recurrence was 2 years (Fig. 12-9, *A* and *B*). Recurrence usually occurs at the margin of the scar. Treatment is conducted with intense coagulation burns.

Subretinal fibrous membrane

Initial improvement of visual acuity, with resolution of serous and hemorrhagic detachment of the sensory retina, following argon laser photocoagulation of the subretinal pigment epithelial neovascular membrane was observed in two eyes; however, after 5 months and 3 years respectively, subsequent visual acuity showed progressive deterioration without recurrence of serous or hemorrhagic detachment of the macula. One of the patients died 20 months after laser treatment and 1 year after recurrent visual impairment. Histopathologic examinations showed a dense fibrous membrane between Bruch's membrane and the sensory retina (Fig. 12-10). This case report provides an explanation for visual loss in the absence of recurrent inflammation or vascular leakage.

SUMMARY

Argon laser photocoagulation does not significantly increase visual acuity over pretreatment levels. However, such treatment properly given does efficiently destroy subretinal neovascularization. Optimal lesions must be applied in order to destroy the neovascular membrane. The most significant points of technique are—

    1. Administration of retrobulbar anesthetic

2. Heavy treatment of the entire frond, which usually is accomplished with 200 μm beam diameter, 0.2- to 0.5-sec exposure, at 400 to 500 mW power
3. Close follow-up at intervals of 3 to 5 days until the neovascular frond is destroyed

If the edge of the neovascular frond is within 300 μm of the fovea, treatment presents a very definite hazard to foveal vision and should be attempted only in the most experienced hands and on only the best-informed patient.

Even though the funduscopic appearance is improved in most eyes treated, a randomized control study is needed to evaluate the effect of photocoagulation on the ultimate visual results in patients with macular involvement due to presumed histoplasmic choroiditis.

REFERENCES

1. Elliott, J.: Presumed histoplasmic maculopathy; clinical course and prognosis in nonphotocoagulated eyes. In Schlaegel, T. F., editor: International Ophthalmology Clinics, vol. 15, Ocular histoplasmosis, Boston, 1975, Little, Brown and Co.
2. Gass, J. D. M. Photocoagulation of macular lesions, Trans. Am. Acad. Ophthalmol. Otolaryngol. **75:**580, 1971.
3. Gass, J. D. M., and Wilkinson, C. P.: Follow-up study of presumed ocular histoplasmosis, Trans. Am. Acad. Ophthalmol. Otolaryngol. **76:**672, 1972.
4. Giles, C. L., and Falls, H. F.: Amphotericin B therapy in the treatment of presumed histoplasma chorioretinitis, Am. J. Ophthalmol. **66:**101, 1968.
5. Hoefnagels, K. L. J., and Pijpers, P. M.: *Histoplasma capsulatum* in a human eye, Am. J. Ophthalmol. **63:**715, 1967.
6. Hyndiuk, R. A., and Reagan, M. G.: Radioactive depot–corticosteroid penetration into monkey ocular tissues. I. Retrobulbar and systemic administration, Arch. Ophthalmol. **80:**499, 1968.
7. Hyvarinen, L., Lerer, R. J., and Knox, D. L.: Fluorescein angiographic findings in presumed ocular histoplasmosis, Am. J. Ophthalmol. **71:**449, 1971.
8. Krause, A. C., and Hopkins, W. G.: Ocular manifestations of histoplasmosis, Am. J. Ophthalmol. **34:**564, 1951.
9. Krill, E. K., Chisti, M., Klien, B. A., Newell, F. W., and Potts, A. M.: Multifocal inner choroiditis, Trans. Am. Acad. Ophthalmol. Otolaryngol. **73**(2):222, 1969.
10. Little, H. L.: Macular diseases: classification and treatment with argon laser slit lamp photocoagulation, Doc. Ophthalmol. **1:**35, 1973.
11. Little, H. L., and Zweng, H. C.: Photocoagulation au laser a l'argon dans les affections maculaires et les retinopathies diabetiques, Arch. Ophtalmol. (Paris) **32:**789, 1972.
12. Little, H. L., Zweng, H. C., and Peabody, R. R.: Argon slit lamp retinal photocoagulation, Trans. Am. Acad. Ophthalmol. Otolaryngol. **74:**85, 1970.
13. Loosli, C. G.: Symposium on clinical advances in medicine; histoplasmosis; some clinical, epidemiological and laboratory aspects, Med. Clin. North Am. **39:**171-199, 1955.
14. Makley, T. A., Jr., Lond, J. W., and Stephan, J. D.: Presumed histoplasmic chorioretinitis with special emphasis on present modes of therapy, Trans. Am. Acad. Ophthalmol. Otolaryngol. **69:**443, 1965.
15. Maumenee, A. E.: Histoplasmosis; clinical course and description. In Kimura, S. J., and Caygill, W. M., editors: Symposium on differential diagnostic problems of posterior uveitis. Retinal diseases, Philadelphia, 1966, Lea & Febiger.
16. Maumenee, A. E.: Discussion of previous papers, Trans. Am. Acad. Ophthalmol. Otolaryngol. **72:**374, 1968.
17. O'Connor, R.: Experimental ocular histoplasmosis. In Schlaegel, T: F., editor: International Ophthalmology Clinics, vol. 15, Ocular histoplasmosis, Bostom, 1975, Little, Brown and Co.
18. Patz, A., Maumenee, A. E., and Ryan, S. J.: Argon laser photocoagulation, Trans. Am. Acad. Ophthalmol. Otolaryngol. **75:**569, 1971.

19. Ryan, S.: Histological correlates of presumed ocular histoplasmosis. In Schlaegel, T. F., editor: International Ophthalmology Clinics, vol. 15, Ocular histoplasmosis, Boston, 1975, Little, Brown and Co.

20. Schlaegel, T. F., Jr.: Personal communication, 1975.

21. Schlaegel, T. F., Cofield, D. B., Clark, C., and Weber, J. C.: Photocoagulation and other therapy for histoplasmic choroiditis, Trans. Am. Acad. Ophthalmol. Otolaryngol. **72:**355, 1968.

22. Schlaegel, T. F., Weber, J. C., Helveston, E., et al.: Presumed histoplasmic choroiditis, Am. J. Ophthalmol. **63:**919, 1967.

23. Schwarz, J.: Mycotic infection, Arch. Ophthalmol. **49:**587, 1953.

24. Smith, J. L., and Singer, J. A.: Experimental ocular histoplasmosis. I. The natural course of primary infection of the rabbit eye; III. experimentally produced retinal and choroidal lesions; VI. Fluorescein fundus photographs of choroiditis in the primate, Am. J. Ophthalmol. **58:**3, 413, 1021, 1964.

25. Smith, R. E., Knox, D. L., and Jensen, A. D.: Ocular histoplasmosis, Arch. Ophthalmol. **89:**296, 1973.

26. Spaeth, G. L.: Absence of so-called histoplasma uveitis in 134 cases of proven histoplasmosis, Arch. Ophthalmol. **77:**41, 1967.

27. Van Metre, T. W., Jr., and Maumenee, A. E.: Specific ocular uveal lesions in patients with evidence of histoplasmosis, Arch. Ophthalmol. **71:**314, 1964.

28. Walma, D., Jr., and Schlaegel, T. F., Jr.: Presumed histoplasmic choroiditis: a clinical analysis of 43 cases, Am. J. Ophthalmol. **57:**107, 1964.

29. Watzke, R. C., and Leaverton, P. E.: Light coagulation in presumed histoplasmic choroiditis, Arch. Ophthalmol. **86:**127, 1971.

30. Wong, V., and Green, R.: Koch's stulates and experimental ocular histoplasmosis. In Schlaegel, T. F., editor: International Ophthalomology Clinics, vol. 15, Ocular histoplasmosis, Boston, 1975, Little, Brown and Co.

31. Woods, A. C., and Wahlen, H. E.: The probable role of benign histoplasmosis, Am. J. Ophthalmol. **34:**564, 1951.

32. Zweng, H. C., Little, H. L., and Peabody, R. R.: Laser photocoagulation and retinal angiography, St. Louis, 1969, The C. V. Mosby Co.

13
CYSTOID MACULAR EDEMA

Cystoid macular edema was defined in Chapter 6 as an extracellular accumulation of fluid in the retinal layers, with coalescence of the fluid into thin-walled compartments, especially in the outer plexiform layer. This occurs in the macula, due to extravasation of serum, plasma, or rarely whole blood from dilated perifoveal capillaries in occlusions of the central retinal vein and its temporal branches, due to increased intraluminal pressure generated by the occlusion; in diabetic retinopathy, due to circulatory factors, poor perfusion of tissue secondary to impaired rheology probably being a large factor; in inflammatory diseases of the peripheral retina and ciliary body, as seen in pars planitis or occasionally after xenon arc photocoagulation of peripheral retinal disease; and after cataract extraction. The reason for leakage from the perifoveal capillaries is unknown in the latter two categories.

Argon laser photocoagulation treatment of microcystic macular edema in diabetic retinopathy and in retinal vein occlusions is discussed in Chapters 14 and 16 respectively. We have no experience, and know of none, in the direct photocoagulation treatment of microcystic macular edema in peripheral retinal and ciliary body inflammations. Diathermy[11] and cryocoagulation of areas of inflammation have been used in the latter circumstance, with some claims of success.[3]

Cystoid macular edema following cataract surgery (Irvine-Gass syndrome) was first described by S. R. Irvine[5] and further delineated by Gass and Norton.[1,2] In 1971 A. R. Irvine et al.[4] reported that fluorescein angiography performed between the fourth and sixteenth week after cataract surgery showed cystoid macular edema in 40% of eyes. In their opinion, an inflammatory process is the main cause.

CLINICAL ASPECTS

Onset of cystoid macular edema occurs from weeks to months or even several years after cataract surgery. Microcysts are seen in the macula, especially on slit-lamp funduscopy. At times, flecks of blood and swelling of the nerve head are present, two findings seen especially in severe cases, indicating greater dilation of macular and nerve head capillaries. Vision can vary from a difficult 20/20 to

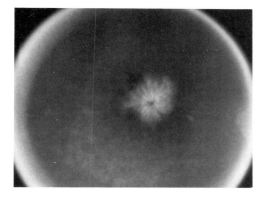

Fig. 13-1. Fluoroangiogram of left eye of 65-year-old white woman with microcystic macular edema 6 months after cataract extraction. Delayed-phase photograph shows typical pattern of accumulation of dye in microcystic spaces, giving a "petaloid" appearance.

20/400. Even when distance vision, as measured by the Snellen chart, is relatively good, patients complain of problems while reading. Gass and Norton found both eyes involved in about one half of their patients with bilateral cataract extraction. Vitreal traction on the macula, originally considered a major factor in the etiology of this disease, is found relatively infrequently.[5,6,9,10] However, adhesion of the vitreous to the cataract wound is seen frequently but not in a majority of cases; this finding is associated with a longer course and a worse visual prognosis.[5] Evidence of low-grade inflammation in the form of inflammatory cells in the posterior vitreous is very common but not invariable. Fluorescein angiography shows a typical "petal" pattern due to septae in the outer plexiform layer formation, formed by compaction of the fibrils between the fluid-filled spaces (Fig. 13-1). Some leakage of fluorescein is often seen from nerve head capillaries, even when there is no clinical nerve head swelling.

NATURAL COURSE

As reported by Gass and Norton,[2] resolution of microcystic macular edema occurred in approximately 72% of the eyes observed (46 of 64). Clearing occurred between 1 and 36 months after onset. Of those that cleared, 50% did so within 6 months of onset, and 13% within 6 more months; thus almost two thirds cleared in 1 year. However, there was a difference between eyes with and without vitreous to the cataract wound; 60% of eyes with vitreous cleared (12 of 25), versus 80% without (31 of 39). Furthermore, the average time of clearing was 25 weeks in eyes without vitreous incarceration, versus 65 weeks with.

Visual prognosis was good overall in the series reported by Gass and Norton. After resolution of macular edema, which occurred in 46 eyes, 33 (80%) had visual acuity of 20/25 or better; however, comparable vision was present at the end of follow-up in three (17%) of the 18 eyes in which edema did not clear. Therefore, their report makes plain that eyes with vitreous incarceration have a worse prognosis than those without. Furthermore, vitreous surgery was done in nine of the 25 eyes reported as having vitreous in the wound, making comparison with natural history more difficult.

Inasmuch as some inflammation is present in the great majority (but not all) of these eyes, and because macular edema is seen in eyes with prolonged cyclitis, steroids are suggested as a therapeutic solution; however, there is no evidence that steroids are more than temporarily effective.

Vitrectomy in eyes with vitreous to the cataract wound, to reduce intraocular inflammation due to constant tugging on the whole vitreous body by the strand to the wound (not to relieve nonexistent traction on the macula), is a therapeutic approach that is being explored.[8]

Because of the adverse effect of levo-epinephrine on some maculas in aphakic eyes,[7] glaucoma in eyes with microcystic macular edema should be controlled by other medications.

TREATMENT

In view of the relatively benign course of macular edema in most eyes, only observation with fluorescein angiography is indicated for at least 6 months. If the edema has not cleared in that time, and especially if it has worsened, a course of steroid therapy should be considered. We recommend that four injections of 40 mg of triamcinolone acetonide (Kenalog) be given retrobulbarly approximately 1 month apart. Before each injection, the patient should be reexamined with fluoroangiography to determine if there has been any improvement; if so, the injection is postponed for 1 month.

Photocoagulation therapy in *persistent* microcystic macular edema after cataract extraction is experimental and should be carried out only in centers equipped to administer treatment and evaluate results carefully. Only a controlled study will determine the role, if any, of argon laser photocoagulation in this disease.

REFERENCES

1. Gass, J. D. M., and Norton, E. W. D.: Cystoid macular edema and papilledema following cataract extraction, Arch. Ophthalmol. **76:**646-661, 1966.
2. Gass, J. D. M., and Norton, E. W. D.: Follow-up study of cystoid macular edema following cataract extraction, Trans. Am. Acad. Ophthalmol. Otolaryngol. **73:**665-682, 1969.
3. Gills, J. P., Jr.: Combined medical and surgical therapy for complicated cases of peripheral uveitis, Arch. Ophthalmol. **79:**723-728, 1968.
4. Irvine, A. R., et al.: Macular edema after cataract extraction, Ann. Ophthalmol. **3:**1234, 1971.
5. Irvine, S. R.: A newly defined vitreous syndrome following cataract surgery, Am. J. Ophthalmol. **36:**599-619, 1953.
6. Jaffe, N. S.: Vitreous traction at the posterior pole of the fundus due to alterations in the vitreous posterior, Trans. Am. Acad. Ophthalmol. Otolaryngol. **71:**642-651, 1967.
7. Kolker, A. E., and Becker, B.: Epinephrine maculopathy, Arch. Ophthalmol. **79:**552-562, 1968.
8. Michels, R. G., Machemer, R., and Mueller-Jensen, K.: Vitreous surgery; history and current concepts, Ophthalmic Surg. **5:**13, 1974.
9. Reese, A. B., Jones, I. S., and Cooper, W. C.:

Macular changes secondary to vitreous traction, Trans. Am. Ophthalmol. Soc. **64:**123-134, 1966.

10. Tolentino, F. I., and Schepens, C. L.: Edema of posterior pole after cataract extraction, Arch. Ophthalmol. **74:**781-786, 1965.

11. Welch, R. B., Maumenee, A. E., and Waler, E. H.: Peripheral posterior segment inflammation, vitreous opacities, and edema of the posterior pole, Arch. Ophthalmol. **64:**540-549, 1960.

14
DIABETIC RETINOPATHY

Diabetes is one of the four leading causes of blindness in the United States.[23] It is the second leading cause of adult blindness in the United States[26] and the first cause of newly acquired blindness in Great Britain.[33] Because both prevalence of diabetes and life expectancy are increasing, the incidence of blindness due to diabetes has increased from 4.3% in 1940 to 18.4% in 1962.[24] Retinopathy accounts for at least 80% of blindness in diabetes.[5]

Of the approximately four million people with diabetes mellitus in the United States, about 40% have diabetic retinopathy to some degree.[4] Of those with retinopathy, approximately 90% have nonproliferative retinopathy, which never leads to total blindness; of the 10% of patients with proliferative retinopathy, only 7% become totally blind. Nonproliferative retinopathy most frequently occurs with adult-onset diabetes, whereas proliferative retinopathy is most commonly associated with juvenile diabetes. Both forms of retinopathy are related to duration and probably to poor control of diabetes.

CLASSIFICATION OF DIABETIC RETINOPATHY

Of the numerous classifications of diabetic retinopathy, the most detailed are the O'Hare and the Airlie House Classifications;[6] other systems of classification are less complex. Nonetheless, in discussing natural history and response to treatment, one must classify diabetic retinopathy into nonproliferative and proliferative forms of the disease. Extent and location of neovascularization and of macular edema must be considered. We use the following classification, because of its adaptability in evaluating the response of retinopathy to photocoagulation:

Nonproliferative

IA. "Background" diabetic retinopathy without macular edema

IB. Macular edema, with localized intraretinal leakage

IC. Macular edema, with diffuse intraretinal leakage, usually associated with cystoid edema

Proliferative

IIA. Neovascularization in plane of retina

IIB. Neovascularization off optic disc or into the vitreous

180

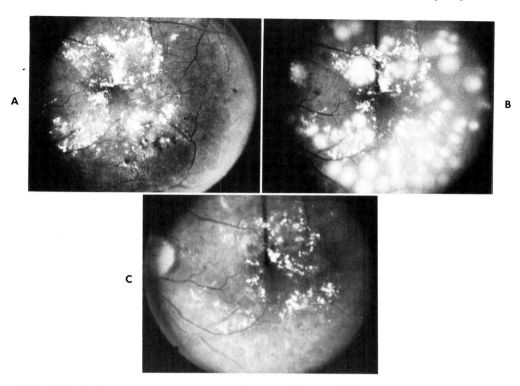

Fig. 14-1. A, Pretreatment appearance of nonproliferative diabetic retinopathy, showing microaneurysms, hemorrhage, macular edema, and circinate exudates. VA, 20/200. **B,** Appearance of left fundus immediately after argon laser photocoagulation to intraretinal vascular leaks. **C,** Resolution of hemorrhage, exudates, and edema 6 months after treatment. VA 20/30.

    IIC. Neovascularization off optic disc or into the vitreous, associated with pronounced fibrous (glial) component

Nonproliferative diabetic retinopathy

In nonproliferative diabetic retinopathy, visual impairment results from any of the following conditions affecting the macula: abnormal permeability of capillaries; microaneurysms leading to macular edema, exudates, and hemorrhage; capillary nonperfusion leading to macular ischemia and edema; and finally, preretinal membrane contracture.

There is little controversy with respect to the role of photocoagulation in the management of nonproliferative diabetic retinopathy in eyes with localized intraretinal macular vascular leaks that impair or threaten loss of central vision.[20,21,30,32,39] Treatment consists of photocoagulating the intraretinal vascular leaks, with intent to reduce macular edema, exudate, and hemorrhage (Figs. 14-1 and 14-2).

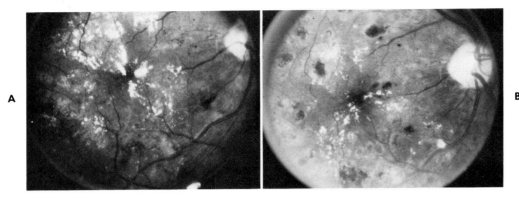

Fig. 14-2. A, Pretreatment appearance of right eye shows hard exudates bordering fovea. VA, 20/30. **B,** Resolution of exudates 6 months after photocoagulation. VA, 20/30.

At the time of treatment, the fluorescein angiogram is reviewed, either with enlargements or with the projected negative of the angiogram, to assist in detection of microvascular leaks. Sometimes fluorescein is given intravenously at the time of photocoagulation, because pooling at leakage points fluoresces when activated by the argon laser beam. With this technique, previously undetected microaneurysms and intraretinal leakage points may be observed while adjacent lesions are being photocoagulated.

The usual settings for argon laser treatment of nonproliferative intraretinal vascular leaks are 50- to 200-μm spot diameters, 200 to 400 mW power, and 0.1- to 0.2-sec exposure. If the ocular media are cloudy due to lens or vitreous opacities, higher power settings and longer time exposures are required. When power levels are sufficiently high, the energy absorbed by the cloudy media is sufficient to cause local index of refraction changes in the media, which tends to diverge the beam; this process is termed thermal blooming. With the Coherent Radiation and Optics Technology laser photocoagulators, the highest incidence occurs at the 100-μm setting; thus, if excessive thermal blooming is observed, other spot sizes should be used. For treatment of small lesions in the presence of cloudy media when using the Coherent Radiation photocoagulator, the 50-μm spot size is more satisfactory than are the 100- or 200-μm spot sizes. With the broader beam vergence of the 50-μm spot, there is less thermal blooming of the beam. For larger leaks, the 500-μm spot size is recommended, with power levels of 500 to 1,000 mW at 0.1 to 0.2 sec.

When treating retinal edema associated with circinate exudation, the leakage points are invariably situated within the ring of exudate. Following moderately intense photocoagulation of the leaks, circinate exudates resolve within 3 to 6 months (Fig. 14-3).

Unsuccessful results in the treatment of nonproliferative diabetic retinopathy

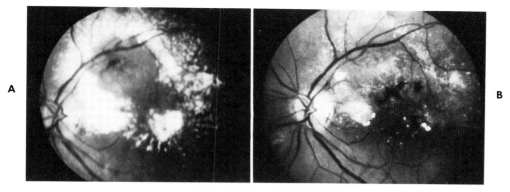

Fig. 14-3. A, Extensive circinate exudative diabetic retinopathy. VA, 20/400. **B,** Resolution of exudates 6 months after photocoagulation to leakage area within center of circinate exudate. VA, 20/200.

occur when insufficiently intense lesions are applied. When inadequately coagulated, intraretinal vascular lesions sometimes leak more profusely, increasing the edema. Satisfactory lesions appear gray to white (Fig. 14-1, *B*). On the other hand, excessive heat with very intense burns may cause preretinal membrane contracture (see Chapter 21).

When treating parafoveal leaks, the 50- or 100-μm spot is used. If the media are clear, the 100-μm spot is preferable because the lesion can be coagulated with only one application. Exposure time for such lesions is reduced to 0.05 sec. Less power is needed when treating near the fovea, because of increased density of pigment granules within the retinal pigment epithelium and because of xanthophil pigment granules within the retina. Typical settings for the treatment of a parafoveal leak is 50-μm spot, 75 mW, 0.05 sec. Leaks within the parafoveal capillary net are treated rarely, because of possible damage to the fovea.

Identification of the fixation point is important when photocoagulating any macular lesion. Some methods used to identify fixation are—
1. Fixation target on both colored and angiographic photography; a minimum of two pictures should be taken to confirm fixation.
2. Visuscope observation.
3. Attenuated fixation beam of argon laser.
4. Anatomic study of macular vessels at time of ophthalmoscopy.

In a randomized control study, Patz et al.[30] found argon laser photocoagulation to be beneficial in the treatment of 63 patients with nonproliferative diabetic retinopathy. Visual results in a 9-month to 3-year follow-up study of the eyes treated with argon laser photocoagulation were 27% improved, 66% unchanged, and 27% worsened; in the untreated eyes, visual results were 10% improved, 27% unchanged, and 63% worsened.

We found similar favorable responses of nonproliferative retinopathy with

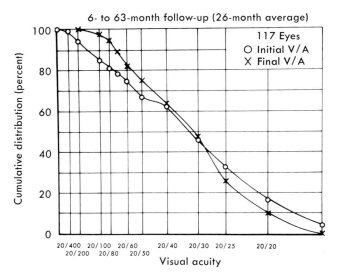

Fig. 14-4. Cumulative distribution of pre- and posttreatment visual acuities for 117 eyes with macular edema due to localized intraretinal vascular leaks (grade IB).

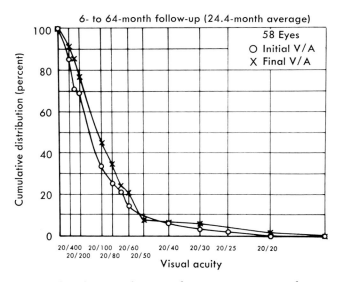

Fig. 14-5. Cumulative distribution of pre- and posttreatment visual acuities for 58 eyes with macular edema due to diffuse intraretinal vascular leaks (grade IC).

localized intravascular leaks within the macula when treated with argon laser photocoagulation (grade IB). We treated 117 eyes in patients whose average age was 57.5 years; duration of follow-up ranged from 6 to 63 months, with an average of 26 months. Of the 117 treated eyes, 75% maintained 20/60 or better vision (Fig. 14-4). In agreement with the Patz study, our results with argon laser photocoagulation of localized leaks preserved pretreatment visual acuity levels in about 65% of eyes, but only improved vision in 25%; thus it is important to diagnose and treat macular leaks before central vision is lost. In contrast to eyes with localized leaks, classified as nonproliferative group IB, the 58 eyes with diffuse macular leaks, classified as nonproliferative group IC, fared poorly with treatment; only 15% of the treated eyes in this group maintained 20/60 or better vision (Fig. 14-5). The average age for the latter group of patients was 62.5 years; the average duration of follow-up was 24.4 months, with a range of 6 to 24 months.

We do not have a randomized control group with which to compare the visual results of the treated eyes. Inasmuch as both initial and final visual acuities of the control group are not tabulated in the Patz et al.[30] or Rubinstein and Myska[32] reports, their control eyes cannot be used for comparison with our treated eyes. However, the control group of Marcus and Aaberg[20] is comparable because patients' visual acuities and ages are similar to those of our treated group who had diabetic macular edema with localized vascular leaks. The average age of the untreated group is 58.8 years and of the treated group is 57.5 years; the average length of follow-up for the untreated group is 20.6 months and for the treated

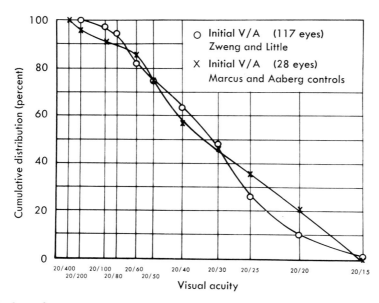

Fig. 14-6. Cumulative distribution of initial visual acuities of treated and of untreated eyes (grade IB).

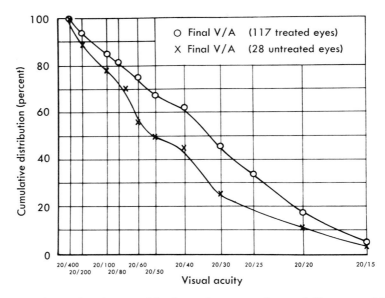

Fig. 14-7. Cumulative distribution of final visual acuities of treated (Zweng and Little) and of untreated (Marcus and Aaberg) eyes (grade IB).

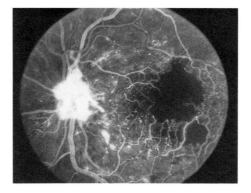

Fig. 14-8. Capillary nonperfusion of macula as seen with fluorescein angiography.

group is 26 months. Figs. 14-6 and 14-7 depict the comparison of visual results of our treated group with the nontreated eyes of Marcus and Aaberg. Visual acuity of their control group is more comparable with the pretreatment visual acuities of our treated eyes than it is to their own group of treated eyes. The data illustrates that the final visual acuities are better in the treated than in the nontreated eyes. This comparison of our treated group with Marcus and Aaberg's untreated group supports the positive visual results with photocoagulation of nonproliferative diabetic maculopathy noted by Patz et al. and by Rubinstein and Myska in their respective randomized control studies.

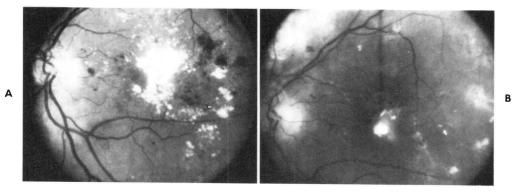

Fig. 14-9. A, Pretreatment appearance of macula, with dense foveal exudate. VA less than 20/400. **B,** Resolution of most of exudate 15 months after photocoagulation; residual hard foveal exudate prevents improvement of VA to better than 20/70 (grade IC).

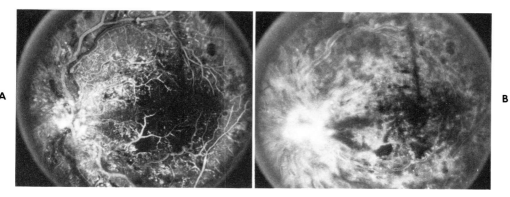

Fig. 14-10. Early-phase **(A)** and late-phase **(B)** fluorescein angiograms of diabetic maculopathy with advanced cystoid edema show diffuse leakage of eye in posterior fundus. In diabetic retinopathy, large cystoid spaces frequently fail to show extensive pooling of dye, suggesting that nonperfusion of macula is also present.

When leaks can be sealed without destruction of the fovea, the visual prognosis is good.

Poor prognostic signs included—
1. Capillary nonperfusion (Fig. 14-8)
2. Foveal hemorrhage
3. Foveal exudates (Fig. 14-9, *A* and *B*)
4. Cystoid edema (Fig. 14-10, *A* and *B*)
5. Preretinal membrane contracture (Fig. 14-11)
6. Diffuse intraretinal leakage and edema (Fig. 14-10, *B*)
7. Hypertensive vascular disease

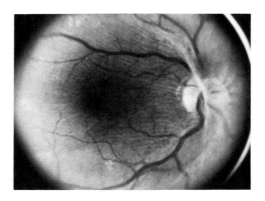

Fig. 14-11. Preretinal membrane contracture with striations through macula in untreated eye with diabetic retinopathy.

To summarize, in selected cases of nonproliferative diabetic retinopathy with localized intraretinal leaks within the macula, photocoagulation maintains or improves visual acuity in approximately 90% of eyes.

Proliferative diabetic retinopathy

In proliferative diabetic retinopathy, visual impairment is caused either by preretinal or vitreal hemorrhage and by retinal detachment produced by abnormal vitreoretinal traction.

Retinal neovascularization is a serious complication of diabetic retinopathy in that it frequently leads to vitreous hemorrhage and traction retinal detachment. It most commonly occurs on the optic disc,[34] probably because of the unique peripapillary capillary plexus (Toussaint, Kuwabara, and Cogan[35]) and the absence of the internal limiting membrane over the optic disc.[37]

The significant role of disc new vessels as the major cause of vitreous hemorrhage was noted by Aiello et al.[2] In their 3-year study, 33 of 72 untreated eyes hemorrhaged; of the eyes that hemorrhaged, 28 (85%) bled from disc new vessels. Patz and Berkow[29] observed that in 59% of cases in which one eye was lost due to proliferative diabetic retinopathy, the second eye had visual loss to 20/200 or worse within 1 year; in 89% of cases, vision in the second eye was 20/200 or worse within 5 years. In a study by Deckert, Simonsen, and Poulsen,[7] 50% of eyes with pre- or peripapillary proliferations became blind within 3 years. These studies indicate that disc neovascularization is a major cause of blindness in diabetes.

That photocoagulation has a role in the management of proliferative diabetic retinopathy has been questioned. It was first employed by Meyer-Schwickerath,[22] who used xenon arc photocoagulation. Irvine and Norton[11] found no significant difference in visual acuities in eyes with proliferative retinopathy treated by xenon arc photocoagulation, compared with an untreated control group. On the other hand, Wessing and Meyer-Schwickerath[36] and Okun[25] reported favorable responses to xenon arc photocoagulation in the management of proliferative diabetic retinopathy. Aiello et al.[2] reported favorable response of disc neovascularization in at least 20% of eyes treated with ruby laser panretinal photocoagulation. In none of these studies were the disc vessels directly coagulated.

Although the visual prognosis is poor for eyes with proliferative retinopathy, particularly when disc neovascularization is present, the natural course of proliferative retinopathy is so extremely variable as to make the prognosis for any single eye unreliable. Thus the evaluation of photocoagulation on the natural course is difficult without a randomized control study. For this purpose, a national collaborative diabetic study is being carried out in a randomized controlled fashion. Early results demonstrate that photocoagulation reduces incidence of blindness, as compared with untreated eyes.[8] Nonetheless, we wish to describe techniques in photocoagulation of disc neovascularization and to present data to support the use of an aggressive approach in the management of retinal neovascularization in proliferative diabetic retinopathy with photocoagulation.

TECHNIQUES FOR PHOTOCOAGULATING DISC NEOVASCULARIZATION

There are three approaches to the management of diabetic disc new vessels. First, there is direct coagulation of the disc vessels, which is seldom used alone because of recurrent neovascularization. This technique can be used with or without identification and coagulation of feeder vessels. Second, panretinal photocoagulation has been shown to be effective in reducing disc neovascularization to some degree in all eyes and totally in about 35% to 40% of eyes treated. Finally, there is the combination of direct coagulation with panretinal photocoagulation, which has been shown to be most effective when properly administered. Details of these techniques used in the management of diabetic disc new vessels follow.

Direct coagulation of neovascular frond

Feeder-frond photocoagulation. Direct coagulation of neovascular fronds requires excellent arterial phase angiograms for identification of feeder vessels and astute observation by the surgeon who studies the fundus in detail under high magnification while studying enlargements of the angiograms (Fig. 14-12) or the projected negative (Fig. 14-13).[18,19,27] Another aid in detection of feeder vessels is observation of afferent corpuscular flow while pressure is applied to the globe by pushing on the fundus contact lens. Once feeder and collector vessels are differentiated, photocoagulation is directed to the feeder vessels. The 50-μm spot is used with power levels of 100 to 250 mW for 0.2 sec. Repeated applications of laser coagulation are directed to the feeder vessel, initially with 100 mW of power; power levels are increased in increments of 25 mW until the blood column in the feeder vessel is interrupted (Fig. 14-14). The beam is then directed to a point more distal on the feeder vessel. This process is continued until the entire feeder vessel is obliterated. Attention is then directed to the distal portion of the

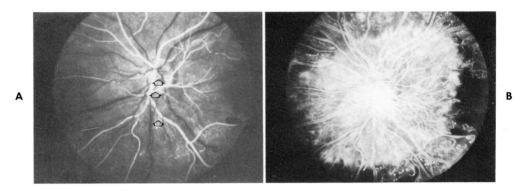

Fig. 14-12. A, Feeder-vessel identification with arterial phase of angiogram. **B,** Appearance of disc neovascularization preceding treatment, as seen on full venous phase of angiogram.

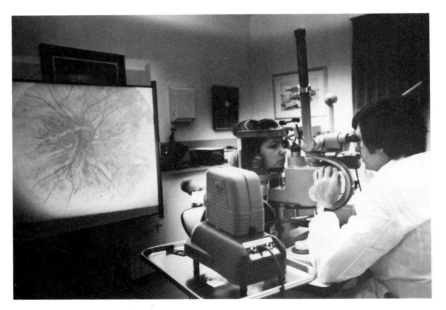

Fig. 14-13. Projection of fluorescein negative to identify feeder vessel. On enlarged projected image of negative, fluorescein appears black rather than white, as in positive prints. (From Little, H. L., Zweng, H. C., Jack, R. L., and Vassiliadis, A.: Am. J. Ophthalmol. **82**(5):675-682, 1976.)

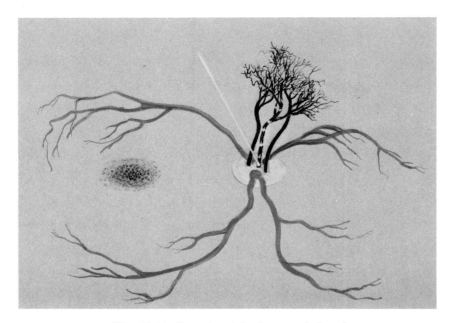

Fig. 14-14. Coagulated feeder vessel closed.

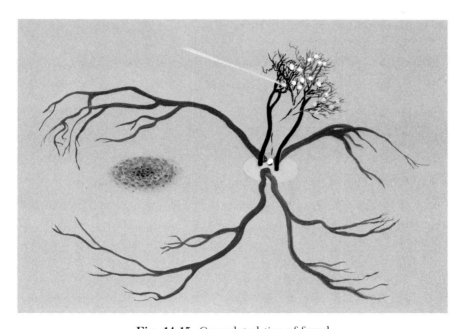

Fig. 14-15. Coagulated tips of frond.

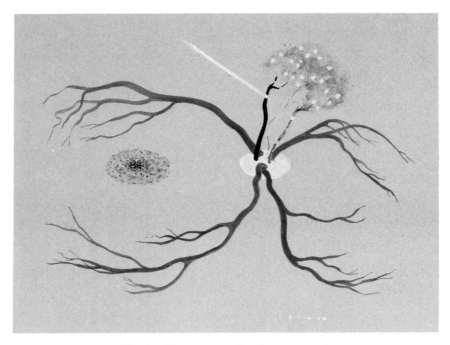

Fig. 14-16. Coagulated collector vessels.

frond. Because the blood flow has been stopped, there is greater absorption by the stagnant blood within the frond; hence the power is reduced to about 150 mW and the spot size is increased to 100 or 200 μm (Fig. 14-15). The efferent vessels (collector vessels) are not photocoagulated for 24 hours, in order to be certain that the feeder vessels have not reopened. If the feeder vessels have reopened, they are re-treated. Once the feeder vessels and the frond have remained closed for 24 hours, the collector vessels can be photocoagulated (Fig. 14-16). As with venous obstruction, venous engorgement and hemorrhage occur if the collector vessel is coagulated first (Fig. 14-17).

Nonfeeder vessel technique. Direct coagulation of the neovascular frond without first treating the feeder vessels was the first technique used for management of disc new vessels,[18] but because of the high incidence of hemorrhage and of recurrent neovascularization, the technique is seldom advocated. When feeder vessels cannot be identified, direct treatment of the frond should not be performed unless involution fails to occur within 3 months after panretinal photocoagulation. In the absence of feeder vessel treatment, the frond is coagulated from its peripheral extent toward its central stalk. The central stalk is treated last in order to avoid the initial coagulation of the efferent vessel, with subsequent engorgement and hemorrhage (Fig. 14-17). Usually the 100- or 200-μm spot size is used, at 0.2 sec with 100 to 300 mW power.

Neovascular fronds are reevaluated and re-treated if they reopen. For this

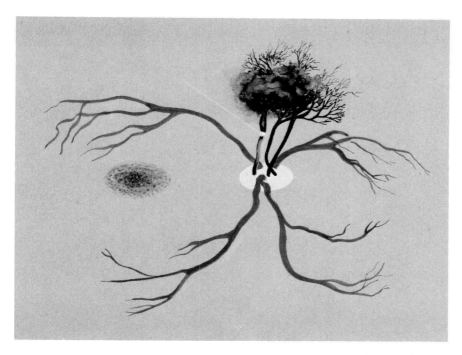

Fig. 14-17. Danger from closing collector vessels before feeder vessel.

reason, repeated evaluations are made 24 hours, 48 hours, and 1 week after treatment.

Experience has shown that focal treatment alone to neovascular fronds is followed by at least 50% incidence of recurrent neovascularization. For this reason, panretinal photocoagulation (PRP) is always recommended when treating disc new vessels. PRP can be used alone or in combination with direct treatment of disc new vessels.

Panretinal photocoagulation (PRP)

Widespread peripheral photocoagulation of the retina in the treatment of diabetic retinopathy was first done by Wessing and Meyer-Schwickerath,[36] using the Zeiss xenon arc photocoagulator, and by Aiello et al.,[2] using the American Optical ruby laser photocoagulator. In both instances, destruction of peripheral retina was planned and carried out because it was often observed that eyes with extensive chorioretinal scars, retinal atrophy secondary to high myopia, or optic atrophy from any cause developed little or no proliferative diabetic retinopathy, compared with the fellow eye not afflicted with any of these pathologic conditions.

It is hypothesized that in diabetic retinopathy the metabolically active retina bordering areas of focal retinal ischemia do not receive sufficient oxygen. The

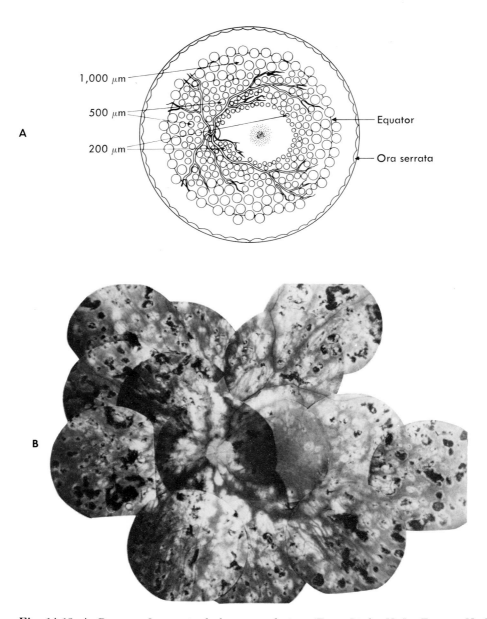

Fig. 14-18. A, Pattern of panretinal photocoagulation. (From Little, H. L., Zweng, H. C., Jack, R. L., and Vassiliadis, A.: Am. J. Ophthalmol. **82:**675-682, 1976.) **B,** Composite photograph of PRP treatment for proliferative diabetic retinopathy (5 years 2 months after PRP treatment).

pathophysiologic response of the hypoxic but viable retina is the elaboration of a vasoproliferative substance that causes the proliferation of new blood vessels on retina and nerve head, which tend to bleed. Furthermore, glial proliferation occurs, probably in response to hypoxia and leakage of plasma and whole blood, producing retinovitreal adhesions, vitreal organization and contracture, and traction retinal detachments, with permanent marked visual loss. In eyes with extensive chorioretinal scars or optic atrophy, the retinal metabolic activity is reduced and the oxygen demand is lessened; furthermore, in these conditions it is possible that, because of reduced numbers of viable cells in the retina, there is insufficient amount of vasoproliferative factor produced to stimulate neovascularization. Therefore it is possible to destroy the poorly perfused hypoxic retina in a carefully planned way with photocoagulation, to preserve central vision and some of the peripheral visual field.

Both Wessing and Meyer-Schwickerath and Aiello et al. reported success with their respective treatment techniques. However, widespread xenon arc photocoagulation often constricts visual fields markedly because of the tendency to give through-and-through burns of the retina, involving the nerve fiber layer.[9] Although ruby laser lesions did not give such field constrictions, the technique produced involution of nerve head new vessels in only 21% of eyes treated.[2]

We use the argon laser photocoagulator, modifying the techniques of Wessing and Meyer-Schwickerath and Aiello et al. for two reasons. On the negative side, use of the argon laser photocoagulator directly to disc vessels is disappointing because recurrent neovascularization occurs in at least 50% of eyes. From a positive point of view, the argon laser instrument allows preselection and precise control of the beam diameter, exposure time, and power, and the slit-lamp delivery system permits very accurate placement of lesions. The technique is as follows:

1. Burns are placed in a tightly spaced pattern, from the edge of the nerve head to the equator (Fig. 14-18); lesions are almost but not quite contiguous (Figs. 14-19 and 14-20).
2. Burns are of moderate intensity, easily seen but not snow white in color.
3. A vertical row of lesions is placed at a distance equal to 4 disc diameters temporal from the fovea, joining the superior and inferior vascular arcades to act as a visual barrier against inadvertent burning of the macula, which is especially helpful when treating the temporal periphery through a mirror of the fundus contact lens (Fig. 14-21).
4. Nonproliferative diabetic retinopathy is treated in the macula and paramacula as deemed necessary.
5. Flat retinal neovascularizations and surrounding areas of capillary nonperfusion are treated focally and heavily.

Because this technique combines widespread peripheral photocoagulation and focal photocoagulation where needed in the macula and paramacula, we call it panretinal photocoagulation (PRP).

Exclusive of treatment to the macula and the area of the maculopapillary

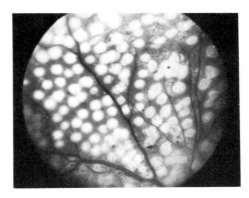

Fig. 14-19. Distribution of 500-μm diameter lesions in midperiphery and of 1,000-μm diameter lesions in periphery.

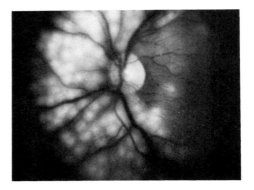

Fig. 14-20. Closely placed 200- and 500-μm diameter lesions extending from margin of optic disease to midperiphery. Normal retinal vessels are avoided in treatment.

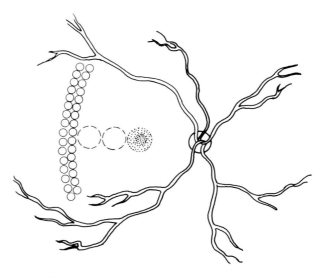

Fig. 14-21. Diagram showing placement of vertical rows of lesions temporal to fovea.

bundle, the following settings are used, but vary depending on the retinal area being photocoagulated:

1. From the edge of the nerve head to 2 disc diameters away from the disc and just inside the temporal vascular arcades: 200-μm beam diameter, 0.05- to 0.1-sec exposure, and 200 to 400 mW power
2. From the edge of the lesions placed around the nerve head to the midperiphery: 500 μm, 0.05 to 0.1 sec, 400 to 800 mW
3. From the midperiphery to the equator: 1,000 μm, 0.05 to 0.1 sec, 1,000 to 2,000 mW

All settings are modified as needed, depending on the clarity of the ocular media. When there is blood in the vitreous cavity, short time exposures are preferable to long ones, because prolonged heating of the blood in the vitreous may induce vitreal contracture.

Initial panretinal photocoagulation requires at least 2,000 lesions, which should be administered over 1 to 2 weeks. Additional lesions are made if the disc new vessels do not atrophy completely. These fill-in lesions are placed between previously treated areas. Scarred areas should not be re-treated, because of the danger of inducing a nerve fiber layer field defect in the retina, thinned because its outer layers are reduced in thickness from previous treatment and because previous treatment has stimulated retinal pigment epithelial hyperplasia; furthermore, patients complain of pain when photocoagulation is directed to pigmented scars. It is not unusual to give 4,000 to 6,000 lesions over 4 to 6 months to retinas in which disc new vessels do not atrophy completely after the first course of PRP.

Complications including increased macular edema, hemorrhage from disc neovascularization, exudative detachment of the retina, and choroidal and ciliary body detachment with compromise of the anterior chamber angle have occurred when all of the panretinal photocoagulation lesions were applied in one treatment session; thus, 3 to 5 treatment sessions are advised, over a period of 5 to 14 days. One approach is to treat one quadrant per session, with at least 1 day between sessions. Either temporal quadrant is treated first, the diagonally opposite nasal quadrant second, the other nasal quadrant third, and the remaining temporal quadrant fourth (Fig. 14-22).

Another technique of treatment is to coagulate the midperipheral areas of nonperfused retina first. One of us (HLL) prefers to photocoagulate from the disc margin superiorly into the midperiphery, including the areas of nonperfusion. This usually requires approximately 200 lesions with the 200-μm spot and 300 lesions with the 500-μm spot setting. In the second treatment session, a similar procedure is done inferiorly. The third session of treatment consists of coagulating the superior peripheral retina 120°, usually with the 1,000-μm spot size. The inferior periphery of 120° is treated on the fourth session. Finally, the temporal periphery of 120° is treated in the fifth session (Fig. 14-23). Between each session of treatment, vision is checked and the retina is examined for exudative de-

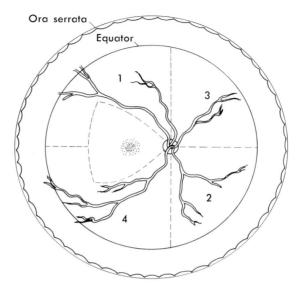

Fig. 14-22. Diagram showing quadrant method of panretinal photocoagulation.

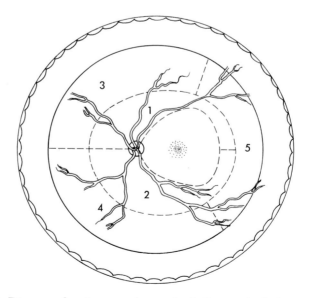

Fig. 14-23. Diagram showing annular method of panretinal photocoagulation.

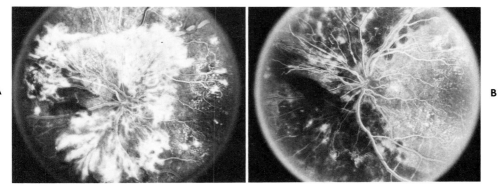

Fig. 14-24. A, Pretreatment angiogram of large neovascular frond off optic disc. **B,** Marked involution of neovascular frond 2 weeks after panretinal photocoagulation.

tachment and increased macular edema. If problems are detected, subsequent treatment is postponed until they are resolved.

Pain may occur during treatment, because the patient usually is not given a retrobulbar anesthetic. If there is pain, the following corrective measures should be considered:

1. Because the peripheral retina is more pain sensitive than is the posterior pole, treat the peripheral areas slowly and intermittently to reduce patient discomfort.
2. Reduce frequency of applications to less than one per sec.
3. Reduce exposure time of coagulation to 0.05 sec, increasing power as needed to obtain desired lesions.
4. Reduce the beam diameter from 1,000 to 500 μm, decreasing power as needed to obtain desired lesions.
5. Interrupt treatment for several minutes.
6. Retrobulbar analgesia is occasionally necessary.

In spite of no direct treatment to the disc new vessels, there can be a surprisingly rapid involution of vessels within a 2-week period (Figs. 14-24, *A* and *B*). This technique minimizes hemorrhage from disc new vessels, simply because these are avoided. With all techniques, patients are treated also with focal photocoagulation to background retinopathy and flat retinal neovascularization.

Combined direct coagulation of disc new vessels with panretinal photocoagulation

The techniques as outlined above have been combined in different chronologic order: direct disc vessel treatment 1 to 6 months prior to PRP, panretinal photocoagulation 1 to 6 months prior to direct treatment, or concurrent direct and panretinal treatment (i.e., each done within the same 4-week period). Visual results indicate that the concurrent treatment technique has the best outcome

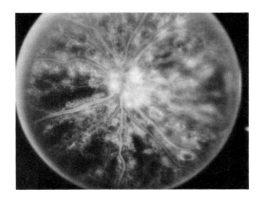

Fig. 14-25. Fluorescein angiogram 4 months after combined feeder-frond and panretinal photocoagulation shows eradication of disc neovascularization; note closely placed chorioretinal laser scars, which spare normal retinal vessels. Compare with Fig. 14-12, B.

(Fig. 14-25) and that the initial direct treatment followed 1 to 6 months later with PRP is least effective of the three sequences.

Panretinal photocoagulation of the retina for diabetic disc new vessels as described here is a relatively safe procedure. However, only if done meticulously as described will results be comparable. For example, we have seen eyes in which this technique was termed a failure, but which have received less than 1,000 lesions. When 2,000 to 3,000 panretinal photocoagulation lesions are applied, disc new vessels are reduced by at least three fourths in about 70% of cases. Because the amount and the vascular engorgement of neovascularization are reduced by PRP, the incidence of hemorrhage and the need for subsequent direct treatment of disc vessels is reduced. Occasionally, the change of disc new vessels into glial tissue makes direct treatment of residual vessels more difficult than if treated originally, because the glial strands may obsure the vessels to be treated.

Based on our experience, recommendations for photocoagulation treatment of disc neovascularization are—

1. Carry out PRP as described above.
2. Follow up on the patient every month.
3. If the disc new vessels have not atrophied 50% in 1 month or 75% in 3 months, additional panretinal photocoagulation is carried out. This is done by filling in coagulations between previously placed lesions by carrying the treatment area anterior to the equator and over previous lesions if coagulation burns can be produced. Intensive PRP must be accomplished before disc vessels are treated directly.
4. If the disc new vessels have not atrophied in 6 months, direct treatment of these vessels is performed using the feeder-frond technique as described by Patz[27] and by us.[15,18]

5. Because the best results are obtained with direct coagulation of disc new vessels and panretinal photocoagulation done concurrently, this technique is recommended when employed by the experienced argon laser surgeon.
6. All eyes, even if quiescent, must be followed up at intervals of no longer than 4 months.

Results

We have treated 248 eyes with argon laser photocoagulation for diabetic disc neovascularization. Patients' ages ranged from 18 to 73, averaging 41 years; 46% were male and 54% were female. Time since diagnosis of diabetes ranged from 1 to 45 years, with median and average of 20 years. The disc neovascularization extended from ½ to 4 disc diameters in width, with minimal to moderate glial tissue. Disc vessels treated in this study included N_1 Fo Ho to N_2 F_2 H_1 by O'Hare Classification.[6] Four techniques evolved sequentially as experience accumulated.* In this retrospective study, treatment was not randomized, nor were fellow eyes used as controls.

All eyes reported were followed up from 12 to 62 months. Evaluation of treatment was based on the pre- and posttreatment ophthalmoscopic appearances, including fluorescein angiograms (Table 14-1) and visual acuities (Table 14-2). Improved appearance was defined as at least a 50% reduction in nerve head neovascularization. A change in vision was defined as at least a 2-line increase or decrease in acuity on the Snellen chart.

---

*References 13-15, 17-19, 27, 38.

Table 14-1. Clinical appearance 12 or more months following first argon laser photocoagulation for diabetic disc neovascularization (May 1969 to February 1974)

	Group I: nonfeeder	Group II: feeder-frond	Group III: PRP and feeder-frond	Group IV: PRP alone
Follow-up (months)	12 to 61	12 to 55	12 to 45	12 to 35
Number of eyes	60	24	73	35
Better	16 (27%)	16 (67%)	62 (85%)	31 (89%)
Quiescent	6 (10%)	3 (12.5%)	31 (42%)*	13 (37%)
No significant change	5 (8%)	0 (0%)	1 (1%)	0 (0%)
Worse	39 (65%)	8 (33%)	10 (14%)	4 (11%)
Hemorrhage per treatment session	6%	5%	5%	3%†

Little, H. L., Zweng, H. C., Jack, R. L., and Vassiliadis, A.: Techniques of argon laser photocoagulation of diabetic disc vessels, Am. J. Ophthalmol. **82**:675-683, 1976.
*Data tabulated through July 1975 show 51% of eyes quiescent in Group III versus 36% of eyes quiescent in Group IV.
†All during focal treatment.

Table 14-2. Visual acuity 12 or more months following first argon laser photocoagulation for diabetic disc neovascularization (May 1969 to February 1974)

	Group I: nonfeeder	Group II: feeder-frond	Group III: PRP and feeder-frond	Group IV: PRP alone
Follow-up (months)	12 to 61	12 to 55	12 to 35	12 to 45
Number of eyes	60	24	73	35
Better (2 or more lines)	5 (8%)	2 (8%)	2 (3%)	4 (11%)
No significant change	19 (32%)	11 (46%)	55 (75%)	23 (66%)
Worse (2 or more lines)	36 (0%)	11 (46%)	16 (22%)	8 (23%)

Little, H. L., Zweng, H. C., Jack, R. L., and Vassiliadis, A.: Techniques of argon laser photocoagulation of diabetic disc vessels, Am. J. Ophthalmol. **82:**675-683, 1976.

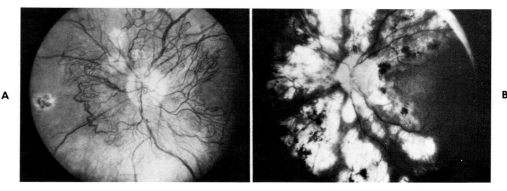

Fig. 14-26. A, Pretreatment appearance of disc neovascularization of 14 years' duration in 23-year-old diabetic woman. **B,** Quiescent appearance of retinopathy 26 months after photocoagulation. (From Little, H. L., Zweng, H. C., Jack, R. L., and Vassiliadis, A.: Am. J. Ophthalmol. **82**(5):675-682, 1976.)

A further evaluation of treatment was afforded by using the concept of quiescence, by which we mean virtually total elimination of disc new vessels for at least 6 months from the last treatment (Fig. 14-26, *A* and *B*). In addition, the quiescent eye showed some optic pallor, decrease in venous engorgement, and resolution of all significant background retinopathy. The goal of photocoagulation therapy is to achieve quiescence in order to remove all vision-threatening pathologic conditions. Quiescence should not be construed as cure, because neovascularization can reactivate at a future time.

With focal photocoagulation, almost two of three patients were worse visually and ophthalmoscopically at the end of the follow-up period, compared with their pretreatment status. Only 10% were quiescent. The incidence of disc vessel hemorrhages during treatment or within 1 week after treatment was high, approximately 15% per treatment session. For these reasons, this technique was deemed dangerous and ineffective and was abandoned.

Feeder-frond photocoagulation was used to minimize hemorrhagic complications of focal coagulation. It was helpful in that the hemorrhage rate fell to 6%. However, again only about one eye in 10 was quiescent, and in 40% of eyes treated by the feeder vessel technique recurrent vessels developed. Vision deteriorated in 46% of the eyes treated with this technique. The 24 eyes in group II represent only 60% of the eyes initially treated by this technique; the remaining 40% were removed from group II before the 12-month follow-up, because of significant recurrent neovascularization, for which they were additionally treated with PRP. The 67% improvement in the clinical appearance of the remaining 24 eyes is therefore misleading, because it excludes the 16 eyes that subsequently received PRP. Of the 40 eyes initially treated with the feeder-frond technique alone, only 40% were improved. This technique alone was judged unsatisfactory and was abandoned.

Feeder-frond with panretinal photocoagulation and panretinal photocoagulation alone, used since July 1971 and January 1972 respectively, gave results that were clearly superior to those obtained with the first two methods. Ophthalmoscopic appearance improved in at least 85% of eyes, and pretreatment vision was maintained in 77% of eyes; 51% of eyes treated with combined feeder-frond and panretinal photocoagulation and 37% of eyes treated with panretinal photocoagulation alone became quiescent. Groups III and IV showed similar and significant improvements in the clinical appearance of the retinopathy. Inasmuch as most patients in this study had 20/40 or better visual acuity immediately before the first treatment, maintenance rather than improvement of pretreatment visual acuity was the main goal of treatment. This was accomplished in 77% and 78% of the eyes treated in groups III and IV, but in only 40% of eyes in group I and 54% in group II.

In addition to comparison of visual acuities (Table 14-2), the cumulative distribution of visual acuities before and after treatment can also be compared. In contrast to data in Tables 14-1 and 14-2, compiled between May 1969 and February 1974, the data expressed by cumulative distribution were collected through July 1975. This evaluation was done on 197 eyes, with follow-up ranging from 1 to 5 years (Figs. 14-27 to 14-30). Visual acuity is read on the abscissa, and the corresponding percentage of people with that respective visual acuity or better are shown on the ordinate. Comparison was made of results from photocoagulation of disc vessels only, panretinal photocoagulation only, and combined photocoagulation of disc neovascularization with panretinal photocoagulation. Except for the 27 eyes that received photocoagulation solely to disc new vessels, only eyes receiving over 1,000 lesions were included. These data illustrate that the cumulative visual acuities are far worse for eyes in which the disc vessels alone are treated (Fig. 14-24). Much better visual results were obtained with panretinal photocoagulation alone (Fig. 14-28). However, best vision resulted from com-

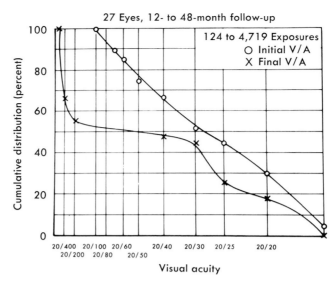

Fig. 14-27. Cumulative distribution of pre- and posttreatment visual acuities when only disc new vessels are treated with direct or feeder-frond technique without panretinal photocoagulation. (From Little, H. L., Zweng, H. C., Jack, R. L., and Vassiliadis, A.: Am. J. Ophthalmol. **82**(5):675-682, 1976.)

bined feeder-frond and panretinal photocoagulation (Figs. 14-29 and 14-30). The latter figure illustrates that the visual results are better when photocoagulation of disc vessels and panretinal photocoagulation are contemporaneous. Furthermore, no significant loss of vision occurred from 1 to 3 years after combined feeder-frond panretinal photocoagulation (Fig. 14-31). When eyes were treated contemporaneously with the latter technique, 57% became quiescent. The incidence of quiescence is higher for eyes with the larger number of exposures (Fig. 14-32).

In discussing the use of PRP versus combined PRP with direct treatment of disc neovascularization, one must first understand the importance of the number of PRP lesions. On studying the results of eyes treated for disc new vessels in which an average of 3,367 PRP lesions were applied using 500- or 1,000-μm spot-size lesions in a 12- to 69-month follow-up, one notes that the visual results are much better than those in which an average of 1,573 lesions were applied (Fig. 14-28, *A* and *B*). Furthermore, the results of eyes treated with more PRP lesions are comparable to those treated with combined PRP with direct treatment of disc new vessels in which the average number of lesions was 3,133 (Figs. 14-28, *B*, and 14-30). The importance of the larger number of PRP lesions in the management of proliferative diabetic retinopathy is further expressed by data in Fig. 14-32.

Prognosis is dependent on the selection of patients to be treated. Eyes with cloudy ocular media due to vitreous hemorrhage should not be treated unless the hemorrhage clears. Patients with massive fibrous elements in the proliferative

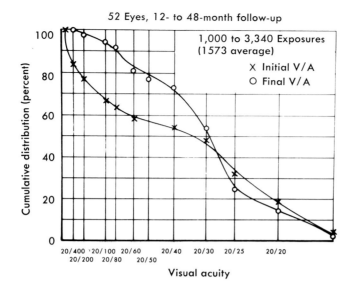

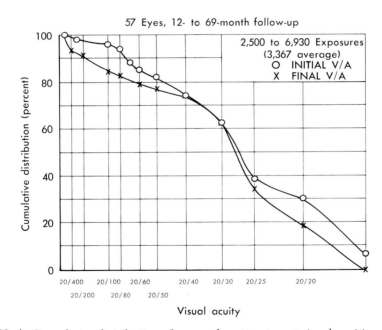

Fig. 14-28. A, Cumulative distribution of pre- and posttreatment visual acuities when disc new vessels are treated by panretinal photocoagulation alone. (From Little, H. L., Zweng, H. C., Jack, R. L., and Vassiliadis, A.: Am. J. Ophthalmol. **82**(5):675-682, 1976.) **B,** Cumulative distribution of pre- and posttreatment visual acuities when disc new vessels are treated by extensive panretinal photocoagulation alone (eyes with more than 2,500 lesions).

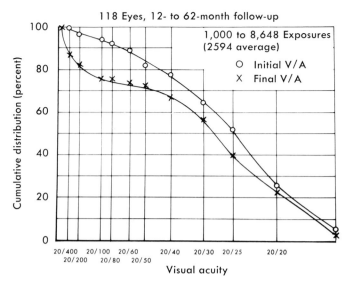

Fig. 14-29. Cumulative distribution of pre- and posttreatment visual acuities when disc new vessels are treated with feeder-frond technique combined with panretinal photocoagulation. (From Little, H. L., Zweng, H. C., Jack, R. L., and Vassiliadis, A.: Am. J. Ophthalmol. **82**(5):675-682, 1976.)

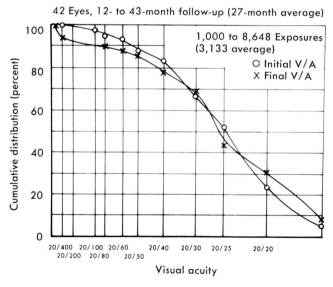

Fig. 14-30. Cumulative distribution of pre- and posttreatment visual acuities when disc new vessels are treated contemporaneously with feeder-frond technique and panretinal photocoagulation. (From Little, H. L., Zweng, H. C., Jack, R. L., and Vassiliadis, A.: Am. J. Ophthalmol. **82**(5):675-682, 1976.)

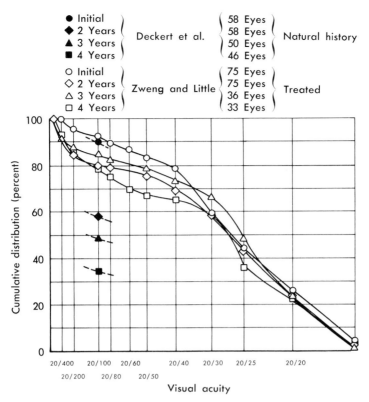

Fig. 14-31. Preservation of visual acuity 1, 2, 3, and 4 years after combined photocoagulation of disc new vessels and panretinal photocoagulation. Note comparison of visual results with untreated eyes.

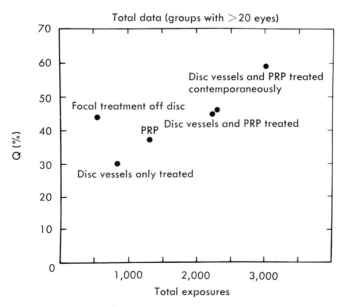

Fig. 14-32. Relationship of total number of exposures to incidence of quiescence.

retinopathy are extremely poor subjects; the argon laser beam cannot be focused on the vessels, due to intervening connective tissue. Clear detailed fluorescein angiograms are essential in visualizing feeder vessels if the feeder-frond technique is to be used. Furthermore, the prognosis is guarded when there is massive vitreous contracture, with hemorrhage along with vitreous base, traction retinal detachment, or extensive areas of preretinal membrane formation. The cases herein reported all had disc neovascularization with no or only moderate glial tissue on the nerve head or along the vascular arcades.

Discussion

Wessing and Meyer-Schwickerath[36] and Aiello et al.[2] reported only 20% involution of disc vessels when using xenon arc and ruby laser disseminated photocoagulation respectively. With argon laser panretinal photocoagulation alone, therefore, it was not anticipated that as high an incidence of involution of disc vessels would be achieved as with panretinal photocoagulation combined with feeder-frond coagulation of new disc vessels. Therefore, the results were a surprise and they deserve special comment.

The involutional effect of panretinal photocoagulation on diabetic retinopathy might result from any of the following factors:[31]

1. Reduction of retinal requirement for oxygen, thus leaving more oxygen for the remaining untreated retina
2. Destruction of hypoxic tissue, producing a vasoproliferative factor
3. Elimination of sluggishly perfused capillaries, thus increasing rate of blood flow in the remaining capillaries
4. Opening of new channels for metabolic transfer by way of photocoagulation-induced openings in the retinal pigment epithelium.

Experience has shown that the more extensive the photocoagulation, the greater and longer lasting is the involutional effect on retinopathy.

An explanation is needed for the difference between the experiences of successful elimination of disc neovascularization (40% of eyes reported here) from those reported by Aiello et al. and Wessing and Meyer-Schwickerath (20%).

Photocoagulation instruments—whether xenon arc, ruby laser, or argon laser—can create pathologic conditions ranging in severity from no demonstrable lesion to extensive destruction; thus, aspects of techniques, such as number, intensity, size, and distribution of lesions, must be compared. Aiello et al.[2] reported marked improvement in proliferative retinopathy in 23 of 80 eyes (21%). Wessing and Meyer-Schwickerath[36] reported definite involution of proliferative retinopathy in 12 of 60 eyes (20%). In Aiello and associates' cases, approximately 600 to 800 2.5° moderately light ruby laser lesions were applied during a 4- to 6-week interval. These lesions were not applied beyond the midperiphery, nor were they intense enough to involve more than the outer segments of the photoreceptors. Probably much less destruction of retina, both in thickness and in total area, was produced by the ruby laser technique than by the technique we have reported here. Wessing and Meyer-Schwickerath placed 200 to 300 moderately heavy xenon arc lesions with 1.5° to 3° spots in one to three sessions. Lesions extended from 2 disc diameters of the macula to the midperiphery. The retinal lesions described with the xenon lesions were much fewer in number (200 to 300) than those reported in this argon laser study (1,200 to 3,000), in which the lesions were placed much closer together and over a greater area of the retina. The difference in the results of photocoagulation on the disc neovascularization obtained in our study and those of Wessing and Meyer-Schwickerath and Aiello et al. is explained by the larger number of lesions, the larger area of retina treated, and the greater density of lesions applied. Hence, the safest method of treating disc new vessels appears to be initial panretinal photocoagulation, with subsequent feeder-frond treatment to residual disc vessels performed 6 weeks after the initial panretinal photocoagulation therapy.

It is important to compare treatment results with the natural course of the disease. Deckert, Simonsen, and Poulsen[7] observed that, of 50 eyes with disc neovascularization in 29 juvenile diabetics, only 47% of eyes had better than 20/100 vision within 3 years. This is in contrast to 85% of 33 eyes with better than 20/100 acuity 3 years following combined panretinal photocoagulation and direct treatment of disc new vessels done by us[18] (Fig. 14-31). This observation is significant to the $P < 0.002$ level (Tables 14-3 and 14-4). Furthermore, one can compare Beetham's[4] 3-year follow-up of 29 patients with proliferative diabetic retinopathy without photocoagulation with 52 eyes treated by us (Fig. 14-33). The

Table 14-3. Diabetic disc neovascularization; 20/100 or worse visual acuity (minimum 3-year follow-up)

	Initial (%)	*≥ 36 months (%)*
Treated eyes (Little and Zweng)	8	16
Untreated eyes (Deckert et al.)	10	52

Table 14-4. Comparison of treated eyes with natural history (3-year follow-up)

	≤ 20/200	*> 20/200*	*Total*
Treated eyes (Little and Zweng)	5	28	33
Untreated eyes	$\frac{26}{31}$	$\frac{24}{52}$	$\frac{50}{83}$

$x^2 = 10.01$.
Significant at $P < 0.002$ level.

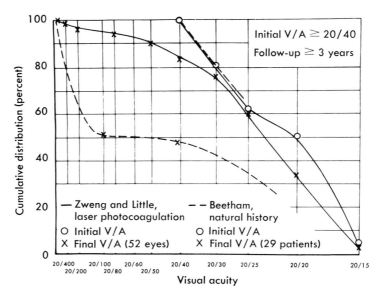

Fig. 14-33. Comparison of visual results of untreated and treated eyes with proliferative diabetic retinopathy after 3-year follow-up.

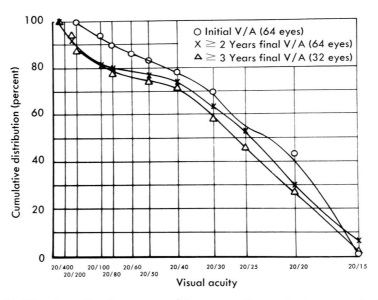

Fig. 14-34. Visual results of eyes treated for noncapillary retinal neovascularization.

Table 14-5. Comparison at 20/100 (3-year follow-up)

	≥ 20/100	≤ 20/200	*Total*
Treated eyes (Zweng and Little)	49	3	52
Untreated eyes (Beetham)	30	28	58
	79	31	110

$x^2 = 22.42$.
Significant at P < 0.001 level.

Table 14-6. Evaluation of clinical appearance

	Treated	*Untreated*
Better	14	0
Quiescent	8	0
Same	0	7
Worse	2	9

Comparison of treated versus untreated eyes in 16 patients after 12 or more months. All eyes initially had visual acuity of 20/100 or better. The worse eye was treated in 11 of the 16 patients. Treatment technique consisted of panretinal photocoagulation in all cases.
$x^2 = 13.9$, df = 1.
Significant at the P = 0.001 level.

initial visual acuity was 20/40 or better in both groups. After 3 years, in Beetham's untreated group only 50% had 20/100 or better; in the treated group, 95% had 20/100 or better (Fig. 14-34). This is statistically significant to P < 0.001 (Table 14-5).

In a nonrandomized study of 16 patients with visual acuities of 20/100 or better in each eye, who had reasonably symmetrical proliferative retinopathy involving both discs, only one eye was photocoagulated. In 11 of the 16 eyes, the eye with the worse proliferative disease was treated. After a 12- to 24-month follow-up, the clinical appearance of the treated eye had improved in 14 of 16 eyes; eight of the 16 eyes became quiescent (Table 14-6). None of the untreated eyes showed improvement in clinical appearance. The visual acuity was better in the treated eyes, but the difference was not statistically significant (Table 14-7). However, the difference of improvement of the retinopathy of the treated eyes was statistically significant to P < 0.001.

Patz and Berkow[29] reported the natural course of proliferative diabetic retinopathy in 27 patients whose vision was 20/200 or less in the worse eye and 20/80 or better in the other. To evaluate further the effect of argon laser photocoagulation, we studied a similar series of 24 patients (Table 14-8). The better eye was treated with feeder-frond and PRP or PRP alone. At the end of 12 months, 59% of the 27 patients in the Patz-Berkow study had reduced vision of 20/200 or less in the better eye, whereas only three of the 24 patients (13%) in our study had a similar

Table 14-7. Evaluation of visual acuity

	Treated	*Untreated*
Better	1	0
Same	13	11
Worse	2	5

Comparison of treated versus untreated eyes in 16 patients after 12 or more months. All eyes initially had visual acuity of 20/100 or better. The worse eye was treated in 11 of the 16 patients. Treatment technique consisted of combined feeder-frond and panretinal photocoagulation in all cases. A two-line or greater change on the Snellen chart justifies change in acuity.
$x^2 = 0.615$, df = 1.
The difference between treated and untreated eyes is not statistically significant.

Table 14-8. Argon laser photocoagulation versus natural course

	Treated *(Little and Zweng)*	*Natural course* *(Patz and Berkow)*
Number of eyes	24	27
≥ 20/80 (initial and final)	21 (87%)	11 (41%)
≥ 20/80 (initial) and ≤ 20/200 (final)	3 (13%)	16 (59%)

Evaluation of visual acuity in the fellow eye (initially ≥ 20/80) after other eye (initially ≤ 20/200) was lost to proliferative retinopathy. No eyes in either study had acuity between 20/80 and 20/200 after 12-month follow-up. Treatment technique consisted of either feeder-frond and PRP argon laser photocoagulation or PRP alone.

reduction with argon laser treatment. These results were highly statistically significant.

NONDISC RETINAL NEOVASCULARIZATION

Of 168 eyes treated for neovascularization in the plane of the retina, 95 eyes have been followed for at least 6 months. All patients were treated with focal argon laser photocoagulation of the neovascular fronds and surrounding nonperfused retina, using 200- and 500-μm spot sizes, 0.2-sec exposure, and 200 to 500 mW power intially; then the individual feeder vessels were treated when identified, with 50- to 100-μm spot sizes for 0.2 sec at 100 to 200 mW. Fig. 14-38 shows the visual outcome 2 and 3 years after treatment of nonpapillary retinal neovascularization. Although such treatment usually eliminates existing new vessels, about 19% of eyes progressed to disc neovascularization during a 1- to 4-year follow-up period. This experience suggests that in cases with extensive retinal neovascularization, panretinal photocoagulation should be done to prevent the development of disc new vessels.

FOLLOW-UP EVALUATION

Follow-up evaluation of patients after treatment is extremely important. Because recurrent neovascularization is a common sequel, all patients treated for proliferative retinopathy should be reevaluated with biomicroscopic fundus examination and with fluorescein angiography or angioscopy every 2 to 4 weeks until all active retinopathy is eliminated and thereafter every 3 to 4 months indefinitely. Close follow-up and early detection of recurrent retinopathy enables the surgeon to repeat photocoagulation before advanced proliferans and hemorrhages occur.

COMPLICATIONS

The four major complications of argon laser photocoagulation of disc neovascularization are hemorrhage, recurrent neovascularization, nerve fiber field defect, and ischemia (thermal) papillitis.[10,14,15,38] Feeder vessel treatment and panretinal photocoagulation have reduced the rate of hemorrhage. Panretinal photocoagulation has minimized recurrent neovascularization. Nerve fiber field defects are avoided by not using over 500-mW power with 500-μm spot diameter in the peripapillary area and by not re-treating in the peripapillary zone once the retina is thin due to previous coagulation. If treatment over a peripapillary atrophic area is necessary, the 50-μm spot should be used to minimize the size of a sector defect that might be produced. Ischemic (thermal) papillitis is prevented by using the 50-μm spot with 100 to 200 mW at short exposures of 0.1 to 0.2 sec. These settings permit treatment of the abnormal vessels, with minimal damage to the underlying or surrounding optic nerve.

Even though the panretinal photocoagulation technique is the safest method employed to treat disc neovascularization, it is not free of complications.[11] When over 1,000 lesions were placed in one session of treatment, the following complications have occurred:

1. Hemorrhage from disc neovascularization occurred in two eyes within 24 hours of treatment, presumably due to increased resistance of blood flow in the retinal circulation, with increased blood flow to the disc vessels.
2. Macular edema frequently occurred and persisted in one eye.
3. Transient exudative retinal detachment has resulted but has subsided, usually within 5 to 7 days.
4. Two eyes developed traction retinal detachment.
5. Transient myopia was a frequent occurrence, lasting from 1 to 7 days; the myopia was attributed to anterior displacement of the iris lens diaphragm, caused by vascular engorgement of the ciliary body.[3]
6. In one eye, panretinal argon laser photocoagulation caused transient angle-closure glaucoma secondary to extensive choroidal effusion, with anterior displacement of the iris lens diaphragm, which resolved after 48 hours.
7. Seizures, resulting from photic stimulation of repeated rhythmical argon laser photocoagulation, occurred in two patients.

Reduction of light sensitivity and impairment of night vision occur invariably following panretinal photocoagulation. The peripheral field loss in patients follow-

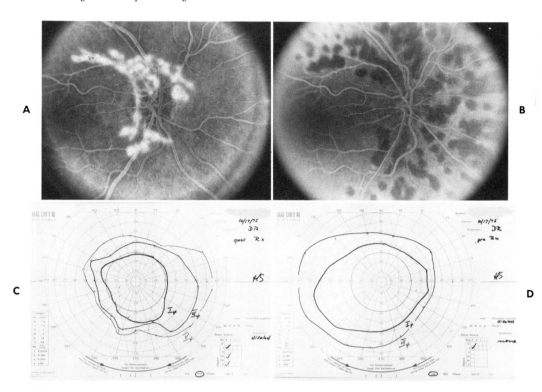

Fig. 14-35. A, Pretreatment angiogram of diabetic disc neovascularization. **B,** Involution of disc new vessels 4 weeks after combined panretinal and disc new vessel treatment. **C,** Same eye as **B.** Moderate constriction of peripheral visual field noted with Goldmann perimetry. **D,** Visual field of patient's untreated eye, for comparison.

ing these extensive multiple panretinal photocoagulation lesions is about 15° in each meridian (Fig. 14-35, *A* to *D*). In patients treated in a similar manner with xenon arc photocoagulation, greater visual field constriction occurs.[8,9]

SUMMARY

In nonproliferative diabetic retinopathy, argon laser photocoagulation of localized intraretinal vascular leaks maintains or improves vision in about 90% of eyes treated. In most cases vision is maintained at pretreatment levels; in only 25% is visual acuity improved. Thus, treatment is recommended before significant loss of central vision occurs.

Preservation of visual acuity and regression of proliferative retinopathy were achieved most frequently with the combined feeder-frond–panretinal photocoagulation technique. Because results are almost as good with panretinal photocoagulation alone and because it is a safer technique, we recommend that panretinal photocoagulation be used initially, except by an experienced argon laser surgeon. Filling in of "skip" areas in the panretinal photocoagulation treatment pattern and re-treatment of lightly treated areas should also be carried out if treatment is indicated. If obvious regression has not begun by 6 weeks and regression of at least 75% of the new vessels has not occurred 6 months after the start of treatment, the feeder-frond technique should be used in addition. Careful monthly follow-up with ophthalmoscopy is required while any active pathologic condition is present; when quiescent, follow-up every 4 months is satisfactory.

Disc new vessels are reduced at least 50% in magnitude in 85% of eyes treated with panretinal photocoagulation, and eliminated in 57% of eyes treated with concurrent photocoagulation of disc vessels and panretinal photocoagulation. A comparison of 16 treated eyes with 16 untreated control eyes indicates that treated eyes fared better ophthalmoscopically but not statistically better visually at a follow-up period of from 1 to 2 years. A comparison of the visual results in 24 eyes in this study was made with 27 eyes in the Patz-Berkow study. At the end of 36 months a significantly greater percentage retained vision of 20/80 or better in the greated series as compared with the untreated group.

A controlled randomized study evaluating the effect of photocoagulation on proliferative diabetic retinopathy, essential to making final conclusions, is in progress. A preliminary report[8] indicates that photocoagulation therapy is definitely beneficial for "extensive neovascularization" on or near the optic disc and also appears to be beneficial for two other groups of eyes when vitreous hemorrhage is present: those with "early new vessels" on or near the optic disc and those with "extensive new vessels" away from the optic disc. Our experience with argon laser photocoagulation strongly indicates that this modality is effective in reducing or eliminating retinal neovascularization when employed with the techniques described in this chapter. *Aggressive treatment* as described and *close follow-up and re-treatment* are essential to obtaining good results.

In the future, therapy for diabetic retinopathy will be directed toward preventing the development of microangiopathy. Therapy will probably be in the form of medication that alters red cell and platelet aggregation, hormones that inhibit growth hormone, and automatic feedback mechanisms that regulate insulin and blood sugar levels. Until these more sophisticated and definitive approaches are available, properly applied photocoagulation seems to be the safest and most effective therapy available for diabetic retinopathy.

REFERENCES

1. Aiello, L.: Personal communication, 1975.
2. Aiello, L., Beetham, W., Marios, C. B., Chazan, B. I., and Bradley, R. F.: Ruby laser photocoagulation in treatment of diabetic proliferative retinopathy: preliminary report. In Goldberg, M., and Fine, S., editors: Symposium on treatment of diabetic retinopathy, U.S. Department of Health, Education and Welfare, publication no. 1890, 1968, pp. 437-463.
3. Baulton, P. E.: A study of the mechanism of transient myopia following extensive xenon arc photocoagulation, Trans Ophthalmol. Soc. U.K. **93:**287, 1973.
4. Beetham, W. P.: Visual prognosis in proliferating diabetic retinopathy, Br. J. Ophthalmol. **47:**611, 1963.

5. Caird, F. I.: Diabetic retinopathy as a cause of visual impairment. In Goldberg, M., and Fine, S., editors: Symposium on treatment of diabetic retinopathy, U.S. Department of Health, Education and Welfare, publication no. 1890, 1968, pp. 41-45.

6. Davis, M. D., Fine, S. L., Goldberg, M. F., McMeel, J. W., Norton, E. W. D., Okun, E., and Wetzig, P.: A note on the O'Hare Classification of diabetic retinopathy. In Goldberg, M., and Fine, S., editors: Symposium on treatment of diabetic retinopathy, U.S. Department of Health, Education and Welfare, publication no. 1890, 1968, pp. 21-24.

7. Deckert, T., Simonsen, S. U. E., and Poulsen, J. E.: Prognosis of proliferative retinopathy in juvenile diabetics, Diabetes **16:**728, 1967.

8. Diabetic Retinopathy Study Research Group: Preliminary report on effects of photocoagulation therapy, Am. J. Ophthalmol. **81:**383, 1976.

9. Frank, R. N.: Visual fields and electroretinography following extensive photocoagulation, Arch. Ophthalmol. **92:**591, 1975.

10. Goldberg, M., and Herbst, R.: Acute complications of argon laser photocoagulation, Arch. Ophthalmol. **89:**311, 1973.

11. Irvine, A., and Norton, E.: Photocoagulation for diabetic retinopathy, Am. J. Ophthalmol. **71:**437, 1971.

12. Little, H. L.: Complications of argon laser retinal photocoagulation: a five year study. In Zweng, H. C., editor: International Ophthalmology Clinics: Recent advances in photocoagulation, Boston, 1976, Little, Brown and Co.

13. Little, H. L.: Argon laser therapy of diabetic retinopathy. In Francois, J., editor: Symposium on light coagulation, Doc. Ophthalmol. Proc. Ser. **1:**77-84, 1972.

14. Little, H. L.: Preventing complications in argon laser retinal photocoagulation. In Francois, J., editor: Symposium on light coagulation, Doc. Ophthalmol. Proc. Ser. **1:**87-95, 1972.

15. Little, H. L., and Zweng, H. C.: Complications of argon laser photocagulation, Trans. Pac. Coast Otoophthalmol. Soc. **53:**115, 1971.

16. Little, H. L., and Zweng, H. C.: Photocoagulation au laser a l'argon dans les affections maculaires et les retinopathies diabetiques, Arch. Ophtalmol. (Paris) **32:**789, 1972.

17. Little, H. L., and Zweng, H. C.: Argon laser photocoagulation of disc neovascularization in diabetic retinopathy, Trans Pac. Coast Otoophthalmol. Soc. **54:**123, 1973.

18. Little, H. L., Zweng, H. C., Jack, R. L., and Vassiliadis, A.: Techniques of argon laser photocoagulation in the treatment of diabetic disc new vessels, Am. J. Ophthalmol. **82:**675-683, 1976.

19. Little, H. L., Zweng, H. C., and Peabody, R. R.: Argon laser slit lamp retinal photocoagulation, Trans Am. Acad. Ophthalmol. Otolaryngol. **74:**85, 1970.

20. Marcus, D. F., and Aaberg, T. M.: Argon laser photocoagulation treatment of diabetic cystoid maculopathy, Am. ˙J. Ophthalmol. (In press.)

21. Merin, S., Yanko, L., and Ivry, M.: Treatment of diabetic maculopathy by argon laser, Br. J. Ophthalmol. **58:**85, 1974.

22. Meyer-Schwickerath, G.: Light Coagulation, St. Louis, 1969, The C. V. Mosby Co.

23. McDonald, G. W.: Diabetic source book, U.S. Public Health Service, publication no. 1168, 1964, p. 34.

24. Newell, F. W.: The problem of diabetic retinopathy in vascular complications of diabetes mellitus. In Kimura, S., and Caygill, W. M., editors: St. Louis, 1967, The C. V. Mosby Co., p. 36.

25. Okun, E., and Johnston, G. P.: Role of photocoagulation in the treatment of proliferative diabetic retinopathy: continuation and followup studies (359 eyes of 283 patients). In Goldberg, M., and Fine, S., editors: Symposium on treatment of diabetic retinopathy, U.S. Department of Health, Education and Welfare, publication no. 1890, 1968, pp. 437-463.

26. Patz, A.: Diabetic blindness, American Association of Workers for the Blind, 1969.

27. Patz, A.: A guide to argon laser photocoagulation, Surv. Ophthalmol. **16:**249, 1972.

28. Patz, A.: In Proceedings of laser photocoagulation symposium, Albi, France, May 1974. (In press.)

29. Patz, A., and Berkow, J.: Visual prognosis in advanced diabetic retinopathy. In Goldberg, M., and Fine, S., editors: Symposium on treatment of diabetic retinopathy, U.S. Department of Health, Education and Welfare, publication no. 1890, 1968, pp. 87-91.

30. Patz, A., Schatz, H., Berkow, J. W., Gittelsohn, A. M., and Ticho, U.: Macular edema:

an overlooked complication of diabetic retinopathy, Trans. Am. Acad. Ophthalmol. Otolaryngol. **77:**34-42, 1973.

31. Peyman, G. A., Spitznas, M., and Straatsma, B. R.: Chorioretinal diffusion of peroxidase before and after photocoagulation, Invest. Ophthalmol. **10:**489, 1971.
32. Rubinstein, K., and Myska, V.: Pathogenesis and treatment of diabetic maculopathy, Br. J. Ophthalmol. **58:**76, 1974.
33. Sharkey, T. P.: Diabetes mellitus: present problems and new research. VII. Retinopathy, J. Am. Diet Assoc. **58:**528, 1971.
34. Taylor, E., and Dobree, J. H.: Proliferative diabetic retinopathy: site and size of initial lesions, Br. J. Ophthalmol. **54:**11, 1970.
35. Toussaint, D., Kuwabara, T., and Cogan, D. G.: Retinal vascular patterns. II. Human retinal vessels studied in three dimensions, Arch. Ophthalmol. **65:**575, 1961.
36. Wessing, A., and Meyer-Schwickerath, G.: Results of photocoagulation in diabetic retinopathy. In Goldberg, M., and Fine, S., editors: Symposium on treatment of diabetic retinopathy, U.S. Department of Health, Education and Welfare, publication no. 1890, 1968, pp. 569-592.
37. Wise, G. N.: Retinal neovascularization, Trans. Am. Ophthalmol. Soc. **54:**729, 1956.
38. Zweng, H. C., Little, H. L., and Hammond, A. H.: Complications of argon laser photocoagulation in diabetic retinopathy, Trans. Am. Acad. Ophthalmol. **78:**195, 1974.
39. Zweng, H. C., Little, H. L., and Peabody, R. R.: Further observations on argon laser photocoagulation of diabetic retinopathy, Trans. Am. Acad. Ophthalmol. Otolaryngol. **76:**990, 1972.

15
RETINAL NEOVASCULARIZATION

Retinal neovascularization refers to the growth of new vessels arising from the retinal or ciliary vessels, occurring either on the optic disc or on the retina. The proliferation of these newly formed vessels frequently extends into the vitreous cavity, and intraocular hemorrhages resulting in blindness may occur.

Michaelson's[53,54] work on the development of retinal vessels in fetuses helps one to understand the pathogenesis of retinal neovascularization in disease states. His studies were made on retinas of human and cat fetuses; 50% India ink had previously been injected into the heart, the carotid artery, or the ophthalmic artery of each fetus. He concluded that (1) vessels grow in the retina by the process of budding from the parent vessels at the disc, (2) formation of capillaries is preeminently a function of the retinal vein, and (3) there exists a growth factor that affects growth of retinal blood vessels.

These conclusions were based on the following observations:
1. No retinal vessels were seen before the hyaloid vessels were present.
2. The earliest retinal vessels were seen proceeding from the edge of the disc, adjacent to the hyaloid artery, and passing from the disc into the retina, with subsequent progression to the periphery.
3. Capillary growth occurs predominantly from the veins and in many places from the side of the vein distal to the neighboring artery.
4. Proliferation ceases around arteries; that is, there is a capillary-free zone around arteries.
5. There is absense of capillary proliferation at arterial venous junctions.

These observations strongly suggest the presence of an extravascular intraretinal substance, associated with hypoxia of the retinal tissue, that stimulates new vessel formation. This substance is either inhibited or absent in areas adjacent to arteries. Furthermore, there is a capillary-free zone at the fovea and in the outer retinal layers, which are adjacent to the choroidal blood supply.

In summary, the early embryologic retina is satisfactorily nourished by dif-

218

fusion from the choroidal circulation and from the primary vitreous; however, as the primary vitreous regresses and the retina thickens, the innermost layer of the retina becomes relatively anoxic. At this point, budding from the parent retinal vessel to the disc is stimulated. The gradient of anoxia stimulates orderly development of the retinal vessels. Because of the greater concentration of the stimulating factor about the veins, capillary proliferation occurs only from the veins. Other investigators have presented evidence of the association of new formation of retinal vessels with retinal hypoxia.[1-4,59,60,77,78]

The demonstration of a factor capable of affecting the budding of new vessels in the developing retina and the demonstration of the close association between retinal veins and the capillary system are significant in the appreciation of certain diseases of the retina. Whenever it is possible to trace a connection between newly formed vessels (retinal, disc, preretinal, or intravitreous) and associated larger retinal vessels, the larger retinal vessel is almost always a vein. These findings strongly suggest that the capacity of the retinal vessels to form new vessels persists throughout life.

PATHOLOGIC PHYSIOLOGY OF RETINAL NEOVASCULARIZATION

Two prerequisites seem essential to retinal neovascularization: the presence of retinal hypoxia and viable retinal capillary endothelium.[44] Neovascularization does not occur after central retinal artery occlusion, when the retina is totally anoxic, or after central retinal vein occlusion, presumably because of loss of viable retinal capillary endothelium. Proliferation of new vessels frequently occurs at the margin of ischemic areas, bordered by viable capillaries; however, it can occur at areas removed from the vascular insult, such as on the optic disc or on the iris (as in rubeosis iridis).

Two mechanisms by which retinal hypoxia occurs are changes within blood, causing abnormal blood flow (hemorrheodynamics) and changes of the blood vessels, producing obstruction with impaired flow.[44,45] We have observed retinal neovascularization in the following conditions, listed according to mechanism by which hypoxia is most likely produced:[44]

Changes in blood elements
Diabetes mellitus
Eales's retinal vasculopathy
Sickle cell diseases (SS and SC)
Thalassemia
Leukemia (chronic myelocytic)
Polycythemia
Dysproteinemia (macroglobulinemia)
Sarcoidosis
Inflammatory diseases (pars planitis and Still's disease)

Changes in blood vessels

Branch retinal vein obstruction

Hypertension (associated with branch vein occlusion)

Ocular hypoxia syndrome (carotid insufficiency, aortic arch disease, carotid-cavernous fistula)

Radiation retinopathy

Retrolental fibroplasia

Coats' disease

Preretinal scar formation (intraocular foreign body)

In addition to these conditions, Wise[77] also included malaria as a cause of retinal neovascularization.

Inasmuch as moderate aggregation of erythrocytes is a physiologic phenomenon under conditions of reduced strain rates (velocity), and because the rate of retinal capillary perfusion is reduced with either arterial or venous obstruction,

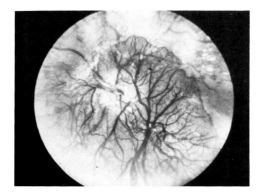

Fig. 15-1. Proliferative diabetic retinopathy with neovascularization extending off optic disc.

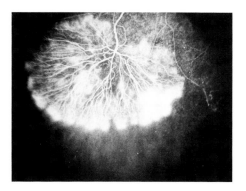

Fig. 15-2. Fluorescein angiogram of neovascular frond in midperipheral retina in patient with Eales's disease. Note noncapillary perfusion distal to frond.

one would anticipate increased aggregation of erythrocytes in the listed conditions that reduce blood flow. If blood flow is retarded or if the pressure gradient across the microcirculation is reduced (by decreased arterial pressure, elevated venous pressure, or increased resistance at the terminal arterioles) rates of shear in the capillaries and postcapillary venules fall. This causes increased aggregation of red cells in the presence of normal blood constituents. This phenomenon occurs in retinal artery and retinal vein occlusions, carotid insufficiency, Takayasu's disease, and carotid-cavernous fistula. In the presence of aggregation, the efficiency with which individual red cells transmit oxygen to the metabolically highly active retina is impaired. Thus, altered hemorrheodynamics causing hypoxia can result from changes in blood or from changes in blood vessels that reduce rate of flow. Sludged flow leads to retinal hypoxia, with subsequent development of microaneurysms and retinal neovascularization.

The above-listed conditions have one underlying common denominator: the reduction of oxygen concentration within the retina. This seems to be the underlying cause of all retinal neovascularization.

There are similarities in all cases of retinal neovascularization. In each there is usually an avascular or reduced vascular zone surrounding the neovascularization; the avascular zone with associated retinal hypoxia stimulates neovascularization.

The location of neovascularization may vary. Proliferative diabetic retinopathy most frequently occurs off the optic disc (Fig. 15-1) or the major arcade of vessels.[71] In hemoglobin SS and SC retinopathy and in Eales's retinal vasculopathy, the neovascularization is usually in the middle or far peripheral retina (Fig. 15-2). Differences in hemorrheodynamics may account for the central or peripheral location of neovascularization. In accordance with Kloti's experimental embolic occlusions, small aggregations of erythrocytes and nonflexible red cells would be expected to occlude the peripheral retinal and paramacular arterioles; large aggregates would be expected to interfere posteriorly nearer to the sources of the blood supply to the retina.[39]

Fluorescein retinal angiography

Fluorescein retinal angiography is an important aid in detecting retinal neovascularization. Detection and photocoagulation of arterial feeders is useful in an attempt to prevent hemorrhage of neovascular tufts.[46,49,50]

Eyes with retinal neovascularization should be studied with indirect and direct ophthalmoscopy and with the Goldmann contact lens, using the slit-lamp biomicroscope. A fundus drawing is customarily made, using the indirect ophthalmoscope to obtain the broad fundus details. The direct ophthalmoscope and contact lens are then used for high-magnification studies to delineate fine detail. With intravenous fluorescein angiography, coupled with indirect ophthalmoscopy using a Kodak Wratten 47A filter attached to the indirect ophthalmoscope, the entire retina can be scanned to search for small retinal neovascular tufts that might otherwise be overlooked. Fluorescein angioscopy provides an excellent means of localizing the less obvious neovascular tufts, as well as a superb means by which to followup on patients once they have been treated, in search of newly developed neovascular tufts on subsequent examinations.

Recent experiences with argon laser photocoagulation in the treatment of neovascular fronds have shown that better results can be obtained if the surrounding zone of retinal nonperfusion and the arterial feeder leading to the neovascular tuft are treated before coagulating the entire frond. Such arterial feeders are best localized by directing the fundus camera toward the site of the tuft under question and by taking rapid-sequence photographs, beginning 8 sec after injection of the fluorescein into the antecubital vein. The photographs are then enlarged by projection of the negative of the angiogram for high-magnification viewing. With this technique, the small arterial feeders to the large neovascular tuft can be identified. Without this technique, the arterial feeders are easily overlooked, because of their small size and their sometimes lateral location to the tuft.

DISEASE ENTITIES ASSOCIATED WITH RETINAL NEOVASCULARIZATION
Changes in blood elements

Diabetes mellitus
Pathogenesis diabetic retinopathy. Evidence indicates that diabetic retinopathy occurs as a result of impaired oxygen transfer to the retina. This tissue is most susceptible to hypoxia, because of its unique vascular anatomy and its high metabolic activity. Altered hemorrheodynamics in the microcirculation seem to play a major role in the production of focal ischemia and retinal hypoxia.[45,47,48] Abnormal red cell aggregation is observed in diabetics with proliferative retinopathy.[45] The increased resistence to flow, caused by the clumped red cells, may impair oxygen transfer. Increased red cell aggregation in diabetics is associated with changes in plasma proteins, including elevation of fibrinogen and alpha-2 globulins and reduction of albumin.[45] Increased levels of these large plasma proteins probably bind red cells into aggregates that cause sludging in the microcirculation and increased resistance to flow.[20] In the presence of endothelial damage, platelet adhesion and platelet release of adenosine diphosphate (ADP) might occur, increasing the red cell aggregate resistance to shear.[43] Focal occlusions of the distal arterioles then occur. In areas of ischemia, there is endothelial and pericyte loss, but endothelial hyperplasia occurs in zones of hypoxia. In hypoxic zones at the margins of focal ischemia, microaneurysms and retinal neovascularization develop in association with micro- and macrovascular shunts. Protein and lipid exudates from leakage of plasma and hemorrhage occur as a result of impaired capillary permeability.

Diabetic retinopathy can possibly be prevented by rigid control of blood sugar levels, which results in decreased production of growth hormone secretion, accompanied by reduced protein synthesis, with amelioration of red cell aggregation and improved hemorrheodynamics in the microcirculation.[29,31,45]

Diabetic retinopathy. Retinal neovascularization may be classified into two groups: rete mirabile, or the proliferation of newly formed capillaries on the retinal surface, and retinitis proliferans, which is the proliferation of newly formed retinal vessels and their supporting tissue into the vitreous cavity. Both can occur in the absence of previous vitreous hemorrhage. Because massive vitreous hemorrhage sometimes occurs and clears without development of retinitis proliferans, the old theory that retinitis proliferans results from previous vitreous hemorrhage is not tenable. The prolonged retinal circulation time in diabetics with retinopathy probably is caused by increased red cell aggregation, with sludging and generalized venous stasis. Retinal hypoxia and foci of retinal ischemia occur with subsequent retinal neovascularization. Possibly the increased thickening of the capillary basement membrane in diabetics contributes to impaired diffusion and retinal hypoxia.[67] The attenuation of retinal arterioles is a common and striking finding in diabetic retinopathy. The prolonged retinal circulation time is influenced also by the increased resistance to arterial flow because of arteriolar attenuation. Possibly venous dilation is an early manifestation of reactive hyperemia, caused by relative obstruction of the postcapillary venules by increased red cell aggregation and altered blood rheology.

Microaneurysms are globular or saccular dilations of capillaries connecting the deep and superficial retinal capillary plexuses. They occur in the inner nuclear layer and range in size from 30 to 90 μm in diameter. Most frequently associated with diabetic retinopathy, they may also occur in retinal vein occlusion, pulseless disease, carotid insufficiency, macroglobulinemia, pernicious anemia, carcinoma with anemia, glaucoma, hypertension, arteriolar sclerosis, Eales's disease, and radiation retinopathy. Rarely they may occur in the peripheral retina in otherwise normal individuals.

There is controversy over the relationship of microaneurysms and retinal neovascularization. Wise[77] states that the globular and saccular buds are not aneurysms but are abortive attempts at neovascularization in response to a retinal tissue factor that is intimately associated with tissue hypoxia. Cogan and Kuwabara[10] and Ashton[2] disagree with this hypothesis; they believe that the occurrence of intraretinal neovascularization is extremely rare.

Cogan and Kuwabara[10] state that the initial pathologic condition is loss of mural cells (pericytes), with subsequent loss of tonicity of the capillary and dilation-produced microaneurysm. They suggest that increased blood flow to the microaneurysm shunts blood from adjacent capillaries, with subsequent obliteration of the surrounding capillaries. This shunt hypothesis is probably incorrect, because blood flow through the microshunts and microaneurysms (as measured by Kohner[42]) is usually sluggish. Ashton,[2] on the other hand, believes that the primary pathologic condition is occlusion of the capillaries associated with endothelial proliferation, and subsequent development of shunt vessels and microaneurysms to provide collateral circulation.

Diabetic retinopathy ranks among the four leading causes of acquired severe visual impairment in the United States.[58] Because of the significant role of diabetic retinopathy in the production of blindness, we have treated patients with diabetic retinopathy with photocoagulation, particularly with the argon laser. Again it is emphasized that the initial treatment of proliferative retinopathy consists of coagulating the midperipheral extensive zones of capillary nonperfusion by means of panretinal photocoagulation. Subsequent feeder-frond photocoagulation technique is directed to residual neovascular areas. (For examples and techniques of treatment of proliferative diabetic retinopathy, see Figs. 15-1 and 15-3 and Chapter 14.)

Eales's disease. Eales' disease (first described by Henry Eales in 1880) is a clinical entity characterized by retinal perivenous sheathing associated with neovascularization and vitreous hemorrhages.[17] The bilateral condition usually begins in the third decade of life and predominates in males. Perivasculitis and venous stasis is followed by retinal neovascularization in the involved venules. It usually occurs in the peripheral retina (Fig. 15-2), even though phlebitis and neovascularization rarely develop on the optic disc.

Lyle and Wybar[52] have reported a condition that possibly represents a type of Eale's disease, in which there is an apparent vasculitis of the central retinal vein. The condition occurs in young adults and is similar to retinal vein thrombosis, with engorged vessels, papilledema, and retinal hemorrhage; however, it differs from vein occlusion in that there is absence of associated arteriolar disease and improvement with systemic steroids.

The etiology of Eales's disease is unknown. Elliott[19] postulated that the vasculopathy is caused by a hypersensitivity reaction related to the tuberculin antigen and recommended treatment with steroids. Possibly it is a disease that involves an abnormal constituent in plasma proteins, which would account for the altered blood rheology with secondary retinal neovascularization, as occurs in macroglobulinemia and probably in diabetes.[45]

We have successfully treated 12 eyes in eight patients with Eales's disease with argon laser photocoagulation. Lesions with a broad beam of 500 or 1,000 μm are made in the nonperfused zone surrounding the frond; a 50-μm beam is directed to the arterial feeder vessels, and the 100- and 200-μm beams are used to treat the neovascular fronds. The vascular fronds have been obliterated and recurrent hemorrhages have stopped in all eyes treated.

Sickle cell disease. Sickle cell anemia was first described by James Herrick[35] in 1910. Sickle cell disease is a general term used to describe conditions characterized by the presence of hemoglobin S, including sickle cell trait without anemia, sickle cell anemia, and sickle cell hemoglobin in combination with other abnormal types of hemoglobin, such as hemoglobin C. It is a hereditary disease peculiar to blacks and their descendants. Various surveys of American blacks indicate the following incidence of abnormal hemoglobin: 8%, sickle cell trait; 0.4%, sickle cell anemia; and 0.1% to 0.2%, sickle cell hemoglobin C disease.[57]

Hemoglobin S is chemically and immunologically different from normal adult hemoglobin A, as noted on hemoglobin electrophoresis. In the oxygenated state, hemoglobin S has approximately the same solubility as hemoglobin A. In the deoxygenated state, the solubility of hemoglobin S is significantly less than hemoglobin A, forming elongated crystallike structures that cause distortion of the erythrocytes, producing the characteristic sickled appearance of the cell. These rigid sickled erythrocytes cannot change shape to easily pass through capillaries and venules; thus stasis, thrombosis, and hemorrhage result. In some instances, subsequent retinal neovascularization occurs, with its sequelae of hemorrhage and traction retinal detachment.

Funduscopic changes in sickle cell anemia were first described by Cook[11] in 1930. The classic picture of sickle cell C retinopathy has been described by Hannon[30] and by others,[28,56] and more recently by Goldberg and others.[23-27,70,74] Welch and Goldberg[74] have described the following fundus findings in hemoglobin SS, SC, and AS diseases. The prototype appearance of the fundi in SS disease includes tortuosity of veins, peripheral black disc-shaped scars, designated by them as "black sunburst sign," obliterated peripheral vessels associated with dilated arteriolar segments, through which fluorescein fails to flow, and rarely retinitis proliferans. The salmon patch, seen ophthalmoscopically in sickle cell disease, is an intraretinal hematoma; furthermore, the black sunburst, noted ophthalmoscopically, probably results from dissection of intraretinal hemorrhage into the subretinal space, with subsequent hyperplasia of the retinal pigment epithelium.[62] The prototype for SC disease includes the formation of arteriovenous fans projecting into the vitreous, which Welch and Goldberg designate as the "sea fan sign," the obliteration of peripheral venules and arterioles, and in some cases the presence of the black sunburst sign.[74] In regard to the significance of retinal hypoxia in the stimulation due to vascularization, the retina surrounding the sea fan vascular tufts is nonperfused on fluorescein angiography. Patients with hemoglobin AS (sickle cell trait) generally have normal fundi, with the rare exception of the black sunburst sign, retinal artery occlusion, and possibly retinal vein thromboses.

In hemoglobin SS and SC diseases, the peripheral neovascularization probably results from small distal arteriole and capillary occlusions; because sickling is increased by hypoxia, the less vascular peripheral retina is more vulnerable. Blood of patients with SC disease enters the central retinal artery without difficulty, and probably no significant abnormal rheologic problem occurs until the rigid sickle cells reach the terminal arterioles in the peripheral retina and in the macula. The SC and SS cells are rigid, making them likely to obstruct end arterioles and capillaries, even in the absence of reduced oxygen.[40] Goldstone et al.[27]

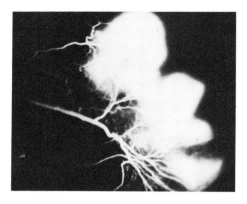

Fig. 15-3. Fluorescein angiogram of equatorial neovascular frond in patient with hemoglobin C disease.

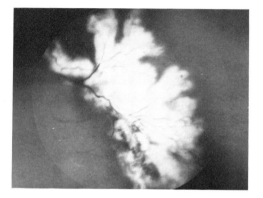

Fig. 15-4. Appearance of frond (Fig. 15-3) immediately after argon laser photocoagulation. Lesions should be applied to distal portion of frond and to surrounding zone of poor capillary perfusion.

also documented total inability of sickle cell blood to pass through a millipore filter with 5- and 8-μm pores.

Because of the recurrent vitreous hemorrhages associated with neovascular areas, commonly in SC and rarely in SS disease, argon laser photocoagulation is indicated in the management of these diseases. Photocoagulation is carried out in an attempt to obliterate the neovascular tufts, to prevent recurrent vitreous hemorrhages. We have treated five eyes in three patients with SC disease. In all instances the tufts were successfully obliterated by treating the arterial feeders and subsequently treating the entire neovascular tuft (Figs. 15-3 to 15-5). In addition, the surrounding zones of capillary nonperfusion were treated with larger spot sizes.[44,51]

Thalassemia. Thalassemia is an inherited disorder in which there is a defect

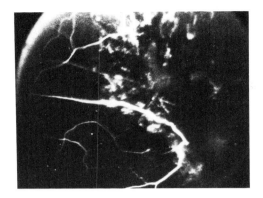

Fig. 15-5. Fluorescein angiogram of frond (Fig. 15-3), showing obliteration of newly formed vessels, noted 3 months and 3 years after argon laser photocoagulation.

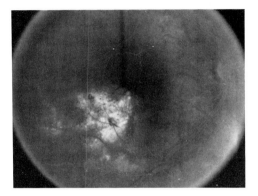

Fig. 15-6. Microaneurysms with leakage of fluorescein on angiography, and early cystoid macular edema in man with thalassemia minor.

in the rate of hemoglobin synthesis.[32] It occurs in individuals living in countries bordering the Mediterranean or in their descendants. Thalassemia major (Cooley's anemia), which is the homozygote form of the disease, causes death in the first decade of life. The heterozygous form, thalassemia minor, is compatible with normal development and life span. Retinal hemorrhage may rarely occur in thalassemai minor.[15] Thalassemia can also occur in combination with the sickle cell hemoglobinopathies.

We have seen two cases of thalassemia minor in which there were bilateral microaneurysms with surrounding circinate exudates. In both, the lesions were temporal to the macula and were associated with scattered hemorrhages and retinal edema (Fig. 15-6). Retinal neovascularization was not seen. Because of the macular edema, the leaking microaneurysms were treated with argon laser pho-

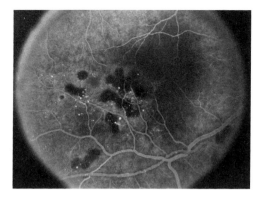

Fig. 15-7. Eye in Fig. 15-6 after argon laser photocoagulation. Note regression of leakage and persistence of a few scattered microaneurysms.

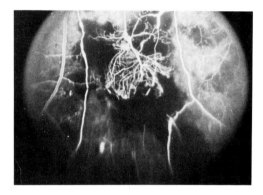

Fig. 15-8. Midperipheral neovascular frond in 44-year-old man with chronic myelocytic leukemia.

tocoagulation (Fig. 15-7). Focal coagulation technique was used, as described in the treatment of nonproliferative diabetic retinopathy (see Chapter 14).

Leukemia (chronic myelocytic). The presence of retinal neovascularization in association with leukemia is an extremely rare phenomenon. We saw a 42-year-old man whose initial complaint was impaired vision due to vitreous hemorrhages associated with retinal neovascularization. Medical workup showed that the patient had chronic myelocytic leukemia. He was treated with busulfan (Myleran), which arrested the leukemia, dropping the white blood cell count from 600,000 to 10,000/mm³ However, because of the recurrent vitreous hemorrhages in both eyes, associated with retinal neovascularization with prominent neovascular tufts extending from the retinal surface into the vitreous, the patient was considered for argon laser photocoagulation. Because of the severe preretinal hemorrhages obscuring most of the fundus view in the right eye, this eye could not be treated. In the left eye, fluorescein angiographic studies demonstrated a midperipheral neovascular frond (Fig. 15-8). The feeder vessel was obliterated, after which the entire neovascular tuft and the surrounding nonperfused retina were treated with the argon laser. No complications ensued in the 12-month follow-up after treatment.

Presumably the retinal neovascularization in this case is a result of impaired retinal circulation, due to the increased viscosity of the blood flow due to macroglobulins and to the high leukocyte count, resulting in retinal hypoxia and new formation of retinal vessels. Because the leukocyte count is reduced to normal and the circulation has improved, further development of retinal neovascularization is not anticipated, unless there is an increased dysproteinemia.

Two similar cases of retinal neovascularization in chronic myelocytic anemia have recently been reported.[22,55]

Polycythemia. In polycythemia, there is venous engorgement, peripheral retinal hemorrhages, and microaneurysm. We have seen scattered microaneurysms peripheral to the equator, but no definite neovascularization. In this condition, red cell aggregation is a function of a very high hematocrit level. Photocoagulation has not been indicated in the management of any of our cases of polycythemia.

Dysproteinemia. Macroglobulinemia and cryoglobulinemia are diseases of the reticuloendothelial system. Macroglobulinemia was first described by Waldenström[73] in 1944. The disease usually is seen in men over 50 years of age. It is characterized by the presence of inordinate amounts of abnormally high molecular weight globulins in the plasma. In contrast to normal gamma globulins, having a molecular weight of about 150,000, the molecular weight of globulins in macroglobulinemia is over 1,000,000.[69]

The initial complaints are malaise, fatigue, weight loss, bleeding tendencies, visual impairment, and central nervous system involvement, with aphasia and hemiparesis.[12,13] Lymphadenopathy, hepatosplenomegaly, and purpura occur. The fundus shows engorgement of the discs and retinal veins, sausagelike dilation of the retinal veins, with increased viscosity of the blood flow, punctate and flame-shaped retinal hemorrhages, cotton-wool exudates, retinal vein thromboses, and retinal neovascularization.[12,13,16] Microaneurysms have been demonstrated histologically with the use of trypsin digestion techniques.[6] Multiple myeloma and leukemia must sometimes be ruled out, because these diseases frequently are associated in patients with macroglobulinemia.

The sedimentation rate is increased, the albumin-globulin ratio is reversed, a biologically false-positive serology may be present, and there is anemia. A positive Sia test, manifested by the formation of a milky precipitate when several drops of the patient's serum are placed in distilled water, suggests the diagnosis.[66] In macroglobulinemia and cryoglobulinemia, marked stasis, noted with the slit-lamp, occurs in the conjunctival vessels when a tube of ice water is placed against them.[13] Plasma protein electrophoresis demonstrates the presence of abnormal proteins, but centrifugation is the specific test for the diagnosis of macroglobulinemia, based on determining the rate of settling of protein components measured in Svedberg units.

The natural course of the disease includes progressive pancytopenia, increasing hemorrhagic diathesis, and death from cerebrovascular accident. This course and the fundus picture can be reversed with plasmapheresis, penicillamine, and chlorambucil.[16] Penicillamine depolymerizes the macroglobulin molecules into smaller molecules, whereas chlorambucil directly affects the reticuloendothelial cells responsible for the production of the abnormal globulins. Because therapy is different from that for central retinal thromboses, the correct diagnosis is important. If there is underlying leukemia, Hodgkin's disease, or collagen disease, it is treated accordingly.

Sludged flow in the retinal circulation in macroglobulinemia is a well-recognized syndrome.[76] In a patient with macroglobulinemia, who exhibited venous engorgement and sludged flow, in vitro rheoscopic studies of the blood showed severe aggregation of red cells, even at high strain rates.

The use of argon laser photocoagulation is usually unnecessary in the management of macroglobulinemia, because there usually is only venous engorgement and retinal hemorrhages. Only rarely does one find the development of retinal neovascularization (Fig. 15-9) with recurrent vitreous hemorrhages which would necessitate argon laser photocoagulation. The use of fluorescein angiography is of help in detecting the areas of retinal neovascularization that need to be treated. We have not treated any patients with dysproteinemia with argon laser photocoagulation.

Sarcoidosis and other inflammatory diseases. Retinal neovascularization rarely occurs in association with retinal inflammatory diseases. The diagnosis of pars planitis is made if there are inflammatory cells in the vitreous and a "snow bank" of inflammatory cells over the inferior pars plana.[5,38,75] We have seen two cases of pars planitis in which there has been associated retinal periphlebitis. In

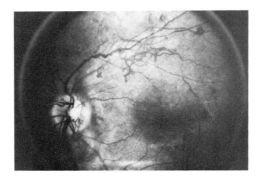

Fig. 15-9. Retinal neovascularization along superotemporal arcade in patient with macroglobulinemia.

one case the neovascularization was on the optic disc, and in the other it occurred in the peripheral retina.

Another unusual occurrence of retinal neovascularization was seen in a 12-year-old girl with Still's disease in which there was keratopathy, anterior iridocyclitis with posterior synechia, cataract formation, and inflammatory cells in the vitreous. The patient developed recurrent vitreous hemorrhages in the left eye, with resultant total loss of vision in that eye. There was a large area of retinal neovascularization extending off the right optic disc. Because of the recurrent vitreous hemorrhages in the right eye, argon laser photocoagulation was directed to the retinal neovascularization extending off the right optic nerve. Photocoagulation could not be done until the area of band keratopathy had been temporarily removed with edetate disodium (Sodium Versenate). Following argon laser photocoagulation to the areas of proliferative retinopathy extending off the right optic nerve head and to the surrounding midperiphery, the patient has had no subsequent vitreous hemorrhages.

A third inflammatory disease that has been associated with retinal neovascularization is sarcoidosis. A 42-year-old woman with sarcoidosis but no evidence of uveitis had two vitreous hemorrhages caused by retinal neovascularization superior and temporal to the right macula (Fig. 15-10). The neovascularization and the surrounding zone of poor capillary perfusion were treated with 500-μm diameter lesions. The neovascularization disappeared without recurrence after 1 year.

Retinal neovascularization occurring in patients with chronic ocular inflammatory disease (pars planitis and Still's disease) and with systemic inflammatory disease (sarcoidosis) can be explained on the basis of altered blood rheology. Fahraeus[20] observed that chronic inflammatory diseases were associated with clumping of red cells, attributed to increased numbers of the large molecular weight plasma proteins (fibrinogen and globulins). As in sarcoidosis, this can be associated with a reduced level of serum albumin.

The treatment of retinal neovascularization associated with inflammatory

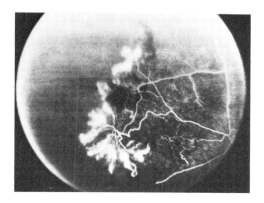

Fig. 15-10. Midperipheral retinal neovascularization in patient with Boeck's sarcoidosis.

diseases consists of attempting to reduce the inflammation with local or systemic steroids and to eradicate neovascularization by photocoagulating areas of new vessel formation and retinal capillary nonperfusion.

Changes in blood vessels

Retinal vein occlusion. Branch venous obstruction is a common cause of retinal neovascularization. In this condition, retinal oxygen tension is sufficiently reduced to reactivate the latent capacity for veins and capillaries to form new vessels, without lowering the oxygen tension to the point of producing retinal necrosis. On the contrary, central vein occlusion and arterial obstruction cause ischemia infarction and retinal necrosis, thus destroying capillary endothelial cells, which respond to the hypoxic stimulus, or destroying highly metabolic retinal cells, which produce the metabolic products that stimulate neovascularization. However, hypoxia without necrosis can occur with an attenuated arterial supply. This is seen in pulseless disease and in carotid insufficiency, with the subsequent development of new-formed vessels. Rarely, such a condition may also occur with arterial attenuation in hypertensive retinopathy.

After venous obstruction, neovascularization is stimulated by relative retinal hypoxia. Poor perfusion of retinal capillaries peripheral to the point of venous obstruction results in hypoxia of the metabolically active retina. Capillary dilation and microaneurysm formation occur at the proximal margins of the poorly perfused retina. Retinal neovascularization may occur in the area of the venous occlusion or on the optic disc.

Vascular proliferation into the vitreous is related to the integrity of the inner limiting membrane of the retina. Its absence over the disc explains the frequent occurrence of retinal neovascularization extending into the vitreous at the disc. With pathologic changes of the internal limiting membrane, vascular proliferation is no longer restricted, and vitreous involvement occurs in areas overlying the retina.

Proliferative retinopathy occurs in about 25% of eyes with a branch retinal vein thrombosis. Neovascularization may extend off the optic disc as well as off the occluded retinal vein. Because of recurrent vitreous hemorrhages in this condition, patients can be treated with argon laser photocoagulation, in an attempt to obliterate the neovascular tufts and to prevent subsequent hemorrhage. Segmental panretinal photocoagulation with the 500- and 1,000-μm spot sizes is directed to the retinal quadrant of the occluded vein. If involution of the neovascular frond has not occurred within 6 months, direct photocoagulation to the neovascular frond is performed, using the feeder-frond technique with the 50-μm spot. This approach in the management of retinal neovascularization following branch retinal vein occlusion has been successful in 90% of eyes treated. In 28 of 31 eyes with retinal neovascularization after branch retinal vein occlusion, we have successfully eradicated the new vessels with argon laser photocoagulation.

Hypertensive retinopathy. Retinal neovascularization is seldom observed in hypertensive retinopathy. When it does occur, it is usually caused by an occlusion of a branch of the central retinal vein. However, hypoxia without necrosis can occur with a slowly attenuated arterial supply in hypertensive retinopathy. We have not treated any cases of retinal neovascularization in hypertensive retinopathy in the absence of a branch retinal vein occlusion.

Ocular hypoxia syndrome. According to Shimizu and Sano,[65] pulseless disease was first reported by Takayasu in 1908 as a condition with progressive obstruction of the carotid or subclavian artery by panarteritis in young Japanese females. Amarosis fugax is the usual first complaint. Eye signs are peripheral arteriovenous anastomoses, rosarylike swelling of the veins, optic atrophy, cataract, ciliary injection, corneal edema, iris atrophy, uveitis, rubeosis iridis, glaucoma, retinal neovascularization, and vitreous hemorrhage.[18,34,41,68] A similar clinical picture of the ocular hypoxia syndrome has been reported in syphilitic aortitis; atherosclerosis of the aortic, subclavian, and bracheocephalic arteries; and carotid-cavernous fistula.[14,18,34] Myriad microaneurysms have been demonstrated in pathologic specimens obtained from patients with ocular hypoxia syndrome.[14,37,63]

Progressive arterial occlusion in this disorder reduces oxygen tension in the retina to a point where relative retinal hypoxia exists, thus stimulating retinal neovascularization. In contrast, in central retinal artery occlusion there is a sudden retinal anoxia, retinal cell death, and lack of development of retinal neovascularization.

We have seen one patient in whom the left eye was blind as a result of the ocular hypoxia syndrome. End stage disease in this eye included rubeosis iridis, cataract, and vitreous hemorrhage. The right eye had retinal neovascularization, severe arterial attenuation, optic atrophy, and vitreous hemorrhage. Because of the retinal neovascularization demonstrated on fluorescein angiography and funduscopic examination, and because of the history of recurrent vitreous hemorrhages, argon laser photocoagulation was directed to the areas of neovascularization in the fundus of the right eye. Multiple attempts at coagulation were not entirely successful, because of overlying blood and scar formation that prevented focusing the beam on the neovascular tufts. In spite of repeated applications of argon laser photocoagulation, the patient continued to have prognosive loss of vision, because of optic nerve and retinal ischemia.

Radiation retinopathy. Schlaegel[64] and Flick[21] have noted histopathologic changes in vessels of the inner retinal layers in atomic bomb casualties. In clinical practice, radiation retinopathy is seen in patients who have received ocular radiation for retinoblastoma or inadvertent ocular radiation in the treatment of carcinoma of the lid, sinuses, and nasopharynx. Howard[36] found no evidence of radiation retinopathy among retinoblastoma patients treated with 3,500 rads in divided doses; however, in cases requiring a second course of the same dose of radiation, 71% developed radiation retinopathy. A 3- to 18-month latent period elapsed before the vascular changes were evident.

The characteristic clinical findings of radiation retinopathy are sheathing and occlusion of the arterioles, microaneurysms, telangiectases, retinal neovascularization, retinal pigment epithelial atrophy, papilledema, retinal exudates and hemorrhages, and rarely vitreous hemorrhages;[7,9,36] in addition, cataracts and rubeosis iridis may be present. Fluorescein angiography assists in the visualization of the retinal microaneurysms, telangiectases, and neovascularization. Presumably, the retinal neovascularization is stimulated by the relative hypoxia produced by arteriolar narrowing.

We have treated two patients with radiation retinopathy in association with previous irradiation therapy for nasopharyngeal carcinoma and for carcinoma of the antrum. One was a 45-year-old Oriental woman, in whom microaneurysms and cystoid macular edema were noted 6 years after irradiation for a nasopharyngeal carcinoma (Fig. 15-11). Because of associated macular edema and retinal hemorrhages, argon laser photocoagulation was performed. Visual acuity dropped from 20/30 to 20/200; however, 8 months after photocoagulation, visual acuity was 20/30, and the macular edema, microaneurysms, and telangiectasia had resolved (Fig. 15-12). The second patient was a 50-year-old man with rete mirabile–type retinal neovascularization, who was successfully treated with argon laser photocoagulation 5 years after radiation therapy.

Retrolental fibroplasia. Terry[72] first described the condition of retrolental fibroplasia (RLF) in 1942. Clinical findings consist of bilateral ocular disease in premature infants, usually with a history of oxygen therapy. RLF has four stages: the prodomal stage, with arterial atresia and venous engorgement; a proliferative stage, with peripheral retinal neovascularization occurring 4 to 8 weeks after the infant is removed from the incubator; a regressive stage documented by no signs of progression over a 2-week interval; and a cicatricial stage manifested by total retinal detachment, with white vascular retrolental mass.

Infrequently in the practice of ophthalmology, a syndrome of arrested retrolental fibroplasia is seen. Such cases show temporal traction of the retinal vessels, noted in the posterior pole as the vessels leave the optic disc, lattice degeneration in the peripheral retina, abnormal vitreous haze, and vitreal retinal adhesions. Patients are prone to retinal detachments; therefore, they should be followed up with repeat dilated fundus examinations over their lifetimes.

Patz[60] in 1952 showed that the earliest clinical evidence of retrolental fibroplasia in premature infants given oxygen therapy is arterial spasm. He subjected newborn kittens and puppies to 70% oxygen, which produces 100% arterial oxygen tension. The kittens were exposed to these oxygen levels for prolonged times and were noted to develop endothelial nodules of retrolental fibroplasia in the retinas and budding of the capillaries into the vitreous. These findings were associated with marked arterial or vasospasm. Ashton and collaborators[4] found the vasospasm inversely proportional to the time and to the concentration of oxygen. Less than 35% concentration of oxygen had little effect on the newborn kittens. These workers noted that the vasoproliferation does not occur during the

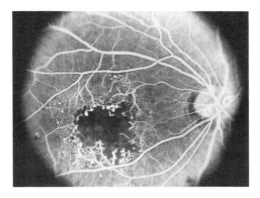

Fig. 15-11. Capillary nonperfusion of macula, with cystoid edema and surrounding microaneurysm and capillary dilation 8 years postirradiation for nasopharyngeal carcinoma.

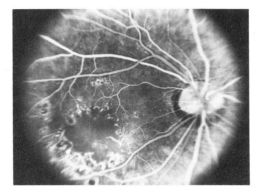

Fig. 15-12. Post–argon laser photocoagulation of leaking microaneurysm in irradiation retinopathy.

hyperoxic stage, but after removing the animals from the hyperoxic environment.

The features of the vasoproliferative phase of RLF suggest a vasoformative factor elaborated by hypoxic retina. The stimulus is probably identical to the normal stimulus for embryologic retinal vascularization and for pathologic neovascularization, resulting in vein occlusions, diabetes, and Eales's disease.

Hyperoxia of an infant in an incubator initially produces an arterial obliteration, leading to RLF. After obliteration of the retinal arterioles, the retina recieves its oxygen from the hyperoxygenated choroidal blood supply while the infant is still under high concentrations of oxygen. Once removed from this environment, a state of retinal hypoxia exists, because the choroidal oxygen tension is reduced and the peripheral retinal arterioles are obliterated. Thus, the setting for retinal neovascularization is present.

We recommend that patients suspected of having retrolental fibroplasia be observed with serial examinations on a weekly basis beginning 4 weeks after removal from the incubator. If proliferative retinopathy is noted, the patient should be observed biweekly. If retinal neovascularization increases, argon laser photocoagulation to the areas of proliferative retinopathy is indicated. Payne and Patz[61] reported success in treating cases of retrolental fibroplasia with nonregressive proliferative retinopathy with the argon laser. Photocoagulation is rarely indicated, because the vessels usually undergo spontaneous involution; hence, close observation is mandatory. The best treatment of retrolental fibroplasia is prevention.

Coats' disease. This disease has been recognized since Coats[8] published his classic paper in 1908; yet the etiology of this syndrome is unknown. Coats' disease consists of yellowish exudation in the external retinal layers and beneath the sensory retina, associated with fusiform irregular dilations of the retinal vessels, retinal neovascularization, and retinal hemorrhages. In some instances, small to massive exudative retinal detachments are present. If the diagnosis can be made before massive exudative retinal detachment occurs, photocoagulation can cure the disease. Xenon arc photocoagulation and in some instances penetrating diathermy have been used in the management of this disease. More recently, argon laser photocoagulation has been introduced in the treatment of this disease entity. We have treated 12 cases of Coats' disease with argon laser photocoagulation. The areas of retinal neovascularization in the peripheral retina and the adjacent areas of poorly perfused retina were identified with angiography (Fig. 15-13). These areas were totally obliterated with photocoagulation, resulting in subsequent scar formation and loss of the abnormal fluorescence in 11 of the 12 eyes. The surrounding retinal exudates and the edema have subsided. One interesting observation in one of the cases was the accumulation of lipid material in the macula in the weeks following photocoagulation of the abnormal peripheral vessels. This subsequently resolved over a 6-month follow-up, without further sequelae.

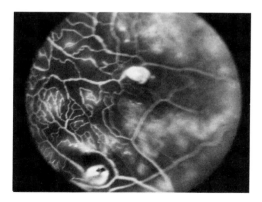

Fig. 15-13. Retinal macroaneurysm, telangiectasia, neovascularization, and capillary nonperfusion in Coats' disease.

In one case, the eye was photocoagulated with xenon arc photocoagulation, with the child under general anesthesia and in the supine position. Four years following treatment, there was recurrent retinal telangiectasia and neovascularization, associated with rubeosis iridis, vitreous hemorrhage, and cataract. There was marked involution of rubeosis and regression of retinal neovascularization 8 weeks after applying partial-penetrating diathermy 360°, combined with an encircling silicone band placed to alleviate vitreoretinal traction.

In the treatment of Coats' angiomatosis retinae, both argon laser and xenon arc photocoagulating systems give excellent results. Successful results are largely dependent on (1) early diagnosis, (2) extensive photocoagulation of abnormal vessels and areas of capillary nonperfusion, using medium to large spot sizes (500 to 1,000 μm), moderately intense lesions, and (3) early and prolonged followup. If extensive areas of retina are to be treated, photocoagulation should be done in different sessions, in order to avoid exudative retinal detachment and angle-closure glaucoma (see Chapter 19).

Preretinal scar formation. Another condition in which retinal neovascularization with vitreous hemorrhage may develop is scar formation following a penetrating intraocular injury. This was observed in a 21-year-old man, following removal of a nonmagnetic intraocular foreign body. The foreign body was removed successfully, and visual acuity of 20/30 was preserved. However, because of extensive preretinal scar formation extending into the vitreous in the interior fundus, in which there was proliferation of newly formed vessels, the patient was referred for argon laser photocoagulation. The vessels were well visualized with funduscopic and slit-lamp examination and were better outlined with fluorescein angiography (Fig. 15-14). The vessels were treated on three separate occasions, using argon laser photocoagulation, without hemorrhage or complications. The vessels were obliterated, and the vitreous hemorrhaging ceased (Fig. 15-15).

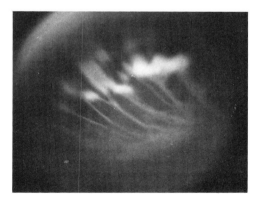

Fig. 15-14. Extreme peripheral retinal neovascularization extending into vitreous cavity 6 months following intraocular foreign body injury.

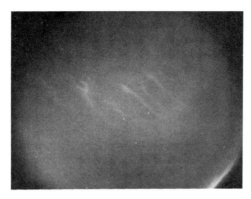

Fig. 15-15. Regression of neovascular frond (Fig. 15-14) following argon laser photocoagulation.

Twelve months after the last treatment, the patient showed no further retinal neovascularization or recurrent hemorrhages.

Discussion

Michaelson's[53,54] observations on the development of retinal vasculature in infants, Ashton's[1,3] and Patz's[59,60] experimental work on animals and retinal tissue culture, using hyper- and hypoxic environments, and Wise's[76,77] clinical studies of cases of retinal neovasculariation all indicate the close relationship of retinal neovascularization to retinal hypoxia. Our studies and their results on photocoagulation applied to anoxic retina peripheral to new vessels support the above data indicating the role of retinal hypoxia in the development of retinal neovascularization.

TREATMENT
General approach

Treatment consists of altering the underlying cause of retinal hypoxia responsible for stimulating retinal neovascularization. When possible, this includes controlling the underlying medical condition responsible for the changes in blood content or in blood vessels that produce retinal ischemia and hypoxia. Such therapeutic approach will prevent recurrence of neovascularization. Furthermore, drugs that reduce levels of plasma and serum macroglobulins and red cell aggregation, such as prednisone, low molecular weight dextran, and fibrinolysin, may play a larger therapeutic role in the future.

Photocoagulation

Once retinal neovascularization is present, photocoagulation provides the best current method to eliminate it, regardless of the underlying cause. Experiences with argon laser photocoagulation in the treatment of neovascular fronds have shown that best results can be obtained if the surrounding zone of retinal capillary nonperfusion and the arterial feeder leading to the neovascular tuft are treated before coagulating the entire frond.[50] Fluorescein angiography is used to identify the nonperfused zones and the areas of neovascularization. The arterial feeders are localized by directing the fundus camera toward the site of the tuft under question and by taking rapid-sequence photographs, beginning 8 to 10 sec after injection of the fluorescein into the antecubital vein. The photographs are then enlarged by projection of the negative of the angiogram for high-magnification viewing. With this technique, the small arterial feeders to the large neovascular tuft can be identified. Without this technique, the arterial feeders are easily overlooked, because of their small size and their sometimes lateral location to the tuft.

When the entire tuft is treated without first treating the arterial vessels, venous engorgement of the tufts and hemorrhage may occur, due to closure of efferent vessels. With the technique of obliterating the arterial feeder first, the tuft becomes less plethoric. At this point, the entire tuft can be coagulated, with less risk of hemorrhage or engorgement of the frond (Fig. 15-16). The incidence of hemorrhage and the number of required treatments per patient have geen significantly reduced by this procedure. In eyes with extensive midperipheral and peripheral zones of capillary nonperfusion, panretinal photocoagulation is made 360°, extending from the posterior pole to beyond the equator, in an attempt to prevent the development of other areas of retinitis proliferans.[50] Frequently, neovascular fronds will undergo involution following treatment of their surrounding zones of capillary nonperfusion in the absence of direct treatment to the frond (Figs. 15-17 and 15-18). Furthermore, when the nonperfused zones are not photocoagulated, recurrent neovascularization is a frequent occurrence (Fig. 15-19).

The effect of photocoagulation on retinal neovascularization is made directly by coagulative necrosis of the treated vessels and indirectly by eliminating the

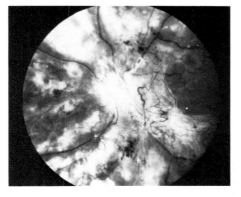

Fig. 15-16. Involution of disc neovascularization (Fig. 15-1) 3 months after feeder-frond technique combined with panretinal photocoagulation.

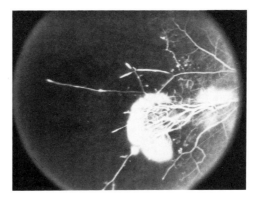

Fig. 15-17. Fluorescein angiogram of midperipheral neovascular frond with surrounding zone of capillary nonperfusion.

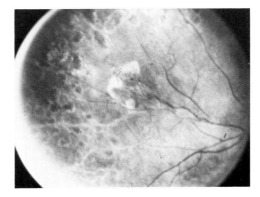

Fig. 15-18. Regression of neovascular frond (Fig. 15-17), following coagulation of nonperfused capillaries surrounding frond. No coagulation was applied directly to tuft.

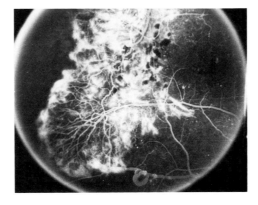

Fig. 15-19. Recurrent neovascularization distal to insufficient coagulation, which did not incorporate nonperfused capillary bed.

stimulus for neovascularization. The latter effect may result from any or a combination of the following mechanisms: (1) elimination of poorly perfused capillaries, with increased rate of blood flow in the remaining capillaries; (2) destruction of hypoxic retina, with its anerobic metabolic by-products presumably responsible for stimulating vasoproliferation; (3) reduction of retinal requirement for oxygen, leaving more oxygen for the remaining untreated retina; (4) opening new channels for metabolic transfer by means of photocoagulation-induced openings in the retinal pigment epithelium; and (5) destruction of underlying choriocapillaris, which had sustained hypoxic retina with impaired retinal circulation.

SUMMARY

Retinal neovascularization occurs in many pathologic conditions and threatens loss of vision by hemorrhage. Retinal hypoxia and viable retinal capillary endothelium must be present for retinal neovascularization to occur. The causes of retinal ischemia and hypoxia are secondary to impaired blood flow, resulting either from changes in blood content (blood cells or large proteins that bind cells) or in blood vessels. The pathologic physiology of specific diseases is discussed. The rationale for treatment of the underlying disease and for photocoagulation of the areas of retinal neovascularization and the retinal zones of poor capillary perfusion are presented.

REFERENCES

1. Ashton, N.: Oxygen and the growth and development of retinal vessels: in vivo and in vitro studies, Am. J. Ophthalmol. **62:**412-435, 1966.
2. Ashton, N.: Vascular complications of diabetes mellitus, St. Louis, 1967, The C. V. Mosby Co.
3. Ashton, N., and Cook, C.: Direct observation of the effect of oxygen on developing vessels: preliminary report, Br. J. Ophthalmol. **88:**433, 1954.
4. Ashton, N., Ward, B., and Serpell, G.: Effects of oxygen on developing retinal vessels with particular reference to the problem of retrolental fibroplasia, Br. J. Ophthalmol. **38:**397, 1954.
5. Brockhurst, R. J., Schepens, C. L., and Okamura, I. D.: Uveitis. II. Peripheral uveitis: clinical description, complications and differential diagnosis. III. Peripheral uveitis: pathogenesis, etiology and treatment, Am. J. Ophthalmol. **49:**1257, 1960; **51:**19, 1961.
6. Carr, R. E., and Henkind, P.: Retinal findings associated with serum hyperviscosity, Am. J. Ophthalmol. **56:**23, 1963.
7. Chee, P. H. Y.: Radiation retinopathy, Am. J. Ophthalmol. **66:**860, 1968.
8. Coats, G.: Forms of retinal disease with massive excretion, R. Lond. Ophthalmol. Rep. **17:**440, 1908.
9. Cogan, D. G.: Ocular effects of radiation, N. Engl. J. Med. **259:**517, 1958.
10. Cogan, D. G., and Kuwabara, T.: Vascular complications of diabetes mellitus, St. Louis, 1967, The C. V. Mosby Co.
11. Cook, W. C.: A case of sickle cell anemia with associated subarachnoid hemorrhage, Am. J. Med. **11:**541, 1930.
12. Coyle, J. T., Frank, P. E., Leonard, A. L., and Weiner, A.: Macroglobulinemia and its effect upon the eye, Arch. Ophthalmol. **65:**99, 1961.
13. Donders, P. C.: Marcoglobulinemia of Waldenstrom with cryoglobulinemia, Ophthalmologica **135:**324, 1958.
14. Dowling, J. L., and Smith, T. R.: Ocular study of pulseless disease, Arch. Ophthalmol. **64:**236, 1960.
15. Duke-Elder, S.: System of ophthalmology. X. Diseases of the retina, St. Louis, 1967, The C. V. Mosby Co., pp. 398-399.
16. Duke-Elder, S.: System of ophthalmology. X. Diseases of the retina, St. Louis, 1967, The C. V. Mosby Co., pp. 400-406.
17. Eales, H.: Case of retinal hemorrhage as-

sociated with epistoxis and constipation, Birm. Med. Red. **9:**262, 1880.

18. Ehrenfeld, W. K., Hoyt, F., and Wylie, E. J.: Embolization and transient blindness from carotid atheroma: surgical considerations, Arch. Surg. **93:**787, 1966.

19. Elliott, A. J.: Recurrent intraocular hemorrhage in young adults (Eales' disease) with continuous subconjunctival therapy with hydrocortisone, Trans. Am. Ophthalmol. Soc. **56:**383, 1958.

20. Fahraeus, R.: Suspension-stability of the blood, Acta Med. Scand. **55:**1, 1921.

21. Flick, J. J.: Ocular lesions following the atomic bombing of Hiroshima and Nagasaki, Am. J. Ophthalmol. **31:**137, 1968.

22. Frank, R. N., and Ryan, S. J.: Peripheral retinal neovascularization in chronic myelogenous leukemia, Arch. Ophthalmol. **87:**585, 1972.

23. Galinos, S. O., Asdourian, G. K., Woolf, M. B., Stevens, T. S., et al.: Spontaneous remodeling of the peripheral retinal vasculature in sickling disorders, Am. J. Ophthalmol. **79:**853, 1975.

24. Goldberg, M. F.: Classification and pathogenesis of proliferative sickle retinopathy, Am. J. Ophthalmol. **71:**649, 1971.

25. Goldberg, M. F.: Natural history of untreated proliferative sickle retinopathy, Arch. Ophthalmol. **85:**428, 1971.

26. Goldberg, M. F.: Retinal vaso-occlusion in sickling hemoglobinopathies, The 30th Proctor Lecture, San Francisco, 1975.

27. Goldstone, J., Schmid-Schonbein, H., and Wells, R.: The rheology of red blood cell aggregates, Microvas. Res. **2:**273, 1970.

28. Goodman, G., Von Sollman, L., and Holland, M. G.: Ocular manifestations of sickle-cell disease, Arch. Ophthalmol. **58:**655, 1957.

29. Hall, K., and Luft, R.: Advances in metabolic disorders, vol. 7, Growth hormone and somatomedin, New York, 1974, Academic Press, Inc.

30. Hannon, J. F.: Vitreous hemorrhages associated with sickle cell–hemoglobin C disease, Am. J. Ophthalmol. **42:**707, 1956.

31. Hansen, A. P.: Normalization of growth hormone hyper-response to exercise in juvenile diabetics after "normalization" of blood sugar, J. Clin. Invest. **50:**1806, 1971.

32. Harrison, T. R.: Harrison's principles of internal medicine, vol. 2, New York, 1970, McGraw-Hill, Inc., pp. 1629-1632.

33. Harrison, T. R.: Harrison's principles of in-

ternal medicine, vol. 2, New York, 1970, McGraw-Hill, Inc., p. 1657.

34. Hedges, T. R.: The aortic arch syndrome, Arch. Ophthalmol. **71:**28, 1964.

35. Herrick, J. B.: Peculiar elongated and sickle-shaped red corpuscles in a case of severe anemia, Arch. Intern. Med. **6:**517, 1910.

36. Howard, G. M.: Ocular effects of radiation and photocoagulation, Arch. Ophthalmol. **78:**7, 1966.

37. Hoyt, W. F., and Spencer, W. H.: Personal communication, 1969.

38. Kimura, S. J., and Hogan, M. J.: Chronic cyclitis, Arch. Ophthalmol. **71:**193, 1964.

39. Kloti, R.: Experimental occlusion of retinal and ciliary vessels in owl monkeys, Exp. Eye Res. **6:**393, 1967.

40. Klug, P. P., Lessing, L. S., and Radice, P.: Rheological aspects of sickle cell disease, Arch. Intern. Med. **133:**577-590, 1970.

41. Knox, D. L.: Ischemic ocular inflammation, Am. J. Ophthalmol. **60:**995, 1965.

42. Kohner, E.: Dynamic changes in the microcirculation of diabetics as related to diabetic microangiopathy, Acta Med. Scand. [Suppl.] **578:**41, 1975.

43. Kwaan, H. C., Colwell, J. A., Cruz, S., et al.: Increased platelet aggregation in diabetes mellitus, J. Lab. Clin. Med. **80:**236, 1972.

44. Little, H. L.: Retinal neovascularization, Trans. Pac. Coast Otoophthalmol. Soc. **57:**161-179, 1976.

45. Little, H. L.: The role of abnormal hemorheodynamics in the pathogenesis of diabetic retinopathy, Trans. Am. Ophthalmol. Soc. **74:**573, 1976.

46. Little, H. L.: Controversy in ophthalmology. The use of photocoagulation in the management of diabetic retinopathy, Philadelphia, W. B. Saunders Co. (In press.)

47. Little, H. L., Sacks, A. H., Krupp, M., Johnson, P., et al.: Abnormal hemorrheology in the pathogenesis of diabetic microangiopathy, International Congress on Diabetes. Brussels, 1973.

48. Little, H. L., Sacks, A. H., and Zweng, H. C.: The role of altered blood rheology in pathogenesis of diabetic retinopathy. Proceedings of XXII Congress International D'Ophthalmologie, Paris, 1974, **1:**321, 1976.

49. Little, H. L., and Zweng, H. C.: Argon laser photocoagulation of disc neovascularization in diabetic retinopathy, Trans. Pac. Coast Otoophthalmol. **54:**123, 1973.

50. Little, H. L., Zweng, H. C., Jack, R. L., and

Vassiliadis, A.: Techniques in argon laser photocoagulation of diabetic disc new vessels, Am. J. Ophthalmol. **82:**675-683, 1976.

51. Little, H. L., Zweng, H. C., and Peabody, R. R.: Argon laser slit-lamp photocoagulation, Trans. Am. Acad. Ophthalmol. Otolaryngol. **74:**85-97, 1970.

52. Lyle, K. T., and Wybar, K.: Retinal vasculitis, Br. J. Ophthalmol. **45:**778, 1961.

53. Michaelson, I. C.: The mode of development of the retinal vessels and some observation on its significance in certain retinal diseases, Trans. Ophthalmol. Soc. U.K. **68:**137, 1948.

54. Michaelson, I. C.: Retinal circulation in man and animals, Springfield, Ill., 1954, Charles C Thomas, Publisher.

55. Morse, P. H., and McCready, J. L.: Peripheral retinal neovascularization in chronic myelocytic leukemia, Am. J. Ophthalmol. **72:**975, 1971.

56. Munro, S., and Walker, C.: Ocular complication in sickle cell haemoglobin C disease, Br. J. Ophthalmol. **44:**1, 1960.

57. Myerson, R. M., Harrison, E., and Lohmuller, H. W.: Incidence and significance of abnormal hemoglobins, Am. J. Med. **26:**543, 1959.

58. National Advisory Eye Council: Interim report on support for vision research, U.S. Department of Health, Education, and Welfare, (National Institutes of Health), publication no. 76, p. 1098.

59. Patz, A.: The role of oxygen in retrolental fibroplasia, Trans. Am. Ophthalmol. Soc. **66:**940-985, 1968.

60. Patz, A., Eastham, A., Higginbotham, D. H., and Kleh, T.: Oxygen studies in retrolental fibroplasia, Am. J. Ophthalmol. **36:**1511, 1953.

61. Payne, J. W., and Patz, A.: Treatment of acute retrolental fibroplasia, Trans. Am. Acad. Ophthalmol. Otolaryngol. **76:**1234-1246, 1972.

62. Romayananda, N., Goldberg, M. F., and Green, W. R.: Histopathology of sickle cell retinopathy, Trans. Am. Acad. Ophthalmol. Otolaryngol. **77:**652-676, 1973.

63. Sanders, M. D., and Hoyt, W. F.: Hypoxic ocular sequelae of carotid-cavernous fistulae, Br. J. Ophthalmol. **53:**82, 1969.

64. Schlaegel, T. F.: Ocular histopathology of some Nagasaki atomic-bomb casualties, Am. J. Ophthalmol. **30:**127, 1947.

65. Shimizu, K., and Sano, K.: Pulseless disease, J. Neuropathol. Clin. Neurol. **1:**37, 1951.

66. Sia, R. H.: Simple method for estimating quantitative differences in globulin precipitation test in kala-azar, Chin. Med. J. **38:**35, 1924.

67. Siperstein, M. D., Unger, R. H., and Madison, L. L.: Studies of muscle capillary basement membranes in normal subjects, diabetic, and prediabetic patients, J. Clin. Invest. **47:**1973, 1968.

68. Smith, J. L.: Unilateral glaucoma in carotid occlusive disease, J.A.M.A. **182:**683, 1962.

69. Spalter, H.: Abnormal serum proteins and retinal vein thrombosis, Arch. Ophthalmol. **62:**868, 1959.

70. Stevens, T. S., Busse, B., Lee, C. B., Woolf, M. B., et al.: Sickling hemoglobinopathies: macular and perimacular vascular abnormalities, Arch. Ophthalmol. **92:**455, 1974.

71. Taylor, E., and Dobree, J. H.: Proliferative diabetic retinopathy: site and size of initial lesions, Br. J. Ophthalmol. **54:**11, 1970.

72. Terry, T. L.: Fibroplastic overgrowth of persistent tunica vasculosa lentis in infants born prematurely, Am. J. Ophthalmol. **25:**1409, 1942.

73. Waldenström, J.: Incipient myelomatosis or "essential" hyperglobulinemia with fibrinogenopenia—a new syndrome, Acta Med. Scand. **117:**216, 1944.

74. Welch, R. B., and Goldberg, M. F.: Sickle-cell hemoglobin and its relation to fundus abnormality, Arch. Ophthalmol. **75:**353, 1966.

75. Welch, R. B., Maumenee, A. E., and Whalen, H. E.: Peripheral posterior segment inflammation vitreous opacities, and edema of the posterior pole, Arch. Ophthalmol. **64:**540, 1960.

76. Wells, R.: Syndromes of hyperviscosity, N. Engl. J. Med. **283:**183, 1970.

77. Wise, G. N.: Retinal neovascularization, Trans. Am. Ophthalmol. Soc. **54:**729, 1956.

78. Wise, G. N., Dollery, C. T., and Henkind, P.: The retinal circulation, New York, 1971, Harper & Row, Publishers, p. 285.

16
RETINAL
VEIN OCCLUSIONS

CLINICAL FINDINGS

Retinal venous obstruction was first described as retinal apoplexy by Liebreich in 1854 and later as hemorrhagic retinitis by Leber in 1877; von Michel in 1878 first recognized that obstruction of the central retinal vein was its cause.[5] Leber described the manifestations of branch retinal vein obstruction.

The syndrome consists of venous engorgement, superficial and deep retinal hemorrhages corresponding to the retinal vascular bed drained by the obstructed vein, retinal edema, and cotton-wool patches of retinal ischemia. In central retinal vein occlusion, these findings are seen in all four quadrants of the retina, and there is associated edema of the optic disc. With central vein occlusion and with temporal branch vein occlusions, there is almost always the presence of macular edema. When macular edema is moderately severe, cystoid changes are observed with fundus biomicroscopy and fluorescein angiography. With time—rarely before 8 weeks' duration—lipid and proteinaceous exudates, preretinal membrane contracture, cystoid macular edema, lamellar macular hole, proliferative retinopathy, and, in central vein occlusions, rubeosis iridis and hemorrhagic glaucoma may occur. Exudative retinal detachment may occur in the early phase of the syndrome, and rhegmatogenous or traction retinal detachment can occur many months to years later.[8,11,22]

FLUORESCEIN ANGIOGRAPHIC OBSERVATIONS

The fluorescein angiographic appearance of retinal vein occlusion has been well documented.[3,7,21] The findings include prolonged circulation time in the involved sectors of the retina; pooling and leakage of fluorescein from the tributaries, venules, and capillaries distal to the occlusion; late staining at the site of the occlusion and of the vein distal to the occlusion; areas of capillary nonperfusion; and pooling of dye in the macula, suggesting early cystoid edema.[1-3] After weeks to months, subsequent changes noted on angiography, in addition to those

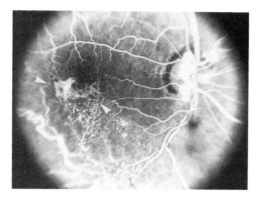

Fig. 16-1. Venous to venous collateral channels temporal and nasal *(arrows)* to macula noted 2 years after inferior temporal branch vein occlusion. Neovascularization present on optic nerve head.

noted, include dilated collateral channels, cystoid macular edema, and microaneurysms. Within months to years after branch retinal vein occlusion, retinal neovascularization may occur (Fig. 16-1).

The acute phase of retinal vein occlusion has been produced experimentally in animals by obstruction of the central retinal vein or its tributaries.[6,9,13]

PATHOGENESIS

The pathogenesis of retinal vein occlusion, as documented by Klien and Olwin,[12] results from one of the following mechanisms: (1) occlusion by external compression and secondary endothelial proliferation; (2) occlusion by primary venous disease of degeneration or inflammation; and (3) occlusion by stagnation thrombosis.

In view of these observations, the pathologic physiology of retinal vein occlusion in the following disorders is better understood:

1. External compression occurs in glaucoma, at the margin of the glaucomatous cupped optic disc, and in hypertension with arteriolar sclerosis, at the arteriovenous crossings.
2. Inflammatory diseases of local or systemic origin can cause venous thrombosis.
3. Diabetes, dysproteinemia, polycythemia, and leukemia probably cause stagnation thrombosis by increased blood viscosity. Carotid insufficiency and pulmonary emphysema reduce the rate of circulation, with subsequent stagnation thrombosis.

INCIDENCE

Raitta[20] found that the average age of 464 patients with central retinal vein occlusion was 61.7 years and that 16 cases occurred in patients under the age of

40; she found that the average age of patients with branch vein occlusion was 62.5 years and that only three cases occurred before age 40 years. In contrast to most vascular diseases, which predominate in males, there was no significant sex difference in incidence of retinal vein occlusions. In a study of 301 patients, Ono[19] noted that 85% had tributary vein occlusion and 15% had central retinal vein occlusion. The frequent occurrence of superior temporal branch vein occlusions is attributed to the greater number of arteriovenous crossings in that quadrant.[18] Foster Moore[18] found five cases of bilateral obstruction in a series of 62 patients; that is, 8% incidence of bilateral occlusions. Zweng and Hecker noted an incidence of bilateral ocular vascular accidents (artery and vein occlusions) in 14% of patients studied.[24] The incidence of glaucoma in patients with central retinal vein thrombosis is about 35%; however, there is no increased incidence of glaucoma in patients with tributary vein occlusion.[20] The incidence of retinal neovascularization (preretinal or papillary) following branch retinal vein occlusion ranges from 24% to 42%.[1,8] There is poor documentation of the incidence of retinal neovascularization following central retinal vein occlusion; however, if it occurs, the incidence is much lower than that following branch vein occlusion. The incidence of rubeosis iridis following central retinal vein occlusion varies from 11% to 43%;[4] rubeosis iridis after branch vein occlusion is extraordinarily rare. The specific predilections of rubeosis iridis to follow central retinal vein occlusion and of retinal neovascularization to follow branch retinal vein occlusion remain an enigma.

VISUAL LOSS AND NATURAL COURSE

Visual loss may result from impaired macular function resulting from edema, hemorrhage, altered capillary perfusion, or preretinal membrane contracture; proliferative retinopathy with vitreous hemorrhage; or rubeosis iridis with hemorrhagic glaucoma.

In order to evaluate any form of therapy, one must first understand the natural course of the disease. In a study of 95 consecutive branch vein occlusions, Archer, Ernest, and Newell[1] evaluated visual results as related to efficiency of arterial perfusion, competency of retinal microvasculature, and the extent of nonperfused retina. When the corresponding artery perfused normally and when the capillary bed perfused without leakage, visual acuity was usually unimpaired and complete recovery was the rule. If there was microvascular incompetency manifested by dilated capillaries, microaneurysms, and extravasation of fluid into extravascular spaces, the visual prognosis was less favorable. Finally, if there was impaired arterial perfusion with areas of nonperfused capillaries in addition to microvascular incompetence, the visual prognosis was poor; 21 of 51 eyes in this group developed retinal neovascularization. Furthermore, their evaluation showed that the final visual result was influenced by the site and the completeness of the venous obstruction, the proximity to the fovea (Fig. 16-2), and the age of the patient; younger patients fared better. Michels and Gass[17] invariably found

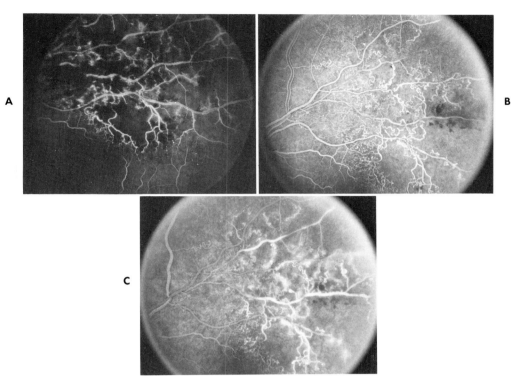

Fig. 16-2. A, Superior temporal branch retinal vein occlusion in 45-year-old woman shows focal areas of nonperfusion with capillary dilation. Areas of edema were restricted to superior temporal macula. VA, 20/20. **B,** With no therapy, VA remained 20/20 after 2 years. Collateral channels noted on angiography. **C,** Hyperfluorescence of tributaries to occluded vein, with capillary distention involving paramacular area, noted on delayed phase of angiogram 2 years after occlusion.

some degree of macular edema in 43 eyes with branch vein occlusion and cystoid changes in 21 (48%) after a 1- to 10-year follow-up. A favorable visual prognosis was observed when the branch occlusion involved one fourth of the macular circumference (3 hours of the clock) or less; in seven of eight eyes with V/A of 20/200 or less, greater than one fourth of the macula was involved.

THERAPY

Any form of therapy should be preceded by a medical and ophthalmologic workup to detect any underlying disease that predisposes to retinal vein occlusion. In macroglobulinemia the use of anticoagulants is contraindicated, but the use of plasmapheresis, penicillamine, and chlorambucil might be indicated. With regard to the use of anticoagulants in central retinal vein occlusion from other causes, Duff, Fall, and Linman[4] found no significant improvement in visual

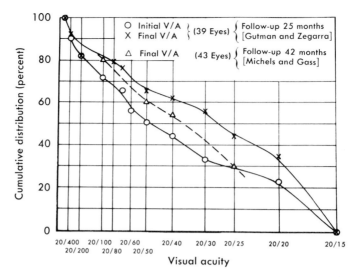

Fig. 16-3. Cumulative distribution of visual acuities in natural history of temporal branch retinal vein occlusions.

acuity in 158 treated cases versus 79 untreated cases; however, the incidence of hemorrhagic glaucoma was reduced from 43% in the untreated group to 9% in the treated group. These observations are in agreement with those of Braend-strup.[2] In patients under 60 years of age, without evidence of systemic vascular disease, and in whom an underlying retinal phlebitis might be present, trial of systemic or retrobulbar steroids seems justifiable.

Inasmuch as the natural course is variable, particularly in branch retinal vein occlusion, and because visual acuity is frequently good (60% ≥ 20/40,[9] 46% ≥ 20/40,[10] 40% ≥ 20/30,[1] and 53% ≥ 20/40[17]) (Fig. 16-3), results of photocoagulation or any other form of therapy are difficult to evaluate. The aim of photocoagulation is to reduce macular edema, eradicate retinal neovascularization, prevent or involute rubeosis iridis in central vein occlusions, and to treat retinal breaks prophylactically.

Material and methods

In an uncontrolled study, we treated 39 eyes with central retinal vein occlusion and 114 eyes with temporal branch vein occlusions, with argon laser photocoagulation. Patients ranged in age from 38 to 84 years (average, 63.7). All patients were referred by ophthalmologists for possible laser treatment; thus, their visual acuities were probably worse than would be expected in a non-screened randomized group with retinal vein occlusions. On the following pages, their final visual results are compared with pretreatment and with final V/A from the natural course of disease, as reported by others.

Central retinal vein occlusion

Of 39 patients with central retinal vein occlusion treated by ALP, 28 were observed for $\geq$ 6 months: 18 were men and 10 were women; six had hypertension, five were diabetic, and one had severe pulmonary emphysema. Macular edema was present in all eyes. Rubeosis iridis was recognized in two eyes. Because vision was poor in most eyes (<20/200 in 15 of 28) and because the long-term visual prognosis is extremely poor for central retinal vein occlusion

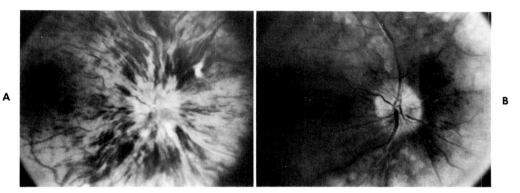

Fig. 16-4. A, Pretreatment funduscopic appearance of central retinal vein thrombosis. **B,** Appearance of fundus 4 weeks post–panretinal argon laser photocoagulation. Note residual hemorrhage and venous engorgement are much less.

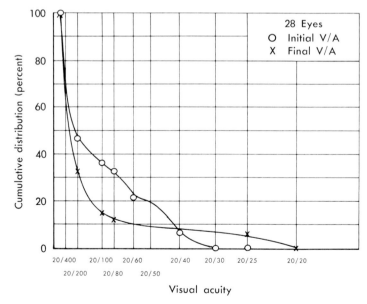

Fig. 16-5. Comparison of pre- and posttreatment visuals results following panretinal photocoagulation for central retinal vein occlusion.

(only 15% to 20% of cases improve spontaneously[4,17]), argon laser photocoagulation was performed. The purpose of treatment was to improve visual acuity by reducing macular edema and to eradicate or prevent the development of rubeosis iridis. Treatment was performed between 1 week and 10 months after the onset of visual impairment; the average time of treatment was 3.4 months after onset of symptoms. Follow-up time ranged from 6 to 39 months, with an average of 16 months.

Treatment consisted of panretinal photocoagulation extending from the disc margin to the equator in all meridians, sparing only the macula and maculopapular bundle. Approximately 2,000 moderately intense photocoagulation burns were placed with the 500- and 1,000-μm spot sizes, using 500 to 2,000 mW power at 0.1 sec.[16] Usually five sessions of treatment were required to complete the applications. Retinal veins and venous collaterals were avoided. In addition, areas of nonperfusion and of capillary leakage, microaneurysm, or questionable areas of neovascularization were treated directly.

Venous engorgement and retinal hemorrhages were markedly reduced in all cases (Fig. 16-4). However, because macular edema persisted in all eyes, vision was not improved. The graph in Fig. 16-5, plotting the cumulative distribution of cases and visual acuity levels pre- and posttreatment, shows little difference between the visual acuities of treated and untreated eyes.

Because of previous experience with involution of rubeosis iridis following panretinal photocoagulation in eyes with diabetic retinopathy[14] (see Chapter 14), two eyes with rubeosis iridis and glaucoma secondary to central retinal vein occlusion were treated. Because of poor pupillary dilation, photocoagulation could not be applied anterior to the midperiphery. Nonetheless, in both eyes the rubeosis regressed but failed to undergo complete involution; the intraocular pressure has remained elevated. The response of rubeosis to panretinal photocoagulation is more favorable in eyes with diabetic retinopathy than in those with central retinal vein occlusions. When not initially present, rubeosis iridis has not developed in any of the 37 eyes treated with panretinal photocoagulation for central retinal vein occlusion.

Temporal branch vein occlusion

We treated 114 patients with temporal branch retinal vein occlusion. Of these, 43 (47%) were men and 48 (53%) were women. Patients ranged in age from 38 to 84 years (average, 63 years). Thirty-four (37%) were taking or subsequently received medication for hypertension. All eyes were treated for macular edema with visual symptoms or retinal neovascularization; cystoid macular edema was observed in 36 eyes (39%). Retinal neovascularization was present in 41 of 91 eyes (45%). Rubeosis iridis was not seen in this group.

Photocoagulation was performed to reduce macular edema, with intent to preserve or improve visual acuity, and to destroy retinal neovascularization. Argon slit-lamp laser photocoagulation was performed, on the average, 16.6 months

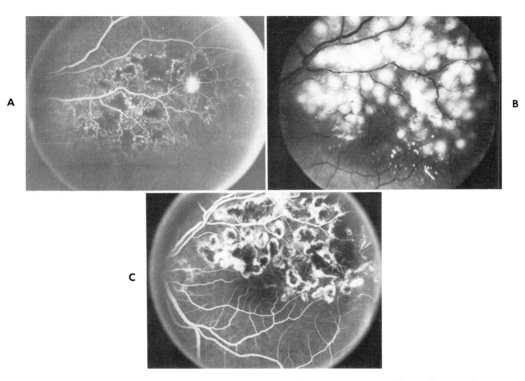

Fig. 16-6. A, Pretreatment fluorescein angiographic appearance of branch retinal vein occlusion, showing impaired circulation with venous engorgement, staining of occluded vessels, capillary leakage of dye involving macula, zones of nonperfused capillaries, and focal area of retinal neovascularization. VA, 20/200. **B,** Photocoagulation is directed to capillary leakage, neovascularization, and area of nonperfusion; normal vessels and collateral channels are avoided in treatment. **C,** Fluorescein angiogram 8 weeks after laser photocoagulation shows reduction of venous engorgement of capillary leakage. VA, 20/50.

after the onset of symptoms (range, from 1 week to 216 months). Eyes were treated an average of 2.7 times, with an average total of 450 lesions. The instrument settings were usually 200 to 500 μm, 300 to 700 mW, and 0.1 to 0.2 sec. Follow-up time ranged from 6 to 58 months, with an average of 19.7 months.

The fluorescein angiogram was used to localize areas of capillary leakage, microaneurysms, neovascularization, and zones of non-perfusion (Fig. 16-6, *A*); the fovea, the major retinal vessels, and collateral channels were avoided in treatment (Fig. 16-6, *B* and *C*). In eyes with retinal neovascularization, whether on the optic disc or in the region of the occluded vessel, panretinal photocoagulation was directed to the sector of retina involved by the occlusion. Involution of neovascular fronds occurred in 74% of eyes following segmental panretinal photocoagulation (Fig. 16-7); however, in fronds with visualized feeder vessels, the feeder vessel and the frond were given treatment additional to segmental panret-

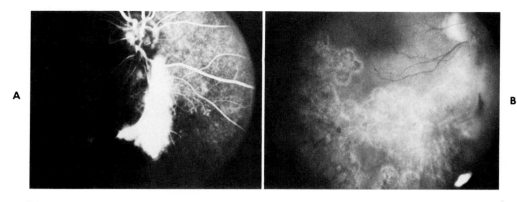

Fig. 16-7. A, Pretreatment angiographic appearance of disc neovascularization following inferior temporal vein occlusion. **B,** Involution of disc neovascularization 3 months after segmental panretinal photocoagulation to involved quadrant.

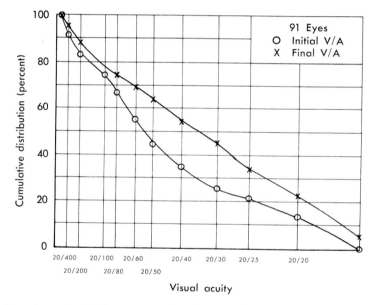

Fig. 16-8. Visual results of 91 eyes treated with argon laser photocoagulation for temporal branch retinal vein occlusion.

inal photocoagulation. Recurrence of the neovascular frond occurred in the early cases when segmental panretinal photocoagulation was not also performed.[15]

RESULTS

Retinal neovascularization was reduced by at least 50% in all eyes treated, and total involution of fronds was observed in 74% of eyes treated for this problem.

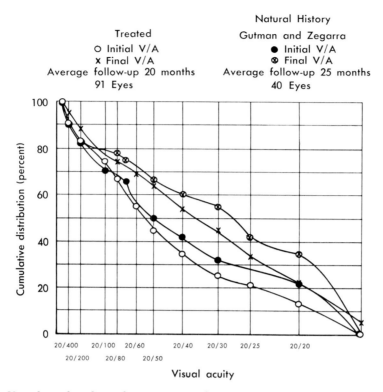

Fig. 16-9. Visual results after tributary vein occlusion, superimposing results of untreated and treated eyes.

Table 16-1. Final visual acuity after temporal branch vein occlusion

	Number of eyes	20/40 or better (%)	20/50 to 20/100 (%)	20/200 or worse (%)
Untreated				
Michels and Gass	43	53	28	19
Gutman and Zegarra	40	60	17	23
Treated				
Little and Zweng	59	52	23	25

Macular edema was reduced in all of the treated eyes, but it was seldom totally resolved.

Visual results of the 91 treated eyes are depicted in Fig. 16-8, which illustrates the cumulative distribution of pre- and posttreatment visual acuities. Of the 91 treated eyes, 55% had 20/40 vision or better at the end of the posttreatment follow-up period. These visual results are similar to those in the natural course of the disease[8,17] (Fig. 16-9 and Table 16-1). *Text continued on p. 259.*

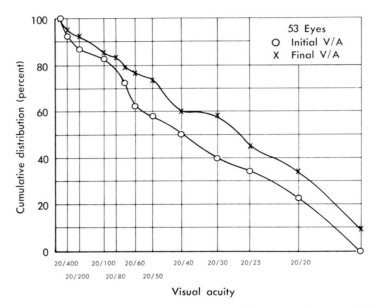

Fig. 16-10. Comparison of pre- and posttreatment visual acuities of eyes with branch vein occlusion but without cystoid macular edema.

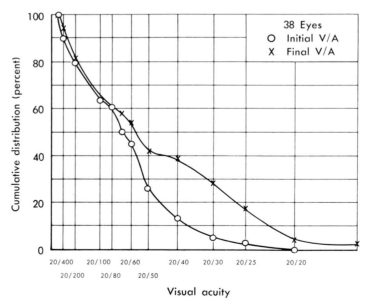

Fig. 16-11. Comparison of pre- and posttreatment visual acuities of eyes with cystoid macular changes.

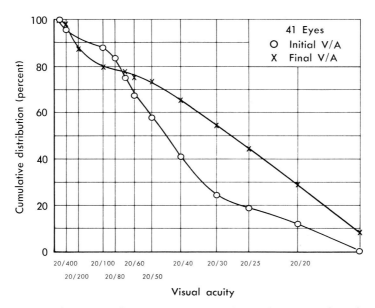

Fig. 16-12. Cumulative visual results when macula involvement is less than 90°.

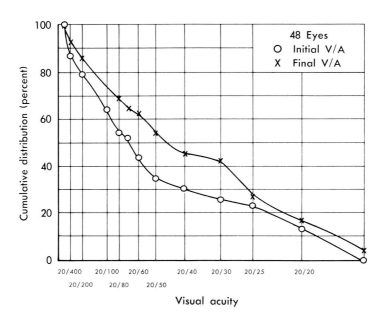

Fig. 16-13. Cumulative visual results when 180° of macula is involved.

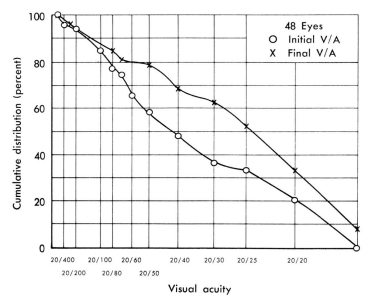

Fig. 16-14. Visual results following laser photocoagulation for branch retinal vein occlusion in patients under 63 years of age.

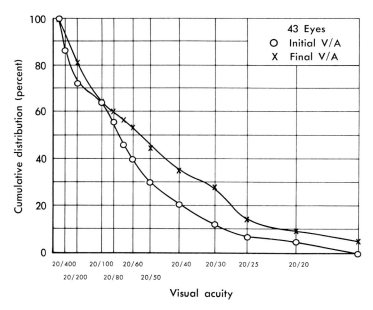

Fig. 16-15. Visual results following laser photocoagulation for branch retinal vein occlusion in patients over 63 years of age.

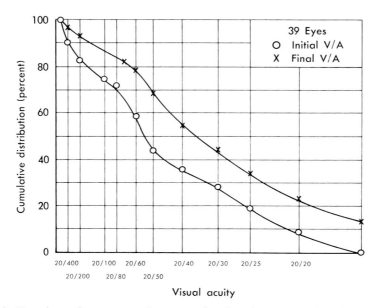

Fig. 16-16. Visual results in eyes photocoagulated within 4 months of venous branch occlusion.

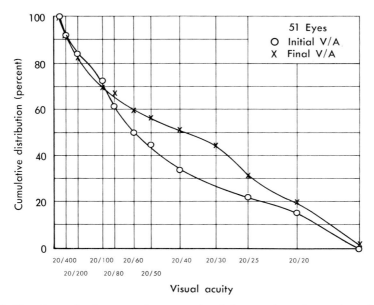

Fig. 16-17. Visual results in eyes photocoagulated longer than 4 months after venous obstructions.

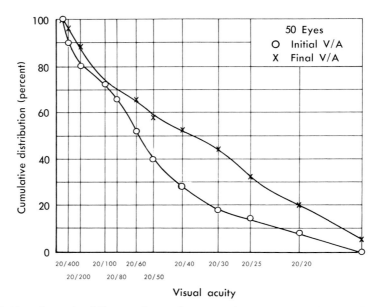

Fig. 16-18. Visual results following laser photocoagulation for branch retinal vein occlusion without neovascularization.

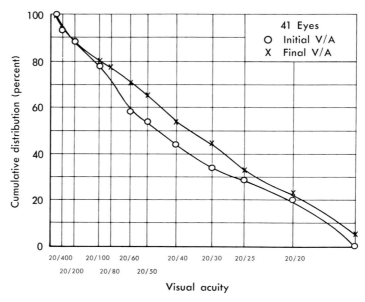

Fig. 16-19. Visual results following laser photocoagulation for branch retinal vein occlusion with neovascularization.

We analyzed our treated patients further from other standpoints: presence or absence of cystoid macular edema (Figs. 16-10 and 16-11), amount of macula involved in the edematous process (Figs. 12-12 and 16-13), patients' ages (Figs. 16-14 and 16-15), length of time that had elapsed between onset of the occlusion—oftentimes a difficult date to ascertain—and treatment (Figs. 16-16 and 16-17), and presence or absence of retinal neovascularization (Figs. 16-18 and 16-19).

The presence of cystoid macular edema gave a poor visual prognosis. Examination of Figs. 16-10 and 16-11 shows that the initial and final visual acuity profile for cystoid macular edema is lower than that for those without. For example, 60% of the eyes without cystoid macular edema ended up seeing 20/40 or better; only 39% with cystoid edema saw as well.

We compared eyes that had one quarter or less of the macula involved (Fig. 16-12) with those that had about one half of the macula involved (Fig. 16-13). Both the initial and final visual acuity profiles are higher for the eyes with lesser macular involvement. The final visual acuity graphs show that for the eyes where less than one quarter was involved, 65% ended with a visual acuity of 20/40 or better, while only 45% ended with 20/40 or better if about half the macula was involved.

The age of the patient appears to be a significant factor in the visual outcome. Figs. 16-14 and 16-15 illustrate the initial and final visual acuity profiles for patients less than or equal to 63 years and those older than 63 years (63 was the average age of the patients). It seems that there is a big difference in the initial and final visual acuities. Forty-eight percent of the younger group saw 20/40 or better before treatment and 68% saw 20/40 or better at the end of follow-up, compared with 20% and 34% respectively in the older group. This was the single most important prognostic factor.

The length of time that elapsed between onset and treatment did not play a major role, although there are indications that the earlier treated eyes did a little better. Fig. 16-16 shows the visual acuities for eyes treated less than 4 months after the vein occlusion, while Fig. 16-17 shows those treated 4 months or longer after the vein occlusion. While the eyes treated earlier had a somewhat higher visual acuity profile than those treated later, the differences are not significant.

Finally, the presence of neovascularization did not seem to play a significant role in the visual outcome of branch vein occlusions. Fig. 16-18 shows the visual acuity profiles for eyes without neovascularization; Fig. 16-19 shows eyes with neovascularization. Although the initial visual acuity profile is somewhat lower for those without neovascularization, all of which had macular edema, the final visual acuity profiles of both groups are almost identical.

SUMMARY

Panretinal photocoagulation for central retinal vein occlusion is followed by reduction of venous engorgement and retinal hemorrhages, but macular edema with impaired vision persists. No eyes with central retinal vein occlusion that we treated by panretinal photocoagulation have developed rubeosis iridis when it was not present at the time of treatment. This is in contrast to an 11% to 43% incidence reported in untreated series.

Argon laser photocoagulation of branch retinal vein occlusion is performed to eradicate retinal neovascularization and to eliminate macular edema. It is successful in the former; however, macular edema, even though reduced, is seldom eliminated. Visual acuities in this group of treated eyes were not significantly better than those of an untreated series (approximately 55% had 20/40 V/A or better).

Visual results of the treated group are probably negatively biased, because in most cases only eyes with progressive visual loss or macular edema were treated.

Nonetheless, because there is little difference in the final visual acuities between eyes treated with argon laser photocoagulation and those reported in natural history studies, a randomized control study is needed to evaluate the visual response of both central and temporal branch retinal vein occlusion to photocoagulation.

REFERENCES

1. Archer, D. B., Ernest, J. T., and Newell, F. S.: Classification of branch retinal vein obstruction, Trans. Am. Acad. Ophthalmol. Otolaryngol. **78:**148, 1974.
2. Braendstrup, P.: Central retinal vein thrombosis and hemorrhagic glaucoma, Acta Ophthalmol. [Suppl.] **35:**1, 1950.
3. Clemett, R. S.: Retinal branch vein occlusion, Br. J. Ophthalmol. **58:**548, 1974.
4. Duff, I. F., Falls, H. F., and Linman, J. W.: Anticoagulant therapy in occlusive vascular disease of the retina, Arch. Ophthalmol. **46:**601, 1951.
5. Duke-Elder, S.: Diseases of the retina. X. System of ophthalmology, St. Louis, 1967, The C. V. Mosby Co., p. 98.
6. Fujino, T., Curtin, V. T., and Norton, E. W. D.: Experimental central retinal vein occlusion, Trans. Am. Ophthalmol. Soc. **66:**318, 1968.
7. Gass, J. D. M.: A fluorescein angiographic study of macular dysfunction secondary to retinal vascular disease. II. Retinal vein obstruction, Arch. Ophthalmol. **80:**550, 1968.
8. Gutman, F. A., and Zegarra, H.: The natural course of temporal retinal branch vein occlusion, Trans. Am. Acad. Ophthalmol. Otolaryngol. **78:**178, 1974.
9. Hamilton, A. M., Kohner, E. M., Rosen, D., and Bowbyes, J. A.: Experimental venous occlusion, Proc. R. Soc. Med. **66:**1045, 1974.
10. Jensen, V. A.: Clinical studies of tributary thrombosis in the central retinal vein, Acta Ophthalmol. [Suppl.] **10:**1, 1936.
11. Joondeph, H. C., and Goldberg, M. F.: Rhegmatogenous retinal detachment after tributary retinal vein occlusion, Am. J. Ophthalmol. **80:**253, 1975.
12. Klien, V. A., and Olwin, J. H.: A survey of the pathogenesis of retinal vein occlusion, Arch. Ophthalmol. **56:**1956.
13. Kohner, E. M., Dollery, C. T., Shakeb, M., Henkind, P., et al.: Experimental branch vein occlusion, Am. J. Ophthalmol. **69:**878, 1970.
14. Little, H. L., Rosenthal, A. R., Dellaporta, A., and Jacobson, D.: The effect of panretinal photocoagulation for rubeosis iridis—a preliminary report, Am. J. Ophthalmol. **81:**804, 1976.
15. Little, H. L., and Zweng, H. C.: Complications of argon laser photocoagulation, Trans. Pac. Coast Otoophthalmol. Soc. **52:**115, 1971.
16. Little, H. L., and Zweng, H. C.: Argon laser photocoagulation of disc neovascularization in diabetic retinopathy, Trans. Pac. Coast Otoophthalmol. Soc. **54:**123, 1973.
17. Michels, R. G., and Gass, J. D. M.: The natural course of retinal branch vein obstruction, Trans. Am. Acad. Ophthalmol. Otolaryngol. **78:**166, 1974.
18. Moore, R. F.: Retinal vein thrombosis. Br. J. Ophthalmol. [Suppl. 2], 1924.
19. Ono, Y.: Acta Soc. Ophthalmol. Jap. **69:**221, 253, 343, 1965.
20. Raitta, C.: Zer Zentralvenen- und Netzhautvenenverschluss, Acta Ophthalmol. [Suppl.] **83:**12, 1965.

21. Wise, G. N., Dollery, C. T., and Henkins, P.: The retinal circulation, New York, 1971, Harper & Row, Publishers.

22. Zauberman, H.: Retinopathy of retinal detachment after major vascular occlusion, Br. J. Ophthalmol. **52:**117, 1968.

23. Zweng, H. C., Fahrenbruch, R. C., and Little, H. L.: Argon laser photocoagulation in the treatment of retinal vein occlusions, Mod. Probl. Ophthalmol. **12:**261, 1974.

24. Zweng, H. C., Little, H. L., and Peabody, R. R.: Laser photocoagulation and retinal angiography, St. Louis, 1969, The C. V. Mosby Co.

17
RUBEOSIS IRIDIS

Treatment of rubeosis iridis and its sequela, neovascular glaucoma, poses a serious problem for the ophthalmologist. Once the fibrovascular membrane, with peripheral anterior synechiae, has caused obliteration of the angle, intractable glaucoma frequently ensues, resulting in blindness and pain despite many months of therapeutic intervention. Attempts to control the pressure with a variety of operative procedures, in particular cyclocryotherapy, have met with mixed success.[3,6,8,9] Similarly, medical therapy often produces very little effect. No attempt has been made to deal with the problem of neovascular glaucoma by eliminating or reversing the fibrovascular membrane.

Involution of rubeosis iridis and angle rubeosis after panretinal argon laser photocoagulation has recently been reported, both retrospectively in patients with diabetes mellitus and disc neovascularization and prospectively in patients with rubeosis iridis from a variety of causes.[13] Experience with panretinal photocoagulation in the management of rubeosis iridis is limited; however, because of the favorable response in 80% of eyes treated, it is worthwhile to describe in detail the results of and rationale for treatment. This data reflects the combined experiences of Rosenthal, Dellaporta, Jacobson, Little, and Zweng; furthermore, this technique has recently been suggested by Jack and Little[10] for the management of aphakic postvitrectomy diabetic patients, in whom there is a 12% incidence of rubeosis iridis.[15]

MATERIALS AND METHODS

Panretinal photocoagulation (PRP) consisted of placing nearly adjacent, moderately intense argon laser photocoagulation lesions from the disc margin to the equator, 360°, except in the area of the macula and papillo-macular bundle. Approximately 1,500 to 3,000 lesions were applied, with spot sizes ranging from 200 to 1,000 μm (see Fig. 14-18). PRP was administered over a 1- to 2-week period, in three to six sessions.

Fifteen eyes of 11 patients were treated. Five patients were women, ranging in age from 45 to 68 years, and six were men, ranging from 49 to 70 years of age. The predisposing conditions leading to the rubeosis iridis in the 11 patients were one old central retinal artery occlusion, one aortic arch syndrome concomitant with diabetes mellitus, one central retinal vein occlusion associated with diabetes mellitus, and eight instances of diabetic retinopathy. The duration of the diabetes ranged from 13 to 40 years. In three additional eyes with rubeosis iridis, sufficient laser burns could not be adequately positioned, due to poor pupillary dilation in two eyes and cloudy media from cataract in one. These three eyes are not included in the study.

RESPONSE OF RUBEOSIS TO PANRETINAL PHOTOCOAGULATION

Of the 15 eyes treated, 12 demonstrated involution of the rubeosis iridis; in three, no involution of iris and angle vessels was observed. In three of the 12 eyes in which treatment was successful, peripheral anterior synechiae (PAS) were observed to regress and angle structures previously obscured became visible. In brown-eyed individuals, the blood-filled iris vessels were replaced by atrophic fibrous strands. In light-eyed individuals, the vessels were no longer visible on slit-lamp examination.

Those eyes in which the rubeosis was observed to involute revealed the following fundus abnormalities: one old central retinal vein occlusion; two instances of background diabetic retinopathy, one with peripheral arteriolar obliteration; and nine cases of vasoproliferative diabetic retinopathy with disc neovascularization. Of the three eyes in which the rubeosis did not disappear after PRP, one had an old central retinal artery occlusion, one had severe retinal ischemia secondary to aortic arch syndrome, and one had background diabetic retinopathy with peripheral arteriolar obliteration.

The intervals from completion of treatment to total involution of the rubeosis iridis ranged from 1 week to 6 months (Figs. 17-1 to 17-4). In those patients treated prospectively, a total or partial response to treatment was documented sooner (4 to 60 days) than in those patients treated for disc neovascularization and in whom it was observed incidentally that there was marked lessening in the number and size of the vessels on the surface of the iris or in the angle (30 to 240 days). The longer time for observed regression in the group treated retrospectively is explained by the more frequent slit-lamp and gonioscopic observations of the rubeosis in the prospectively treated group.

RESPONSE OF GLAUCOMA TO PRP

Of particular interest was the response of intraocular pressure (IOP) to panretinal photocoagulation (Table 17-1). Eyes were categorized into three groups, according to severity of glaucoma and synechia.

Group A

Four eyes with neovascular glaucoma with 360° angle closure from PAS were treated. Three eyes showed no change in iris and angle vessels following PRP,

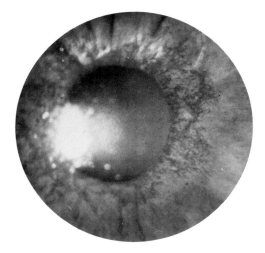

Fig. 17-1. Rubeosis iridis surrounding pupillary margin before panretinal photocoagulation.

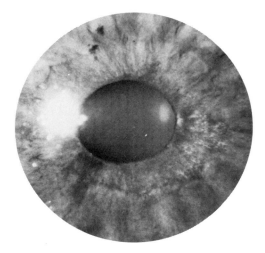

Fig. 17-2. Involution of rubeosis iridis 3 months after panretinal photocoagulation. Note ring of atrophic iris surrounding pupil.

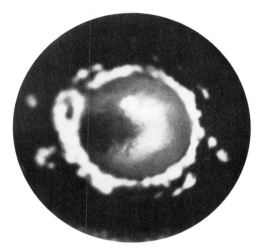

Fig. 17-3. Pretreatment fluorescein angiography of rubeosis iridis diagnosed 4 weeks following vitrectomy and lensectomy in diabetic patient.

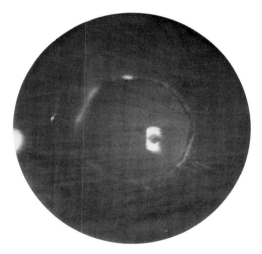

Fig. 17-4. Iris angiography showing involution of rubeosis iridis 4 months after panretinal photocoagulation.

Table 17-1. Effect of panretinal photocoagulation on intraocular pressure

		↑	↔	↓
Group A:	Patients with glaucoma (angle closed 360°)	3*	1	
Group B:	Patients with glaucoma (angle open, with few or many PAS)		1	3
Group C:	Patients without glaucoma (angle open, with few or no PAS)		7	

↑ Increase in IOP after PRP.
↔ IOP controlled on medical therapy or no change in IOP after PRP.
↓ Decrease in IOP on same or less topical antiglaucomatous therapy after PRP.
* Rubeosis iridis failed to involute after PRP.

and the intraocular pressure continued to rise despite maximal medical antiglaucoma therapy. In the fourth eye, the iris and angle vessels completely regressed; however, the angle remained closed. Previous to PRP, the pressure in this eye had been 40 to 50 mm Hg with maximal medical therapy, and the patient had to wear a soft contact lens for bullous keratopathy; this patient after follow-up of 8 months, has been able to discontinue use of the soft contact lens, and with acetazolamide (Diamox) alone, IOP has remained in the 30 to 40 mm Hg range.

Group B

Prior to PRP therapy, pressures in four eyes ranged from 25 to 35 mm Hg with topical antiglaucoma therapy. In all four eyes the angle was open and a few too many PAS were present. All four eyes showed regression of iris and angle vessels following therapy. After PRP, three eyes have shown a reduction in pretreatment intraocular pressure, to less than 20 mm Hg, with the same or less topical medication. One eye continues to have IOP in the low 20's mm Hg, demonstrating a situation similar to that which existed pretreatment; the patient takes 2% pilocarpine every 6 hours.

Group C

In seven eyes of six patients, intraocular pressure was normal, with an open angle and few or no PAS before PRP. All six patients had diabetic retinopathy and bilateral rubeosis iridis. Four of these eyes in four patients showed rubeosis iridis, absolute glaucoma, and light perception (LP) to no light perception (NLP) in the fellow eye. In the fifth patient, the fellow eye demonstrated an elevated IOP and many PAS and was included in Group B. Two additional patients had bilateral rubeosis iridis without PAS. One eye was treated, and the rubeosis involuted; the other eye was followed. Four months after treatment of the first eye, PAS were observed to develop in the second eye. At no time was an increase in IOP recorded. The second eye was then treated with PRP. After PRP in all seven eyes in this group, the angle and iris vessels regressed, the pressure has remained less than 20 mm Hg, and no additional PAS have been observed.

RECURRENCE OF RUBEOSIS IRIDIS

Follow-up of all eyes ranged from 4 to 36 months. In three of 12 successfully treated eyes, a small number of new vessels occurred on the surface of the iris and in the angle. Recurrence occurred in only one of the seven eyes followed over 1 year; rubeosis and glaucoma recurred at 13 months but have been easily controlled with topical medication. In a second eye the recurrence was observed at 4 months; intraocular pressure, which was 50 to 60 mm Hg pretherapy, has been maintained around 35 mm Hg with Diamox, even with the recurrence of rubeosis iridis. IOP in the seventh patient has remained normal, although a few new vessels were observed 7 months posttherapy.

DISCUSSION

Several theories for the pathogenesis of rubeosis iridis have been advanced;[2,4,19] the most widely accepted are—

1. The hypoxic retina produces a metabolite—a vasoformative or vasoproliferative factor—that causes iris and angle neovascularization in addition to the more commonly seen retinal neovascularization.
2. The toxic products of tissue breakdown (e.g., disintegrating hemorrhages) diffuse forward and induce the pathologic vessel proliferation.
3. A specific rubeogenic factor is released from local tissue anoxia, resulting in new vessel growth on the anterior surface of the iris and in the angle.

The observations that PRP prevents the development of rubeosis iridis and subsequent neovascular glaucoma in patients with central retinal vein occlusion[20] and that the new vessels on the iris surface and in the angle disappear in response to PRP[5,7,12] tend to support the theory that the presence of a vasoproliferative factor emanating from distant hypoxic retina causes the development of the new vessels. One could postulate that disseminated photocoagulation eradicates the tendency of the hypoxic retina to elaborate the vasoproliferative factor, thus resulting in the involution of the rubeosis iridis.

The blood-filled channels on the iris and in the angle do not totally disappear, but seem to be replaced by atropic fibrous strands. Iris fluorescein angiography performed by Fetkenhour et al.[7] before and after PRP revealed that the vessels were markedly reduced in size but remained patent, because they continued to leak fluorescein. Additional studies employing rapid-sequence iris angiography will be required to define the fate of the abnormal new vessels.

If the vessels become fibrous strands and fail to carry blood, PRP may be useful in alleviating the hemorrhagic problems of neovascular glaucoma secondary to rubeosis iridis, even when the angle is closed for most of 360° and no dramatic response in the intraocular pressure is observed. PRP may prevent the development of intractable absolute glaucoma, and the symptoms of pain and irritation caused by the breakdown in the blood aqueous barrier may be alleviated. This breakdown may also aggravate glaucoma and bullous keratopathy by compromising whatever degree of angle is functioning and by irritating the corneal epithelium. A brief case summary, courtesy of Dr. Ralph Rosenthal, illustrates this point.[13] Despite 360° angle closure, the patient became far more comfortable after PRP. The anterior chamber became free of proteinaceous material and cells, and the bullous keratopathy somewhat lessened. She was able to discontinue wearing a soft lens for bullous keratopathy. Tension, which was originally in the 50 to 60 mm Hg range, has remained around 35 mm Hg with Diamox alone, and there has been no progression to intractable absolute glaucoma.

Eradication of the blood vessels in the advanced stages may allow for safer operative intervention with another glaucoma surgical procedure, whether it be a filtering operation or cyclodialysis.

Unfortunately, experience with the advanced stages of rubeosis iridis with 360° angle closure have been disappointing; in three of the four eyes treated, the vessels remained and the tension continued to rise.

Because PRP is not uniformly successful in advanced stages of rubeosis iridis, possibly early therapy is advisable as a prophylactic measure. Arguments for early diagnosis and early therapy are—

1. In the present series, treatment of the glaucoma has been successful in three of four eyes with a small number of PAS and elevated intraocular pressure. After resolution of the vessels, less therapy was required to maintain the IOP at less than 20 mm Hg in one eye, and a reduction in pretherapy IOP to less than 20 mm Hg has been achieved with the same topical medications in two eyes.

2. There may be difficulties in administering PRP if either a miotic pupil, bullous keratopathy, significant cataract, hyphema, or vitreous hemorrhage ensue.

3. When an angle commences to close with PAS, the angle closure may rapidly advance to 360°, precluding a beneficial result in the reduction of the IOP by the elimination of the new vessels.

4. Because PRP has been shown to be often successful in eradicating disc neovascularization[1,11,14,14a] and because disc neovascularization is frequently present with rubeosis iridis, one may be killing two proverbial birds with one stone in that the retinal and iris neovascularization can be virtually eliminated with a single therapeutic approach.

5. We have achieved a high degree of success in eliminating the vessels with a mild degree of rubeosis and no glaucoma in seven of seven eyes. In four of these eyes, the fellow eye had developed absolute glaucoma with LP to NLP vision; in a fifth, the fellow eye had a moderate increase in IOP, with many PAS.

Arguments that can be made against the use of prophylactic PRP in early rubeosis iridis are—

1. In many eyes rubeosis of the iris and angle may remain unchanged for several years, or there may be fluctuation in the severity of the neovascularization, without the development of PAS and secondary neovascular glaucoma (24 of 58 eyes in a series reported by Madsen[16]).

2. Spontaneous regression or disappearance of rubeosis has frequently been observed (eight of 37 eyes reported by Ohrt[18] and 15 of 58 eyes reported by Madsen[16]).

3. In diabetic patients who have absolute glaucoma from neovascularization in one eye, the presence of rubeosis in the second eye does not invariably mean the development of PAS and neovascular glaucoma in that eye. Of 30 diabetics studied by Madsen,[17] with rubeosis iridis and hemorrhagic glaucoma in one eye, nine who had rubeosis in the second eye did not develop neovascular glaucoma. In six of these the rubeosis remained stationary for 2 to 6 years; in the other three the rubeosis disappeared.

In light of the latter two important considerations concerning the natural history of the disease, a controlled randomized prospective study in patients with bilateral rubeosis iridis (using one eye as a control) is absolutely required before PRP for eradication of iris and angle neovascularization can be routinely advocated. A reasonable and practical approach to the problem of early therapy may be that once angle vessels are observed to progress to PAS, with partial closure of the angle, PRP should be considered as a means of potentially reversing or halting the progression of the angle closure and development of secondary glaucoma. This should hold true particularly in patients who have lost the fellow eye to neovascular glaucoma.

In addition, we should attempt to predict which patient with neovascularization of the iris and angle will develop neovascular glaucoma. As yet we are unable to do so. It is hoped that additional studies on the natural history of rubeosis iridis will shed some light on this problem.

Finally, the posttreatment observation time reported herein allows only for short-term follow-up to ascertain whether there will be recurrence of the rubeosis and secondary glaucoma. We have observed that in three individuals minimal neovascularization of the iris and angle has recurred in from 4 to 13 months; thus it appears obligatory that these patients be regularly observed for a prolonged period. Iris angiography is an aid in diagnosis and follow-up evaluation, because leakage of fluorescein is sometimes observed on slit-lamp examination in the absence of detectable rubeosis iridis.

SUMMARY

Fifteen eyes of 11 patients with rubeosis iridis and neovascularization of the angle associated with retinal vascular disorders were treated with panretinal photocoagulation. In 12 eyes there was complete regression of the new vessels on the surface of the iris and in the angle. In three of these eyes PAS previously present appeared to regress and angle structures previously obscured became visible. During the follow-up period of from 3 to 36 months, three eyes were observed to develop a small number of new abnormal iris and angle vessels. The arguments for and against PRP therapy in eyes with early rubeosis iridis secondary to circulatory disorders of the retina are discussed.

REFERENCES

1. Aiello, L., Beetham, W., Marios, C. B., Chazan, B. I., and Bradley, R. F.: Ruby laser photocoagulation in treatment of diabetic proliferative retinopathy: preliminary report. In Goldberg, M., and Fine, S., editors: Symposium on treatment of diabetic retinopathy, U.S. Department of Health, Education, and Welfare, publication no. 1890, 1968, p. 437.
2. Anderson, D. M., Morin, J. D., and Hunter, W. S.: Rubeosis iridis, Can. J. Ophthalmol. **6:**183, 1971.
3. Boniuk, M.: Cryotherapy in neovascular glaucoma, Trans. Am. Acad. Ophthalmol. Otolaryngol. **78:**337, 1974.
4. Bresnick, G. H., and Gay, A. J.: Rubeosis iridis associated with branch retinal arteriolar occlusions, Arch. Ophthalmol. **77:**176, 1967.
5. Callahan, M. A., and Hilton, G. F.: Photocoagulation and rubeosis iridis, Am. J. Ophthalmol. **78:**873, 1974.
6. Feibel, R. M., and Bigger, J. F.: Rubeosis iridis and neovascular glaucoma: evaluation of cyclocryotherapy, Am. J. Ophthalmol. **74:**862, 1972.
7. Fetkenhour, C. L., Choromokos, E., and Shoch, D.: Effect of retinal photocoagulation on rubeosis iridis and neovascular glaucoma. Presented at the Association for Research in Vision and Ophthalmology, Sarasota, Fla., April 28, 1975.
8. Hetherington, J. L.: Discussion of three preceding papers, Trans. Am. Acad. Ophthalmol. Otolaryngol. **78:**344, 1974.
9. Hoskins, H. D.: Neovascular glaucoma: current concepts, Trans. Am. Acad. Ophthalmol. Otolaryngol. **78:**330, 1974.
10. Jack, R. L., and Little, H. L.: Photocoagulation after vitrectomy in diabetic patients. In L'Esperance, F. A., Jr., editor: Current diagnosis and management of chorioretinal diseases, St. Louis, 1977, The C. V. Mosby Co.
11. James, W. A., and L'Esperance, F. A.: Treatment of diabetic optic nerve neovascularization by extensive retinal photocoagulation, Am. J. Ophthalmol. **78:**939, 1974.
12. Krill, A. E., Archer, D., and Newell, F. W.: Photocoagulation in complications secondary to branch vein occlusion, Arch. Ophthalmol. **85:**48, 1971.
13. Little, H. L., Rosenthal, R. A., Dellaporta, A., and Jacobson, D. R.: The effect of panretinal photocoagulation for rubeosis iridis: a preliminary report, Am. J. Ophthalmol. **81:**804, 1976.
14. Little, H. L., and Zweng, H. C.: Argon laser photocoagulation of disc neovascularization in diabetic retinopathy, Trans. Pac. Coast Otoophthalmol. Soc. **54:**123, 1973.
14a. Little, H. L., Zweng, H. C., Jack, R. L., and Vassiliadis, A.: Techniques of argon laser photocoagulation of diabetic disc new vessels, Am. J. Ophthalmol. **82:**675, 1977.
15. Machemer, R., and Norton, E. W. D.: A new concept for vitreous surgery. III. Indications and results, Am. J. Ophthalmol. **74:**1034, 1972.
16. Madsen, P. H.: Rubeosis of the iris and hemorrhagic glaucoma in patients with proliferative diabetic retinopathy, Br. J. Ophthalmol. **55:**368, 1971.
17. Madsen, P. H.: Hemorrhagic glaucoma: comparative study in diabetic and nondiabetic patients, Br. J. Ophthalmol. **55:**444, 1971.
18. Ohrt, V.: The frequency of rubeosis iridis in diabetic patients, Acta Ophthalmologica **49:**301, 1971.
19. Schulze, R. R.: Rubeosis iridis, Am. J. Ophthalmol. **63:**487, 1967.
20. Zweng, H. C., Fahrenbruch, R. C., and Little, H. L.: Argon laser photocoagulation in the treatment of retinal vein occlusions, Mod. Probl. Ophthalmol. **12:**261, 1974.

18
PARS PLANA VITRECTOMY

Microsurgical pars plana vitrectomy is becoming widely utilized. The complications of diabetic retinopathy, vitreous hemorrhage and traction retinal detachment, are the most common indications for this procedure. Diabetics received 76% of the first 150 pars plana vitrectomies reported by Machemer and Norton[3] and 51 of 100 consecutive pars plana vitrectomies reported by Michels and Ryan.[4]

Surgeons have commented on the increased success rate of pars plana vitrectomy in patients who previously had received heavy photocoagulation.[1] The reasons for this are related to the decrease in proliferative retinopathy following phocoagulation and the chorioretinal adhesions in the peripheral retina that are formed at the photocoagulation spots.

The uses of argon laser photocoagulation following pars plana vitrectomy in diabetic patients are (1) obliteration of neovascularization, (2) treatment of macular edema and circinate exudates, (3) delimitation of peripheral retinal detachments, (4) surrounding retinal breaks, (5) treatment of rubeosis iridis.

OBLITERATION OF NEOVASCULARIZATION

After pars plana vitrectomy, particularly in juvenile diabetics, many areas of neovascularization may arise from the optic nerve head, the vascular arcades, and the midperipheral retinal vessels. There is a significant risk of recurrent vitreous hemorrhage due to neovascularization, particularly if unrecognized vitreous strands connecting the areas of proliferans to the vitreous base are present. For this reason, in patients in whom active proliferative retinopathy is apparent after the vitreous compartment has been cleared of hemorrhage, we recommend argon laser photocoagulation as soon as the media have cleared sufficiently to allow placement of satisfactory photocoagulation lesions.

To facilitate photocoagulation soon after vitreous surgery, it is useful to avoid removal of the corneal epithelium during surgery. If the corneal epithelium is left intact, photocoagulation can be carried out even within the first few days postoperative. If the corneal epithelium is removed, there is slow regeneration, and often even after weeks or months, placement of a contact lens on the cornea results in sloughing of much of the corneal epithelium.

271

Photocoagulation for neovascularization is carried out in a manner identical to that in patients with diabetic retinopathy who have not had vitrectomy. Focal treatment is carried out to areas of neovascular proliferative fronds, and in addition, areas of nonperfused retina peripheral to the proliferans are photocoagulated with densely packed lesions. In addition, panretinal photocoagulation is performed (see Chapter 14).

TREATMENT OF MACULAR EDEMA AND CIRCINATE EXUDATES

Frequently in older diabetic patients, macular edema or circinate exudates may be apparent in the macular region after vitreous hemorrhage has been cleared with pars plana vitrectomy. In such cases fluorescein angiography should be carried out as soon as the media are clear enough to permit it, and areas of focal leakage and microaneurysms in the center of circinate complexes should be treated with argon laser photocoagulation in a manner similar to that utilized in patients who have not had vitreous surgery[5] (see Chapter 14).

DELIMITATION OF PERIPHERAL RETINAL DETACHMENTS

The production of iatrogenic retinal breaks, particularly peripheral retinal breaks with resultant retinal detachment, is a significant complication of pars plana vitrectomy. Michels and Ryan[4] noted production of retinal tears in 37 of 100 eyes on which they did pars plana vitreous surgery. If such tears are not recognized and treated at the time of surgery, peripheral or total retinal detachments may result. We have treated successfully two peripheral retinal detachments following pars plana vitreous surgery in two diabetic patients with argon laser photocoagulation to delimit the detachments. Both of these patients have been followed up for over 1 year, with no change in the extent of detachment following delimitation. They were treated as described in Chapter 6.

SURROUNDING RETINAL BREAKS

As noted above, iatrogenic retinal tears occur with pars plana vitreous surgery. Retinal breaks in the posterior polar area may result from traction on vitreous bands attaching to the retina posteriorly. Occasionally, tears may occur and the surrounding retina may remain flat. Photocoagulation to surround the retinal breaks may be carried out to reduce the risk of retinal detachment (see Chapter 6).

TREATMENT OF RUBEOSIS IRIDIS

Rubeosis iridis and neovascular glaucoma are recognized complications of pars plana vitrectomy. Rubeosis iridis occurred in 12% of 53 diabetic eyes in a series reported by Machemer and Norton[3] and in 11% of 100 eyes, of which 51 were diabetic, reported by Michels and Ryan.[4] Factors influencing the presence of rubeosis after vitrectomy appear to include the presence of active proliferative retinopathy and surgical aphakia.

The pathogenesis of rubeosis iridis is thought to be the same as that of proliferative diabetic retinopathy; that is, hypoxic retina releases a vasoproliferative or vasoformative factor that causes both retinal and iris neovascularization. The initial observation of the involutional effect of panretinal argon laser photocoagulation on rubeosis iridis was made in 1972 in a patient who had disc neovascularization combined with severe rubeosis iridis. After panretinal photocoagulation was carried out, and concomitant with regression of the disc neovascularization, there was regression and disappearance of the rubeosis iridis. Therefore, a method of treatment that reduces the stimulus to retinal neovascularization might also limit the stimulus to iris neovascularization. To test this hypothesis, a prospective study was carried out by the Palo Alto Retinal Medical Group and the Stanford University Division of Ophthalmology to ascertain the effect of panretinal photocoagulation on rubeosis iridis.[2] As reported by Little et al.,[2] this procedure was successful in 12 of 15 eyes treated by panretinal photocoagulation. Hence, it is recommended in postvitrectomy patients with rubeosis, as well as in eyes with rubeosis iridis from diabetes and retinal venous occlusions.

We have used panretinal photocoagulation as previously described (see Chapter 14) in five eyes with rubeosis iridis and proliferative diabetic retinopathy after pars plana vitrectomy.[1] None had had previous photocoagulation. One eye had severe rubeosis before surgery; the other four developed it after. In four of the five eyes, complete regression of the rubeosis occurred. In the fifth, regression was incomplete, perhaps because the pupil did not dilate well, so photocoagulation could not be done in the retinal periphery. On the basis of this small experience and the experience referred to in Chapters 16 and 17 in successfully treating some eyes with rubeosis from proliferative diabetic retinopathy and retinal vein occlusions with panretinal photocoagulation, we suggest that PRP is beneficial in treating diabetic eyes with rubeosis iridis after pars plana vitrectomy.

REFERENCES

1. Jack, R. L., and Little, H. L.: Uses of argon laser photocoagulation following pars plana vitrectomy. In L'Esperance, F. A., Jr., editor: Current diagnosis and management of chorioretinal diseases, St. Louis, 1977, The C. V. Mosby Co.
2. Little, H. L., Rosenthal, A. R., Dellaporta, A., and Jacobson, D.: The effect of panretinal photocoagulation for rubeosis iridis—a preliminary report, Am. J. Ophthalmol. **81:**804, 1976.
3. Machemer, R., and Norton, E. W. D.: A new concept for vitreous surgery. III. Indications and results, Am. J. Ophthalmol. **74:**1034, 1972.
4. Michels, R. G., and Ryan, S. J.: Results and complications of 100 consecutive cases of pars plana vitrectomy, Am. J. Ophthalmol. **80:**24, 1975.
5. Zweng, H. C., Little, H. L., and Peabody, R.: Further observations on argon laser photocoagulation of diabetic retinopathy, Trans. Am. Acad. Ophthalmol. Otolaryngol. **76:**990, 1972.

19

TUMORS

Photocoagulation of tumors of the fundus of the eye was first carried out by Meyer-Schwickerath and reported by him in his monograph on light and coagulation.[6] In that monograph, he discusses his early results in the treatment of photocoagulation of melanomas of the choroid, choroidal metastases from carcinoma of the breast, retinoblastoma, and angiomatosis retinae (von Hippel–Lindau disease). Although his experience at that time was limited, early results were promising enough to encourage the group at University Eye Hospital (Essen, Germany) to continue their experimentation in the treatment of ocular tumors with photocoagulation.

CHOROIDAL MELANOMAS

Experience with presumed choroidal melanomas treated by photocoagulation has been reported further by Meyer-Schwickerath, and by Vogel and Schmitz-Valckenberg, alone and in collaboration.[4,5,7,8,10] Although photocoagulation of these tumors remains a controversial subject in ophthalmology, their results with a large series of patients indicate that photocoagulation should continue to be given serious consideration as an alternative to enucleation in certain instances. In their most recent report,[11] Vogel and Schmitz-Valckenberg state that no patient in whom they considered the tumor destroyed, as seen on funduscopic and angiographic studies, has died of metastases. They make plain that a considerable period of follow-up will be necessary in order to compare their group with untreated series reported in the literature.

The clinical diagnosis of a melanoma of the choroid is occasionally difficult. Typically, the lesion appears as a slate-gray elevated mass, sometimes with overlying sensory retinal detachment, usually depending on the size of the tumor. It can occur anywhere in the choroid. Lipofusin, an orange pigment, is sometimes seen on the surface. Typically, these tumors do not transilluminate, but for amelanotic tumors, this test can be equivocal. The fluorescein angiogram demonstrates blotchy fluorescence, generally beginning in the venous phase, presumably due to leakage of serum from the vessels in the tumor and to alteration of the

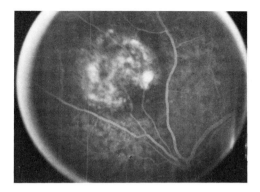

Fig. 19-1. Fluorescein angiogram of tumor in a 54-year-old man, which showed definite growth over a 1-year observation period. Angiogram demonstrates typical mottled fluorescence appearing in venous phase.

integrity of the overlying choriocapillaries (Fig. 19-1). All melanotic lesions should be photographed and measured on succeeding visits to determine whether any growth has occccured. Growth of a suspected melanotic lesion greatly increases the likelihood that it is malignant. If available, a ^{32}P test should be made, but unless done by an ophthalmologist experienced and skilled in this diagnostic technique, a negative finding is not significant. The differential diagnosis includes all pigmented lesions of the fundus. The more common lesions include pigmented nevus, a hemorrhage under the retinal pigment epithelium, inflammatory lesions that have accumulated considerable pigment in the healing phase, choroidal and retinal detachments, congenital hyperplasia of the retinal pigment epithelium, and pigmented hemartomas.

Our experience with presumed melanomas of the choroid is limited to nine cases, one treated with xenon arc photocoagulation and eight with argon laser photocoagulation. We have been interested in applying argon laser light to these tumors, because of the high absorption of the argon wavelengths by both melanin and hemoglobin, two pigments present in relative abundance in most melanomas (see Chapter 1). Follow-up time was 9 years for the eye treated with xenon arc photocoagulation and an average of 15 months for the others (a range from 7 to 27 months). No conclusion is possible on the basis of our experience to date, because much longer follow-up is needed to determine the efficacy of argon laser photocoagulation in these patients, as determined by the all-important tests of lack of metastases, as demonstrated by survival of the patient over a long period of time or, if death does occur from other causes, demonstration by histophathologic examination that the tumor was destroyed. As of this writing, all nine patients are living and well.

We have restricted our selection of presumed melanomas for treatment with argon laser photocoagulation to those that met the following criteria:

1. No evidence of direct extension outside the sclera or of metastatic spread.

2. Lateral measurement no greater than 6 disc diameters, or 9 mm, or 30°.
3. Elevation no greater than 3 diopters, or 1 mm.
4. Location where it is possible to photocoagulate around the tumor entirely, at least to an extent of approximately 1 mm. Melanomas adjacent to the nerve head or so far anterior that photocoagulation cannot be done around the anterior periphery should not be treated with this modality.
5. Lack of significant serous elevation over the tumor. Serous exudate between the tumor and the retina makes photocoagulation of the underlying tumor more difficult. A very small amount of fluid is not significant, but more than that seriously interferes with the photocoagulation process.
6. Media must be clear.
7. Consultative agreement. We never make a diagnosis of malignant melanoma of the choroid unless at least one, and preferably two, colleagues agrees.
8. Patient choice. The patient is, of course, apprised that, in our best judgment, there is a potentially lethal tumor within his eye. He is advised that the traditional method of treating the tumor is enucleation of the eye and that more conservative management (i.e., observation or photocoagulation) is experimental at this time. The patient is given three choices: enucleation, continued observation, or photocoagulation therapy. However, photocoagulation is suggested as one choice only if the tumor meets all criteria listed above. Both patient and spouse, if there is one, must understand the choice at hand, both must participate in the choice, and both must agree that argon laser photocoagulation therapy is the treatment they desire.

In treating presumed melanomas of the choroid, we use the following technique, after the patient has been given a topical anesthetic:

1. *Initial treatment.* The tumor is entirely ringed by a double or triple row of argon laser photocoagulation lesions, using settings of 500-μm spot-size diameter, 0.2- to 0.5-sec time exposure, and 1,000-mW power. The lesions are white and continuous, and must be heavy enough to destroy the choroidal circulation, as evidenced by the appearance of a ring of bare sclera around the tumor on follow-up visits (Figs. 19-2 to 19-4).
2. *Subsequent treatments.* Beginning 2 to 4 weeks after initial treatment, the tumor is treated (settings of 500 μm, 1 to 2 sec, and 1,000 mW). These heavy lesions are also white, and cause coagulative necrosis of the tumor and thrombosing of blood vessels (Fig. 19-5 and 19-6). The parameters used can give vapor bubbles in the retina and vitreous and can cause hemorrhages. Such heavy coagulation should be avoided on initial direct treatment of the tumor; however, on subsequent treatments, the energy delivered to the tumor is increased up to levels that produce bubbles. Subsequent treatment setting of 500 μm, 1 to 2 sec, and 1,500 to 2,000 mW are used at approximately 1-month intervals until the tumor

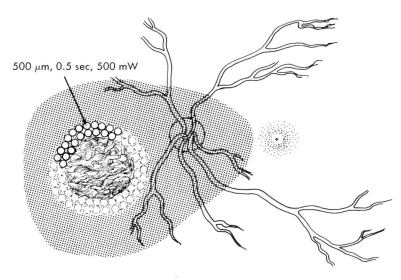

500 μm, 0.5 sec, 500 mW

Fig. 19-2. Drawing representing technique of initial argon laser photocoagulation of presumed malignant melanoma of choroid, showing location and settings of lesions used at first treatment.

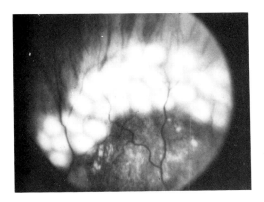

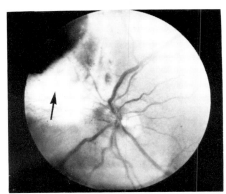

Fig. 19-3   Fig. 19-4

Fig. 19-3. Fundus photograph showing typical appearance of two or three rows of lesions placed in close juxtaposition, completely surrounding tumor before tumor itself is treated. (500-μm spot size diameter, 0.5-sec time duration, 1,000 mW power.)

Fig. 19-4. Fundus photograph of tumor (Fig. 19-1), demonstrating appearance of bare sclera around tumor as a result of heavy treatment *(arrow)*.

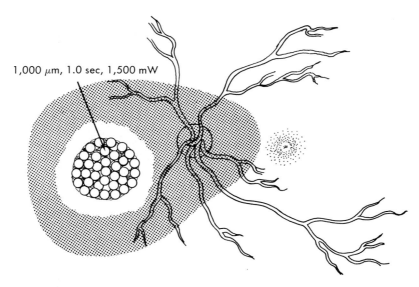

1,000 μm, 1.0 sec, 1,500 mW

Fig. 19-5. Diagram representing technique of direct treatment of malignant melanoma by ALP. This treatment follows initial one by 2 weeks to 1 month. Settings produce very heavy lesions, including vapor bubbles.

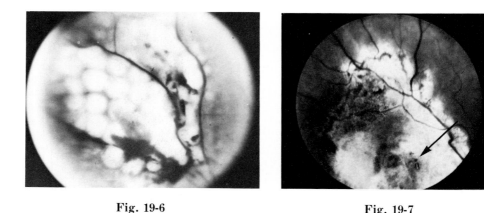

Fig. 19-6   **Fig. 19-7**

Fig. 19-6. Fundus photograph taken immediately after second treatment of tumor (Fig. 19-1). Lesions are heavy, as evidenced by chalk-white appearance. (500 μm, 1 to 2 sec, 1,500 mW.)

Fig. 19-7. Fundus photograph of tumor after series of treatments, showing typical atrophy of retina and avascular pigmentation on sclera *(arrow)*. Denser pigmentation due to photocoagulation.

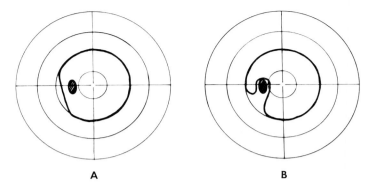

Fig. 19-8. A, Visual field before treatment, showing decreased visual sensitivity in quadrant in which tumor is located. **B,** Postoperative visual field 10 days after first treatment shows inferior temporal quadrant nerve fiber bundle field defect clearly associated with area of heavy treatment. (Same patient as in Figs. 19-1, 19-3, 19-4, 19-6, and 19-7.)

is flat or, preferably, is replaced by an excavation. Often, there remains a faint amount of what appears to be acellular pigmentation on the sclera, marking the site of the previous tumor (Fig. 19-7). Six or seven treatment sessions are usually required.

Follow-up examinations, once the tumor appears clinically to have been destroyed, are given every 3 months. The patient is followed up by his internist concurrently for any evidence of metastases. Visual-field examination shows a nerve fiber layer type of defect peripheral to the tumor (Fig. 19-8).

Apple et al.[1] have demonstrated that a single treatment with argon laser photocoagulation is not sufficient to destroy more than the cells in a surface mantle of photocoagulation. We stress that we do *not* advocate a similar single treatment mode of therapy.

CHOROIDAL HEMANGIOMAS

Hemangiomas of the choroid are usually asymptomatic; if they remain so, they need only to be watched with retinal photography and fluorescein angiography. Typically, these tumors are relatively flat and show an orange-fawn discoloration underlying the retina. There may be some serous exudation under the retina, elevating it; if the serous elevation involves the macula and especially the fovea, central vision is interfered with. Usually, the decrease in vision and degree of metamorphopsia are not severe unless the exudative detachment is high. These tumors are most easily recognized with binocular indirect ophthalmoscopy, because their orange-fawn color is seen beneath the usual serous elevation of the overlying sensory retina. They are usually situated in the posterior fundus. Fluorescein angiography demonstrates very early fluorescence, seen in the arterial phase (Fig. 19-9, *A*). The fluorescence is generally heavy, because of the nature of the tumor, a collection of thin-walled blood vessels with little pigment.

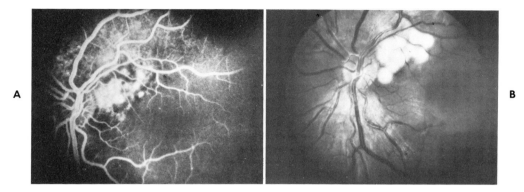

Fig. 19-9. A, Fluorescein angiogram of patient with choroidal hemangioma near disc, showing typical strong fluorescence due to extensive thin-walled blood vessels. VA, 20/50, due to serous retinal elevation extending into fovea. **B,** Photograph showing fundus appearance immediately after treatment. (500 μm, 0.5 sec, 500 mW.)

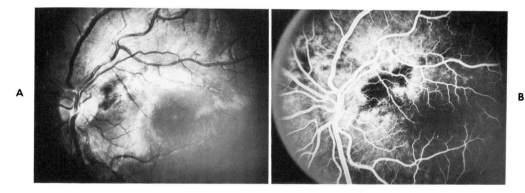

Fig. 19-10. A, Photograph of fundus (Fig. 19-7) 3 months after treatment, showing heavy pigmentation. Sensory retinal detachment has resolved. VA, returned to 20/20. **B,** Fluorescein angiogram of area 3 months after treatment; no fluorescence where highly fluorescent tumor had initially been treated (see Fig. 19-7, *A*). A small amount of residual leakage prompted further treatment, resulting in complete resolution.

Threatened loss of central vision is indication for treatment. Both diathermy and photocoagulation have been used.[2,3,9]

The technique we have used is as follows. The patient is given a topical anesthetic. Then the tumor is treated with heavy lesions of argon laser photocoagulation (Fig. 19-9, *B*). Settings used are 500-μm spot-size diameter, 0.5-sec exposure, and 500 to 700 mW of power. The patient is seen after 6 weeks (Fig. 19-10). Not all the tumor need be destroyed; because symptoms come from the exudative detachment of the sensory retina, destruction of only enough tumor to end that detachment is sufficient. Treatment should not come any closer than 300 μm to the fovea, lest there be photocoagulation damage to the fovea from the relatively heavy lesions used.

The prognosis for argon laser photocoagulation treatment of choroidal hemangiomas is excellent.

RETINAL ANGIOMATOSIS

Angiomatosis retinae (von Hippel–Lindau disease) is a disease entity that initially is manifested by red or orange-red tumors varying in size from barely visible

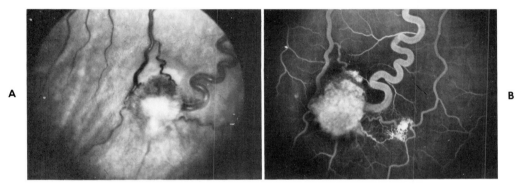

Fig. 19-11. A, Photograph of von Hippel–Lindau tumor, showing feeder and collector vessels. Collector vessel, to right of tumor in photograph, is more dilated and tortuous than is feeder. There is slight local detachment of sensory retina. **B,** Fluorescein angiogram clearly showing feeder and collector vessels and heavy fluorescence of tumor itself.

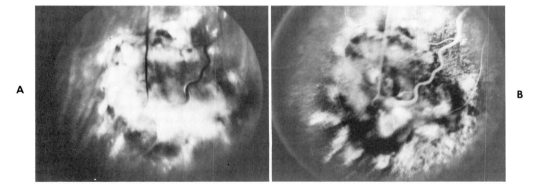

Fig. 19-12. A, Fundus photograph of tumor (Fig. 19-9) after repeated heavy treatments directed to tumor. Feeder and collector vessels not treated. (500 μm, 0.5 sec, 500 mW.) **B,** Fluorescein angiogram of tumor after treatment, showing shrinkage of tumor and also of feeder and collector vessels. Hyperpigmentation due to argon laser photocoagulation.

to large enough to result in massive exudation under the retina, giving retinal detachment. Most typically, both the feeder and collector vessels are extremely dilated and tortuous (Fig. 19-11). There can be some local detachment of the sensory retina, with exudation at the edges of the elevation. These tumors can be found in the course of a routine eye examination, but they more generally are found when macular vision has been impinged on, either by an exudative retinal detachment or by traction on the macular retinal epithelium. Inasmuch as the condition is frequently bilateral and multicentral, both eyes must be carefully examined for other tumors.

Discovery of the lesion is indication for treatment with argon laser photocoagulation. However, if the retina is highly elevated over the angioma, photocoagulation treatment is impossible, and cryotherapy or diathermy must be considered.[12]

The technique of argon laser photocoagulation therapy is direct treatment to the lesion rather than to the feeder vessels. The settings used are 500-μm spot-size diameter, 0.5-sec time exposure, and 500 mW of power. One should attempt to induce gradual shrinkage of the tumor over four to eight sessions of treatment. By inducing increased pigmentation around and on the lesion, there is a greater reaction to treatment and more rapid shrinkage of the tumor (Fig. 19-12). In contrast to the treatment of choroidal melanomas, explosive lesions are not used. Because hemorrhage and exudative retinal detachment frequently occur, intervals of 2 to 4 weeks should elapse between treatment sessions. Every effort must be made to treat with larger spot sizes so that hemorrhage does not occur; therefore, spot sizes smaller than 500 μm should not be used.

REFERENCES

1. Apple, D. E., et al.: Argon laser photocoagulation of choroidal malignant melanoma, Arch. Ophthalmol. **90**:97, 1973.
2. Dufour, R.: Angiome de la choroide simulant un mélanome, Ophthalmologica **127**:249, 1954.
3. MacLean, A. L., and Maumenee, A. E.: Hemangioma of the choroid, Trans. Am. Ophthalmol. Soc. **57**:171, 1959.
4. Meyer-Schwickerath, G.: Lichtkoagulation bucherei des augenarztes, Klin. Monatsbl. Augenheilkd. **33**:70, 1959.
5. Meyer-Schwickerath, G.: Die Moglichkeiten zur Behandlung intraocularer Tumoren unter Erhaltung des Schvermogens, Ber. Dtsch. Ophtholmol. Ges. **63**:178, 1960.
6. Meyer-Schwickerath, G.: Light coagulation, St. Louis, 1960, The C. V. Mosby Co.
7. Meyer-Schwickerath, G.: The preservation of vision by treatment of intraocular tumors with light coagulation, Arch. Ophthalmol. **66**:458, 1961.
8. Meyer-Schwickerath, G.: Malignant melanoma of the choroid treated with photocoagulation; a 10-year follow up. Mod. Probl. Ophthalmol. **12**(0):544-549, 1974.
9. Schepens, C. L., and Schwartz, A.: Intraocular tumors, Arch. Ophthalmol. **60**:72, 1958.
10. Vogel, M. H., and Schmitz-Valckenberg, P.: Treatment of malignant choroidal melanomas with photocoagulation; evaluation of 10-year follow-up data, Am. J. Ophthalmol. **74**:1, 1972.
11. Vogel, M. H., and Schmitz-Valckenberg, P.: Photocoagulation treatment of small malignant melanomas of the choroid. In L'Esperance, F. A.: Current diagnosis and management of chorioretinal diseases, St. Louis, 1977, The C. V. Mosby Co.
12. Weve, H.: Bowman Lecture: Diathermy in ophthalmic practice, Trans. Ophthalmol. Soc. U.K. **59**:43-80, 1939.

20
IRIS AND CONJUNCTIVA

Although photocoagulation has been applied primarily to the posterior segment of the eye, the presence of pigment in the anterior segment makes possible the application of this treatment modality to the front of the eye as well. We have found argon laser photocoagulation useful in treating anterior segment problems.

IRIS
Peripheral iridectomy

Surgical peripheral iridectomy in narrow-angle glaucoma is a well-established procedure, deservedly popular because of its effectiveness and relative safety. Laser peripheral iridectomy, if effective, has several advantages: (1) it does not require an incision that opens the eye, (2) the patient does not require a retrobulbar block anesthetic, and (3) it can be done on outpatients. With these potential advantages, we suggest that laser peripheral iridectomy techniques be evaluated fully to determine if the procedure is as effective as and perhaps safer and simpler than surgical iridectomy.

Early experiments with pulsed ruby and neodymium lasers were very successful in animals, particularly rabbits.[8] Experiments with the argon laser in rhesus monkeys were not encouraging because of the difficulty of obtaining satisfactory iridectomies without lenticular damage. Later application of the ruby laser in humans was found satisfactory in brown eyes but not in blue eyes, and neodymium and argon lasers were found disappointing.[3] More recently, Abraham[1] reported successful argon laser iridectomies using a two-step method. We have used this two-stage technique successfully. L'Esperance has described another technique, which we have not used.[6]

Creation of iris hump (Fig. 20-1). This procedure is done without the use of the corneal diagnostic contact lens. The iris must be treated with 2% pilocarpine or comparable miotic before treatment, one drop every 10 minutes, five times, or humping of the iris will not occur. The beam is applied to the temporal portion of the iris at right angles to the iris, about one third of the distance between the iris root and the pupillary margin, in the 10 o'clock meridian of the right eye and 2 o'clock in the left eye. Parameters used are 200-μm spot size, 0.1- to 0.2-sec ex-

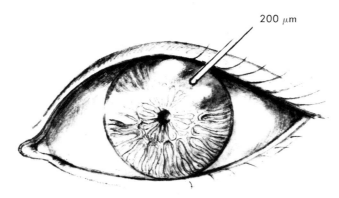

Fig. 20-1. Drawing showing nonpenetrating argon laser application to iris to create elevation on either side of lesion.

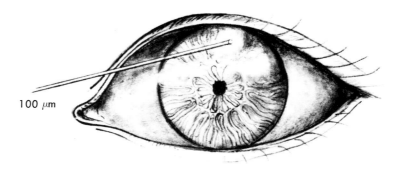

Fig. 20-2. Drawing showing penetrating argon laser application to one of iris elevations.

posure, and 500 mW of power. On either side of the single application, an elevation of the iris (iris hump) usually occurs in the 9 and 11 o'clock meridians in the right eye and 1 and 3 o'clock in the left eye. The elevation is useful to create the iridectomy without serious injury to the lens.

Iridectomy (Fig. 20-2). A diagnostic three-mirror contact lens is placed on the cornea because the applications must be made obliquely by way of one of the peripheral mirrors; thus, when the beam burns through the iris, the beam will not burn the retina, since it is directed peripherally. The treatment is directed to either of the iris elevations previously made. Multiple applications are directed to the top of the elevation, using 50 or 100 μm, 1 sec, and 1,000 to 1,500 mW. Blue irides are definitely easier to penetrate than are brown; hence the need for specifying a range of power settings.

Bubbles appear immediately as the iris tissue is vaporized. If the vapor bubbles remain in the crater but the iris has not yet been penetrated, halt the

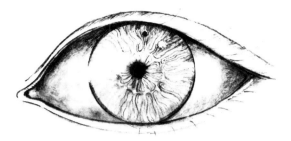

Fig. 20-3. Drawing showing iridectomy made after argon laser photocoagulation application to iris elevation.

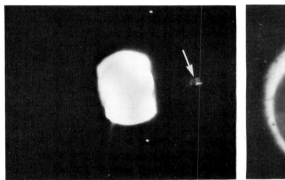 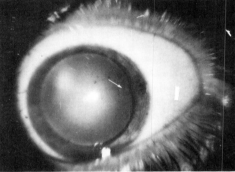

Fig. 20-4   **Fig. 20-5**

Fig. 20-4. Photograph showing peripheral iridectomy *(arrow)*. Light is seen reflected from retina through opening made with argon laser photocoagulation.

Fig. 20-5. Photograph showing dotlike opacity *(arrow)* in anterior lens capsule, which developed during argon laser iridectomy. Opacity has not changed after 1 year.

procedure until the bubbles float out of the crater. Sometimes if the iris appears very thin but no clear iridectomy is made at the time of treatment, examination over the next several weeks will reveal iris atrophy and a functioning iridectomy (Fig. 20-3). However, it is best to see a hole by light reflected through the pupil at the time of the procedure.

The patient's usual antiglaucoma medications are continued until the ophthalmologist is sure that they are no longer needed.

We have created iris iridectomies on nine patients with proved narrow-angle glaucoma (Fig. 20-4). In two patients, both with brown irides, two treatment sessions were required. Postoperatively, the intraocular pressures in the nine eyes did not increase on pupillary dilation, as they had preoperatively.

COMPLICATIONS

We have encountered the following complications of treatment. Corneal burns are usual with the iridectomy settings. When they occur, the beam must be directed around them, since they diffuse the beam. With the settings used, we have noted only epithelial burns, which heal without scarring. Since there is a danger of stromal scarring, however, the ophthalmologist should take care that the beam is not passing through the optical center of the cornea.

In several eyes a dotlike opacity developed on the anterior lens surface at the time of treatment; the opacities have not enlarged (Fig. 20-5).

Iritic reaction is invariable after treatment: iris pigment, flecks of iris tissue, and increased aqueous flare are present at the end of a treatment session. However, in our experience the eye is surprisingly clear the next day. Nonetheless, we suggest the use of topical steroids (1% prednisolone acetate [Pred-Forte]) every 2 hours for a total of six doses on the day of treatment.

Pain is usually mild postoperatively, consisting of an eye or orbital ache. Its duration is about 24 hours.

Laser iridectomy merits full-scale investigation to determine if it should be considered, along with surgical iridectomy, as a valid therapeutic modality in the treatment of narrow-angle glaucoma.

Laser coreoplasty

Optical distortions, or in extreme cases actual occlusion of the pupil, induced by displacement, is treatable in the phakic as well as the aphakic eye by argon laser photocoagulation. The pupillary displacement may be due to trauma (Fig. 20-6, *A*), including surgery, or it may be congenital. Serious interference with vision, from the optical distortion induced by the displaced pupil, is the indication for therapy. The only requirement for treatment is that there be enough iris tissue to respond to the retraction induced by photocoagulation.

The procedure is carried out with the patient under topical anesthesia. Argon laser applications are made about 1 mm from the edge of the pupil. A double row of applications is made, approximating the arc of the pupil. Parameters used are 500 μm, 0.1 to 0.2 sec, 500 mW. During the procedure, there is a gathering of the iris at each coagulation point; the procedure is continued until the pupil is satisfactorily retracted (Fig. 20-6, *B*). Postoperatively, the eye is treated with 1% atropine sulfate solution, one drop three times a day for 1 week. The iris may be re-treated, if necessary.

Iris hemangiomas

Iris hemangiomas are rare, but they can give symptoms of blurred vision, due to intermittent bleeding. These structures are usually difficult to find and often are identified only on a fluoroangiogram (Fig. 20-7, *A*). If a patient complains of blurred vision and erythrocytes are found in the anterior chamber, either as a frank hyphema or as cells dispersed in the aqueous humor, a fluoroangiogram of

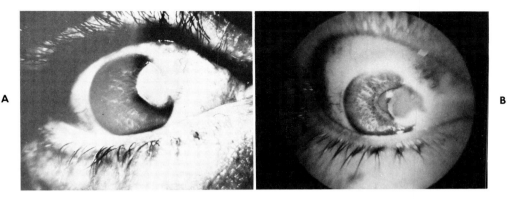

Fig. 20-6. A, Photograph of anterior segment of eye 12 years after penetrating injury. Iris drawn up to adherent leukoma. Lens was thought to be present. VA, light projection. **B,** Photograph immediately after pupillary margin had been treated with argon laser photocoagulation. VA, 20/25.

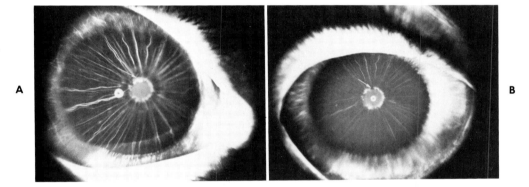

Fig. 20-7. A, Fluoroangiogram of presumed iris hemangioma *(arrow)* at pupillary margin. Patient noted blurred vision 1 week previously. A tiny hyphema was present, with a thin wisp of blood clot adherent to pupil at 11 o'clock. **B,** Fluoroangiogram showing absence of presumed iris hemangioma *(arrow)* 2 weeks after treatment with argon laser photocoagulation.

the anterior segment is indicated. The angiogram must be taken with the pupil at it usual diameter; if the pupil is dilated, the tiny hemangioma is impossible to find. Once the hemangioma is identified, argon laser photocoagulation may be carried out with the patient under topical anesthesia. The parameters used are 50 to 100 μm, 0.1 sec, 100 to 200 mW (Fig. 20-7, *B*). If the structure to be treated is on the pupillary border, great care must be taken to angle the treating beam so the retina is not coagulated. Generally, this can be accomplished by having the patient rotate the eye in such a way that the beam is directed very peripherally.

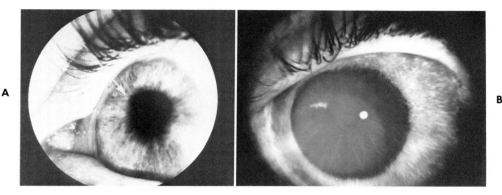

Fig. 20-8. A, Photograph of anterior segment of left eye of 15-year-old girl who had had three discissions of congenital cataract before age 6. A corneovitreal strand had been seen since last surgery. A sheaf of blood vessels was observed for 18 months, growing up strand to cornea. Patient referred for obliteration of vessels before cutting of strand. **B,** Fluoroangiogram showing fluorescence in vessels in vitreal strand.

Iris cysts

Implantation cysts after surgery or trauma, especially if enlarging, may be treated by argon laser photocoagulation.[6] First the posterior and then the anterior walls should be treated, in the same session. However, if the anterior wall is in contact with the cornea, or very nearly so, photocoagulation is dangerous because of potential damage to the corneal endothelium. In such instances, only the posterior wall should be treated. Because the treating beam is focused at the same plane as the viewing optics, the operator must be careful to have the respective walls in sharp focus when treating. Care must be taken not to risk coagulating the retina if the cyst is not lying anterior to the iris. The patient must rotate the eye in such a way that the beam, if it should pass through the cyst, is directed very peripherally. The procedure is done with topical anesthetic. The parameters used are 500 μm, 0.2 sec, 200 to 500 mW. The power is varied to obtain a medium burn. The cyst collapses in days to weeks. Re-treatment may be necessary.

Rubeosis irides

Successful treatment of this disease by panretinal photocoagulation of the retina is discussed in Chapter 17. We have attempted to destroy iris new vessels by direct application of argon laser photocoagulation. Immediate coagulation of vessels occurs, but they recur within 2 weeks.

Vascularized iridocyclitic membranes

Occasionally iridocyclitic membranes, which need to be discissed, are vascularized in the area where discission is required. Argon laser photocoagulation can be used to obliterate the new vessels so that discission can be carried out without hemorrhage.[6] The parameters used are 100 μm, 0.1 sec, and 200 to 300 mW, varying the power to occlude the vessels. Again, the eye must be rotated so that if the beam should pass through the membrane (unlikely in a membrane dense enough to need discission), it will be directed peripherally. Only a short time should pass between the photocoagulation procedure and the planned discission, because the vessels tend to reopen.

Neovascularization of corneovitreal adhesions

Rarely, a strand of vitreous attached to the cornea will become vascularized (Fig. 20-8). Argon laser photocoagulation may be carried out to obliterate the new vessels before the vitreal strand is divided surgically, lest hemorrhage occur at the time of the surgery. Because the new vessels are in a relatively transparent medium, obliterating them requires very accurate placement of the beam; thus, retrobulbar anesthetic is required. The parameters used are 50 μm, 0.1 to 0.2 sec, 200 to 400 mW. Exposures are made repeatedly to interrupt blood flow, to create segments of blood in the vessel. Then the segmented stationary blood is coagulated, occluding the vessel. The vascular strand must be inspected daily for at least 3 days to be certain that the vessels have been destroyed.

CONJUNCTIVA
Hemangiomas

Hemangioma of the conjunctiva is frequently a disfiguring aspect of Sturge-Weber syndrome. As with choroidal hemangiomas, the wavelengths of the argon

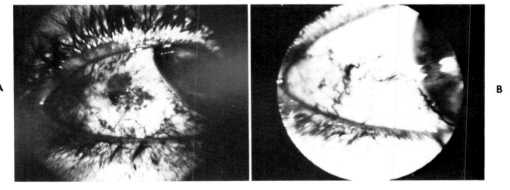

A

B

Fig. 20-9. A, Photograph showing conjunctival hemangiomas in right eye of 12-year-old white girl with Sturge-Weber disease. Eye was under treatment for glaucoma. Photograph taken before treatment with argon laser photocoagulation. **B,** Photograph 15 months after argon laser photocoagulation first given. Three treatments were given: 588 exposures first, 256 after 1 week, and 218 11 months later.

laser photocoagulator are absorbed well by the nubbins and sheets of blood vessels in the conjunctival tumors.

The technique can be carried out with the patient under topical anesthesia, particularly 4% lidocaine (Xylocaine). However, if the patient notes any discomfort from topical anesthetic, subconjunctival injection of 1% or 2% lydocaine *without* epinephrine renders the procedure painless.

The abnormal vessels are treated with repeated exposures of argon laser photocoagulation, using settings of 500 to 1,000 μm, 0.1 to 0.2 sec, and 700 to 1,000 mW. Subconjunctival hemorrhage sometimes occurs but is not an important complication. Treatments are repeated approximately monthly until the cosmetic result is satisfactory to the patient (Fig. 20-9).

Suture removal

Corneoscleral sutures are easily removed with the aid of argon laser photocoagulation. At times, subconjunctival sutures, especially nylon, erode through the conjunctiva and give a scratchy sensation under the upper lid and moderate mucoid discharge (Fig. 20-10). Because only the tip of one arm of the suture is often exposed, removal by scissors or razor blade and forceps is difficult for both patient and ophthalmic surgeon. Settings useful in removing such sutures are 50 μm, 0.05 sec, 1,000 mW. The suture is severed at the point where it emerges from the conjunctiva; the distal end is then lifted off the conjunctiva with forceps. If the exposed suture is only a very short segment (up to 2 mm), often the entire segment is vaporized with treatment.

When corneoscleral sutures are not buried under the conjunctival flap, removal with argon laser photocoagulation is facilitated by using the same settings, directing the beam on one loop of the knot, severing it, and lifting the suture off the limbus.

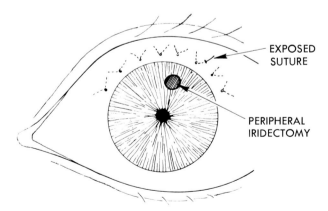

EXPOSED SUTURE

PERIPHERAL IRIDECTOMY

Fig. 20-10. Diagram showing exposed end of corneoscleral suture used in cataract surgery. Suture has eroded through conjunctiva and is irritating to undersurface of upper lid, especially if made of nylon.

OTHER APPLICATIONS

Numerous other applications have been reported. Thus, the argon laser has been used successfully to produce an iridotomy for aphakic pupillary block[2] after cataract extraction. Another application of the argon laser has been for photomydriasis for debilitating pupillary miosis, as proposed and used by L'Esperance.[6] Finally, perhaps the most interesting future application is the use of lasers for modification of angle structures. Originally reported by Krasnov[4] in 1972 and discussed more recently[5] in a 3-year follow-up study, goniopuncture is an interesting approach to the treatment of glaucoma. Although Krasnov has tried other lasers, he reported the Q-switched ruby as the most successful he employed for the goniopuncture procedure. The argon laser has also shown some limited success in similar experimental procedures on the angle structures.[7]

REFERENCES

1. Abraham, R. K., and Miller, G. L.: Outpatient argon laser iridectomy for angle closure glaucoma; a two-year study, Trans. Am. Acad. Ophthalmol. Otolaryngol. **79:**529, 1975.
2. Anderson, D. R., Forster, R. K., and Lewis, M. L.: Laser iridotomy for aphakic pupillary block, Arch. Ophthalmol. **93:**343, 1975.
3. Beckman, H., and Sugar, H. S.: Laser iridectomy therapy of glaucoma, Arch. Ophthalmol. **90:**453, 1973.
4. Krasnov, M. M.: Laseropuncture of anterior chamber angle in glaucoma, Am. J. Ophthalmol. **75:**674-678, 1973.
5. Krasnov, M. M.: Q-switched laser goniopuncture, Arch. Ophthalmol. **92:**37, 1974.
6. L'Esperance, F. A.: Ocular photocoagulation; a stereoscopic atlas, St. Louis, 1975, The C. V. Mosby Co.
7. Ticho, U., and Zauberman, H.: Argon laser applications to the angle structures in the glaucomas, Arch. Ophthalmol. **94:**61, 1976.
8. Zweng, H. C., Paris, G. L., Vassiliadis, A., et al.: Laser photocoagulation of the iris, Arch. Ophthalmol. **84:**193, 1970.

21
COMPLICATIONS

Argon laser photocoagulation provides a new modality for the treatment of retinal and choroidal vascular diseases. We introduced and described the advantages of argon laser slit-lamp photocoagulation at the 1969 American Academy of Ophthalmology.[6] Specifically, the argon laser is ideal for the treatment of retinal vascular lesions and for the coagulation of retinal pigment eipithelium, because the argon wavelengths are highly absorbed by blood vessels and pigment epithelial cells. Thus, retinal vessels can be coagulated, whether they are on the surface of the retina or the disc or are proliferating into the vitreous cavity. Furthermore, the laser burns stimulate retinal pigment epithelium to proliferate sealing of retinal tears, and intense burns can obliterate choroidal vascular lesions underneath the retinal pigment epithelium.

Certain complications have resulted from argon laser retinal photocoagulation of various ocular diseases. These various complications and the means by which many of them can be avoided are discussed on the following pages.

In a 5-year period from May 1969 through February 1974, we used argon laser photocoagulation to treat 1,886 eyes in 1,617 patients. A total of 6,148 treatments were performed, averaging a little over three treatments per eye (Table 21-1). The overall incidence of complications per treatment was 4.5%; the incidence of complications in eyes with diabetic retinopathy was 6% per treatment (Table 21-2). Inasmuch as eyes with diabetic retinopathy were treated an average of 4.6 times, the overall incidence of all complications, including a minute hemorrhage, was 27.8% per eye undergoing treatment for diabetic retinopathy (Table 21-2); however, the incidence of significant complications (i.e., those causing visual impairment or those that interrupted photocoagulation treatment either temporarily or permanently) was 0.44% per treatment, or 2.05% per diabetic eye undergoing multiple treatments.

These figures reflect our overall experience since beginning argon laser photocoagulation in May 1969. The incidence of complications was greatest between October 1970 and June 1971, when we were gaining experience with the more powerful commercially available argon laser photocoagulator just introduced,

292

Table 21-1. Total argon laser photocoagulation experience
(May 1969 to February 1974)

	Number	Percent incidence
Eyes	1,886	
Treatments	6,148	
Patients	1,617	
Eyes with diabetic retinopathy	831	44
Treatments for diabetic retinopathy	3,853	63
Patients with diabetic retinopathy	696	43

Table 21-2. Incidence of complications of argon laser photocoagulation
(May 1969 to February 1974)

	Number	Percent incidence
Total treatments	6,148	
Total complications	262	
Hemorrhages	191	
Incidence per treatment		4.5
Incidence per patient		13.9
Incidence per treatment of diabetics		6.0
Incidence per diabetic patient		27.8
Hemorrhage per treatment		4.4
(significant)		0.44
Hemorrhage per diabetic patient		20.5
(significant)		2.05

Table 21-3. Complications of argon laser photocoagulation per disease
(May 1969 to February 1974)

	Number of eyes	Percent incidence per treatment
Diabetic retinopathy	831	6.0
Senile macular degeneration	278	1.4
Central serous choroidopathy	142	—
Histoplasmic choroiditis	82	4.8
Eales's retinal vasculopathy	11	19.0
Retinal vein occlusions	101	0.9
Retinal tears	143	0.7

based on our prototype.[3,5,9] With improved techniques, the incidence of complications has been reduced significantly, as indicated by comparison of 3.4% incidence of serious complications between May 1969 and December 1971 with 1.7% incidence between January 1972 and February 1974.

The incidence of complications varied according to the disease being treated (Table 21-3). Hemorrhages per disease under treatment ranged from greatest to least frequency as follows: 19% in Eales's retinal vasculopathy, 6% in diabetic retinopathy (1% in nonproliferative retinopathy and 6% in proliferative retinopathy), 4.8% in histoplasmic choroiditis, 1.4% in exudative choroidal macular degeneration, and 0.9% in retinal vein occlusion.

One complication has occurred in the treatment of 143 retinal tears. None has occurred in the treatment of 112 eyes with central serous retinopathy and 30 eyes with diffuse retinal epitheliopathy.

With the exception of hemorrhage and recurrent neovascularization in the treatment of choroidal neovascularization in histoplasmic choroiditis, exudative choroidal macular degeneration, and Eales's retinal vasculopathy, 86% of all complications have occurred in eyes being treated for diabetic retinopathy. Inasmuch as 63% of all treatment sessions were for diabetic retinopathy, one would expect most of the complications to occur in this group; Table 21-4 summarizes the complications of argon laser retinal photocoagulation in the treatment of this disease. Hemorrhage was the most significant complication.

Table 21-4. Complications of argon laser photocoagulation in diabetic retinopathy (May 1969 to February 1974)

	Number of eyes	Percent per treatment
Retinal hemorrhage		
Insignificant	153	4.0
Significant	17	.44
Choroidal hemorrhage	8	.22
Visual-field defect	12	.31
Transient myopia	6	.15
Preretinal membrane contraction	6	.15
Traction detachment	5	.13
Corneal burn	4	.10
Exudative detachment	3	.075
Ischemic papillitis	2	.05
Cystoid macular edema	2	.05
Lenticular opacity	1	.025
Recurrent neovascularization		

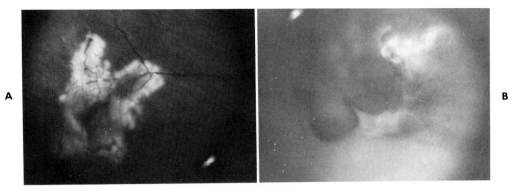

Fig. 21-1. A, Appearance of retinal neovascular frond immediately after photocoagulation. Note obstruction of large venous channel and failure to coagulate nonperfused retina peripheral to neovascular frond. **B,** Large preretinal and vitreal hemorrhage, which occurred 24 hours after photocoagulation of **A.**

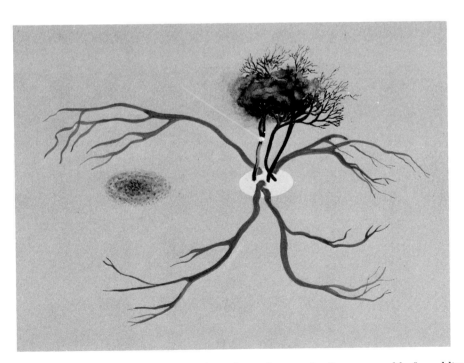

Fig. 21-2. Diagram of hemorrhage resulting from closure of collector vessel before obliterating feeder vessels and neovascular frond.

HEMORRHAGE FROM RETINAL VASCULATURE

Hemorrhage is the most frequent complication of retinal argon laser photocoagulation. It occurs most often from direct photocoagulation of retinal neovascularization, particularly when new vessels on the optic disc are treated (Fig. 21-1). The major cause of hemorrhage in the treatment of disc neovascularization is closure of collector (efferent) vessels before closure of feeder (afferent) vessels that carry blood to the neovascular frond (Fig. 21-2). Because blood is highly absorbent of the argon laser beam, such vascular occlusions produce immediate changes in the hemodynamics of retinal circulation. Sudden closure of venous or efferent channels causes vascular engorgement and hemorrhage; therefore, differentiation of arterial (afferent) vessels from venous (efferent) vessels is essential in reducing the complication of hemorrhage.

Retinal hemorrhage can be avoided by identifying the feeder vessels on arterial-phase angiograms (Fig. 21-3), by projection enlargement of the negative (Fig. 21-4), and by stereoscopic fluorescein angiograms. The feeder vessels, which are usually smaller and less plethoric than the collector channels, are photocoagulated first (Fig. 21-5). After treatment of the feeder vessels, the distal portion of the frond is treated (Fig. 21-6). The collector channels are treated last; larger venous channels should not be coagulated until 24 to 48 hours later, to make certain that the feeder vessels have not reopened.

The least hazardous technique that usually eradicates disc neovascular fronds and reduces the incidence of recurrent neovascularization is panretinal photocoagulation. This technique is employed to exert an indirect involutional effect on neovascularization. It was first suggested by Ámalric, with transcleral diathermy as the treatment modality.[2] It was later employed by Wessing and Meyer-Schwickerath,[7] using xenon arc, and by Aiello et al.,[1] using ruby laser.

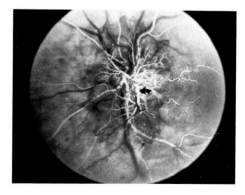

Fig. 21-3. Arterial phase of fluorescein angiogram assists in identification of arterial-feeder vessels *(arrow)* to diabetic neovascular frond off optic disc. (From Little, H. L., Zweng, H. C., Jack, R. L., and Vassiliadis, A.: Am. J. Ophthalmol. **82**(5):675-682, 1976.)

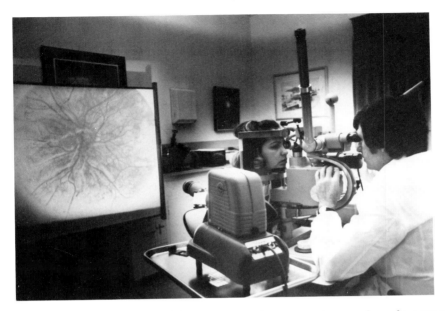

Fig. 21-4. Projection of negative of fluorescein angiogram produces enlarged image with distinct margins; in negative, fluorescein in feeder vessel is black. (From Little, H. L., Zweng, H. C., Jack, R. L., and Vassiliadis, A.: Am. J. Ophthalmol. **82**(5):675-682, 1976.)

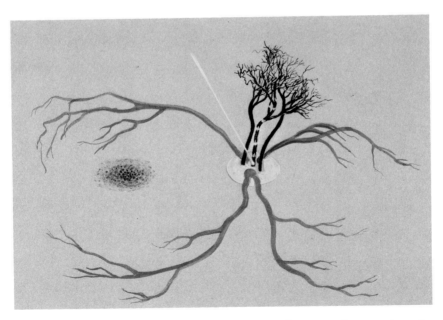

Fig. 21-5. Diagram of coagulation to feeder vessel (50-μm diameter beam).

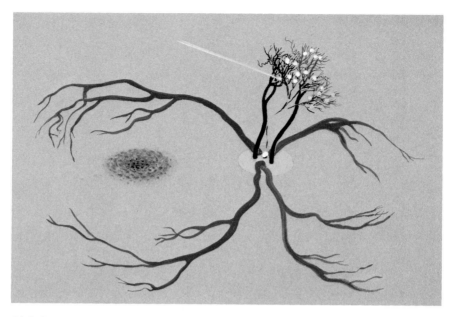

Fig. 21-6. Diagram of coagulation of neovascular frond after first occluding feeder vessel.

The technique consists of inducing an involution of neovascularization by producing diffuse chorioretinal scars similar to extensive chorioretinitis or to retinitis pigmentosa. This technique is discussed in Chapter 14.

HEMORRHAGES FROM CHOROIDAL VASCULATURE

The understanding of power density (see Chapter 1) is important in preventing hemorrhage. Power density is power per unit area. It varies inversely with the size of the photocoagulation beam on the retina. Reduction of the beam diameter from 200 to 100 μm reduces the area four times (area equals πr^2); if the power is unchanged, the power density is four times greater with the 100-μm beam diameter (Fig. 21-7).

In a biologic medium with blood supply, the heat generated in the irradiated area is dispersed by surrounding tissue. A small coagulation spot is cooled more rapidly than a large spot, because the center of the large one is further from the cooling area just outside the lesion (Fig. 21-8). In practice, when the beam diameter is halved, the output power of the laser must be halved.

Choroidal neovascularization is the primary cause of choroidal hemorrhages and hemorrhagic detachments of the retinal pigment epithelium. It occurs in hemorrhagic senile macular degeneration and in histoplasmic choroiditis. High magnification of the choroidal- and arterial-phase angiograms assists in the detection of choroidal neovascularization. Heavy photocoagulation with intense white burns on the entire area of choroidal neovascularization usually eliminates

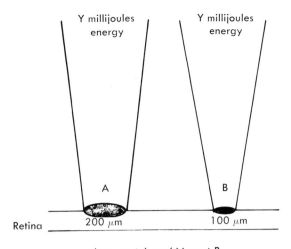

Area spot A = 4 × spot B

∴ Energy density spot B = 4 × spot A

Fig. 21-7. Area of lesions with 200-μm diameter equals four times area of lesion with 100-μm diameter. If same power is used, power density of 100-μm spot lesion is four times power density of 200-μm spot lesion.

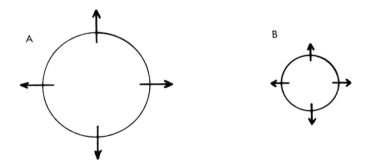

Fig. 21-8. Because of thermal conduction by surrounding tissues in a biologic medium, a small lesion is cooled faster than a large one.

it. Our experiences indicate that the techniques described in Chapters 11 and 12 markedly reduce this complication.

PRERETINAL MEMBRANE CONTRACTURE

Preretinal membrane contracture occurs with some of the disease entities treated with argon laser, particularly diabetic retinopathy, in which macular edema and preretinal striations frequently are present. Therefore, an accurate examination of the macula before treatment is essential.

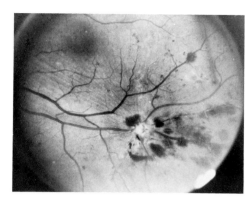

Fig. 21-9. Preretinal membrane contracture, retinal hemorrhage, and branch vein occlusion resulting from intense photocoagulation burn of neovascular frond at an arteriovenous juncture in diabetic retinopathy.

Preretinal membrane contracture has developed in seven eyes (Fig. 21-9). Six instances occurred with treatment of macular lesions or retinal neovascularization in the posterior fundus; one was noted 1 year after treatment of a peripheral retinal tear. Following treatment of preretinal hemorrhage, contracture of the internal limiting membrane has occurred, presumably from increased absorption of the beam by the blood, thus heating the internal limiting membrane and adjacent vitreous.

NERVE FIBER FIELD DEFECTS

Nerve fiber field defects occurred in eight cases (Fig. 21-10, *A*), usually after repeated photocoagulation about the optic disc. In the 2 to 4 weeks following coagulation, the retina becomes thin, and the nerve fiber layer is in closer proximity to the hyperplastic underlying retinal pigment epithelium, which causes absorption of the light and greater heating of the nerve fiber bundles. Under these conditions, it is best to treat over the disc rather than around it. When peripapillary photocoagulation is necessary, it is preferable to treat neovascular areas when the retina is of normal thickness rather than wait until the retina is thin following previous coagulation (Fig. 21-10, *B*). Nerve fiber field loss occurred only once with initial treatment. Nerve fiber field loss can result also from treatment of preretinal blood overlying the nerve fiber layer.

ISCHEMIC (THERMAL) PAPILLITIS

Two cases of ischemic papillitis have occurred from very heavy argon laser photocoagulation directed over the nerve head. Both were observed within 24 hours following coagulation with over 500 mW of power, 1- to 2-sec exposure times, and 200- to 500-μm spot sizes. Both patients had Marcus-Gunn pupillary phenomena and pale swollen nerve heads (Fig. 21-11). Each eye recovered visual acuity within 3 weeks following onset of the papillitis. When treating on the disc,

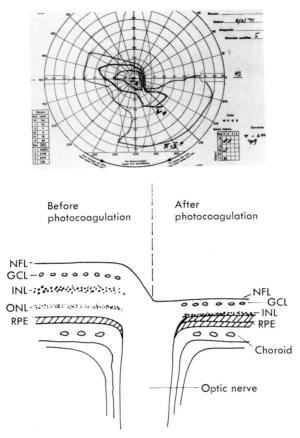

Before
photocoagulation

After
photocoagulation

NFL
GCL
INL
ONL
RPE

NFL
GCL
INL
RPE
Choroid

Optic nerve

Fig. 21-10. Nerve fiber visual field defect resulting from photocoagulation in peripapillary zone where nerve fiber layer is in close proximity to hyperplastic retinal pigment in chorioretinal scar after previous photocoagulation.

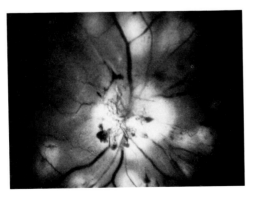

Fig. 21-11. Pale swollen nerve head of thermal papillitis seen 24 hours after intense photocoagulation on nerve head; ischemia resulted from treatment on nerve head. (200- and 500-μm, 400 and 800 mW, 1 sec.)

the beam should be focused on the abnormal vessels. With a beam diameter larger than 100 μm, unnecessary heating of the optic disc is likely to result. Ischemic papillitis should not occur if power levels are kept below 200 mW, spot sizes are kept below 200 μm, and exposure times do not exceed 0.2 sec, and focus of the beam is on the treated vessel rather than the nerve head.

RECURRENT NEOVASCULARIZATION
Retina

Two to 6 months after treatment, recurrent retinal neovascular tufts have developed adjacent to previously treated areas. In at least 40% of eyes with proliferative diabetic retinopathies, with treatment to the frond only, recurrent neovascularization ensues within 6 months (Fig. 21-12). This occurrence alerts the ophthalmologist to the need for continued observation of patients with diseases that make them prone to retinal neovascularization. The stimulus for recurrent proliferation of vessels can be minimized by coagulating areas of poorly perfused retina, noted with fluorescein angiography, which surround the areas of neovascularization; thereby, destruction of poorly perfused hypoxic retina eliminates the stimulus for neovascularization. Panretinal photocoagulation with a minimum of 2,500 medium- to large-diameter lesions is the best method of minimizing recurrent retinal neovascularization.

In addition to recurrent neovascularization on the optic disc, new growth of vessels occurs in the midperipheral or peripheral retina. Midperipheral and peripheral neovascularization occur at the anterior edge of the photocoagulation scars (Fig. 21-13, *A*). Such occurrences can be prevented by extending the panretinal photocoagulation lesions anterior to the equator in all meridians and by treating all areas of poorly perfused capillaries as noted on angiography or angioscopy (Fig. 21-13, *B*).

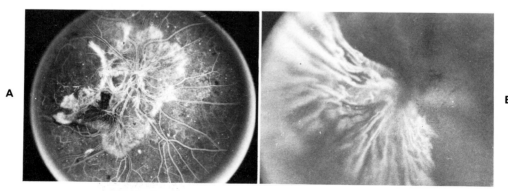

Fig. 21-12. A, Pretreatment appearance of diabetic disc neovascularization in plane of retina. **B,** Increased size of neovascular frond in **A,** which grew into vitreous cavity within 6 months after focal treatment to frond.

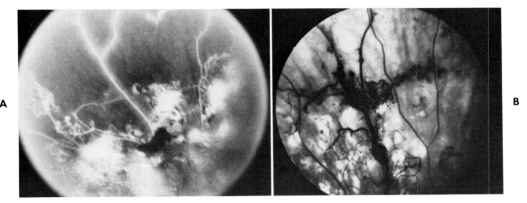

Fig. 21-13. A, Recurrent retinal neovascularization along anterior edge of panretinal photocoagulation lesions. **B,** Fluorescein angiogram depicts area of noncapillary perfusion distal to neovascular frond.

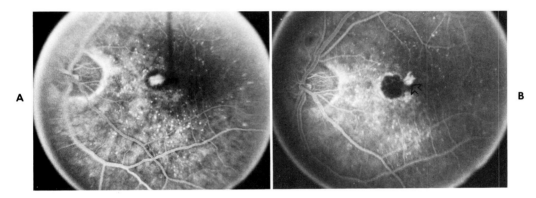

Fig. 21-14. A, Pretreatment angiogram of subretinal neovascular membrane of histoplasmic choroiditis. **B,** Recurrent subretinal neovascular membrane at margin of lesion in **A,** noted 6 weeks after treatment.

Choroid

Recurrent choroidal neovascularization (Fig. 21-14) is a problem that usually results from undertreatment of choroidal neovascularization previously recognized or not. The best management of this complication is its prevention by intense photocoagulation of the area of choroidal neovascularization when first detected. Early detection of recurrent neovascularization is achieved by repeating angiographic studies within 2 weeks of initial treatment. Repeated heavy photocoagulation is indicated. When the choroidal neovascularization is eliminated, follow-up examinations should be made after 1 and 3 months and at 6-month intervals thereafter.

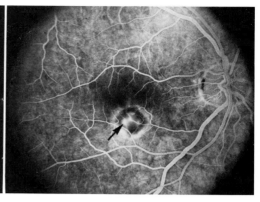

Fig. 21-15. A, Fluorescein angiogram in early venous phase taken 15 days after argon laser photocoagulation was done to destroy subretinal neovascular membrane from presumed histoplasmic choroiditis. Note early diffusion of dye from retinal vessels overlying SRNM and thus also affected by treating beam. Leakage is due to photocoagulation vasculitis. **B,** Dye has leaked more extensively from affected vessels. Leakage follows pattern of vessels, distinguishing it from choroidal neovascularization.

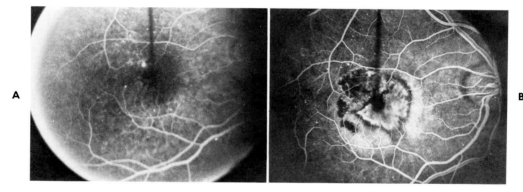

Fig. 21-16. A, Pretreatment angiogram of choroidal macular degeneration with focal pooling of fluorescein beneath retinal pigment epithelium. **B,** Recurrent subretinal neovascular membrane 18 months after photocoagulation of leak in **A.**

Fine and Patz have stressed that recurrent choroidal neovascularization must be distinguished from photocoagulation-induced retinal perivasculitis.[2a] Both conditions have leakage of fluorescein and both occur in the area of photocoagulation. The leaks of retinal vasculitis correspond to the retinal vessels (Fig. 21-15), and the leaks resolve several weeks after treatment. Photocoagulation-induced retinal perivasculitis should not be treated.

The 50-μm diameter beam should not be used when photocoagulating small retinal pigment epithelial detachments, because it is more likely to produce a rupture in Bruch's membrane, with subsequent ingrowth of vessels, than is a larger

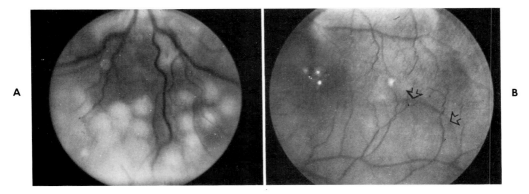

Fig. 21-17. Choroidal and exudative retinal detachment *(arrows)* after extensive panretinal photocoagulation performed in one treatment session. Systemic hypertension predisposes eye to this complication.

beam setting (Fig. 21-16). Fig. 21-16, *A*, shows a focal area of blocked fluorescence adjacent to the area of fluorescence on the pretreatment angiogram. This area of blocked fluorescence probably was caused by hemorrhage beneath the retinal pigment epithelium (RPE) due to a subretinal neovascular membrane (SRNM). To assure deeper penetration in such a case, the 50-μm spot size should not be used; to treat SRNM, always make an intense burn with a 200- or 500-μm spot setting.

MISCELLANEOUS COMPLICATIONS

Although panretinal photocoagulation is the safest method for treating disc neovascularization, it is not free of complications. When over 1,000 lesions were placed in one session of treatment, the following complications have occurred:

1. Hemorrhage from disc neovascularization occurred in two eyes within 24 hours of treatment, possibly from increased resistance of blood flow in the retinal circulation and increased blood flow to the disc vessels.
2. Macular edema occurred and persisted in one eye.
3. Transient choroidal and exudative retinal detachments have resulted from extensive panretinal photocoagulation done in one session of treatment. Systemic hypertension is a predisposing factor (Fig. 21-17).
4. Traction retinal detachment developed in two eyes.
5. Transient myopia was a frequent occurrence, lasting from 1 to 7 days. It was attributed to anterior displacement of the iris lens diaphragm, caused by vascular engorgement of the ciliary body.
6. Transient angle-closure glaucoma caused by choroidal effusion, with anterior displacement of the iris lens diaphragm, occurred in two eyes after extensive panretinal photocoagulation done in one session.
7. Seizures occurred in two patients, from photic stimulation of repeated

rhythmic argon laser photocoagulation; one was a petit mal seizure, and the other was grand mal.[8]

Five cases of corneal burns were seen early in 1971. Four consisted of minor superficial epithelial edema, which cleared within 24 to 48 hours. One patient had an ulceration of the anterior corneal stroma. All occurred from use of the 100-μm spot size, with power levels greater than 500 mW; in the severe burn, the power level was 1W. Exposure times were 1 to 4 sec in all instances.

Elimination of corneal burns has been achieved by changes in the laser and in the optical train that conducts the beam into the eye. The beam diameter at the cornea was altered from 100 to 1,000 μm, while maintaining a 100-μm spot at the retina. The increased corneal beam diameter greatly reduced the energy density of the laser beam at the cornea.

One case of lenticular burn has been documented, in the above patient who had the severe corneal burn. It resulted from settings of 100 μm, 1,000 mW, 1 sec. The lenticular burn consisted of discrete opacities in the anterior cortex. It was observed at the time of coagulation, and no change in the opacity has occurred in a 4-year follow-up.

Since Coherent Radiation has made modifications of its instrument, such corneal and lenticular burns have not been produced. Nevertheless, with this instrument, the 100-μm spot has the smallest beam diameter at the cornea; thus, it is most hazardous with power levels over 400 mW. Furthermore, because of the greater beam vergence with the 50-μm diameter setting, the 50-μm spot is safer and more effective than the 100-μm spot, particularly when applying small retinal lesions in eyes with cloudy media.

SUMMARY

Hazards from use of the argon laser slit-lamp photocoagulator derive from the same properties of the instrument that make it advantageous for the treatment of retinal vascular diseases: the wavelengths are highly absorbed by blood, and the beam can be focused to a small diameter. The operator must become familiar with the dangers involved with argon laser photocoagulation. Complications can be avoided entirely by using applications so light that virtually no effect is obtained, but such an approach, though safe, cannot be called therapeutic.

The most important complications that have occurred at the time of treatment or within 1 week after treatment are described for a wide variety of retinal diseases. The treatment techniques recommended will reduce the incidence and severity of such complications.

REFERENCES

1. Aiello, L., Beetham, W., Marios, C. B., Cha-zan, B. I., and Bradley, R. F.: Ruby laser photocoagulation in treatment of diabetic proliferative retinopathy: preliminary report. In Goldberg, M., and Fine, S., editors: Symposium on treatment of diabetic retinopathy, U.S. Department of Health, Education and Welfare, publication no. 1890, 1968, pp. 437-462.
2. Ámalric, P.: Trial of treatment of exudative diabetic retinopathy, Bull. Soc. Ophthalmol. Fr. **6:**359, 1960.
2a. Fine, S., and Patz, A.: Personal communication, 1975.
3. Goldberg, M., and Herbst, R.: Acute complications of argon laser photocoagulation, Arch. Ophthalmol. **89:**311, 1973.
4. Little, H. L., and Zweng, H. C.: Complications of argon laser retinal photocoagulation, Trans. Pac. Coast Otoophthalmol. Soc. **53:**115, 1971.
5. Little, H. L., and Zweng, H. C.: Complications of argon laser photocoagulation—a 5 year study. In Ámalric, P., editor: Symposium on laser photocoagulation, Twenty-second International Congress of Ophthalmologists, Albi, France, 1974. (In press.)
6. Little, H. L., Zweng, H. C., and Peabody, R. R.: Argon laser slit lamp retinal photocoagulation, Trans. Am. Acad. Ophthalmol. Otolaryngol. **74:**85, 1970.
7. Wessing, A., and Meyer-Schwickerath, G.: Results of photocoagulation in diabetic retinopathy. In Goldberg, M., and Fine, S., editors: Symposium on treatment of diabetic retinopathy, U.S. Department of Health, Education and Welfare, publication no. 1890, 1968, pp. 569-592.
8. Wilson, S.: Personal communication, 1975.
9. Zweng, H. C., Little, H. L., and Hammond, A. H.: Complications of argon laser photocoagulation in diabetic retinopathy, Trans. Am. Acad. Ophthalmol. **78:**195, 1974.

22
IDEAL PHOTOCOAGULATOR

Every photocoagulation system is composed of three elements: the light source, the delivery system, and the operator. The operator is the most variable element, and inexperience, rashness, or carelessness on the part of the operator can destroy vision as surely as can any disease. We are often asked about the likelihood of development of a new "ideal" photocoagulator in the near future. Therefore, we discuss here the elements that might be desirable in such an instrument.

LIGHT SOURCE

The ideal light source has the following characteristics:
1. *Monochromaticity,* necessary only to the extent that the spectral width of the source should be narrower than the width of the absorption band of the targets.
2. *Coherence,* necessary to gain a small spot size. A beam that is spatially coherent permits sharp focusing to a small spot size, especially useful in treating macular disease. A practical limit to how small the spot need be is 50 μm.
3. *Continuous wave,* necessary to give the operator control over length of exposure. For example, 0.05-sec exposure is useful for making lesions of minimal depth, as in treating central serious retinopathy, whereas a 0.5-sec exposure is needed to give deep burns as in treating choroidal and subretinal neovascularization.

Pulsed light sources with exposures in the microsecond or shorter range cannot be easily changed temporally to give the versatility needed to cope with various retinal problems. Production of a hole through the occluded trabecular meshwork into Schlemm's canal to treat open-angle glaucoma, as reported by Krasnov,[1] is the only instance that comes to mind where a very short pulsed light might be superior to a continuous-wave source. This procedure is highly experimental at this time.

The ideal light source, then, should be spatially coherent, relatively narrow in spectral output, and preferably capable of operating in a continuous wave.

The following factors influence the selection of the specific wavelength:
1. The beam must traverse the ocular media well, with minimal absorption, lest the cornea, lens, or vitreous be coagulated. This factor limits the possibilities from 475 to 900 μm (see Fig. 1-12), or a little beyond the visible spectrum on the infrared end.
2. The aiming light should be seen well and be part of the treating beam; thus it should be *in* the visible spectrum, reducing the choice on the red end to 700 μm.
3. The light must be absorbed well by melanin, one of the two pigments available in the eye to change the light energy to heat. With 50% light absorption by melanin as a satisfactory level, all the visible wavelengths are acceptable, but maximum absorption, 70%, occurs in the 500- to 600-μm range (see Fig. 1-12).
4. The light must be absorbed by hemoglobin, the other pigment used in retinal photocoagulation. Here the choice of wavelength is much more critical, because of the precipitous drop in absorption of wavelengths longer than 600 μm (see Fig. 1-13). Reasonably good absorption occurs from 400 to 590 μm, but peak values occur between 525 and 570 μm.
5. A shift from the blue-green to the yellow part of the spectrum makes retinal photocoagulation through the sclerosed lens nucleus easier, because it absorbs considerable blue light.
6. Probably a minor factor is that yellow light is absorbed less by the xanthochromatic pigments in the center of the macula, an area in which photocoagulation is not desirable, than are shorter wavelengths.

A survey of laser light sources emitting wavelengths around 575 μm shows two possibilities. The krypton gas laser has a yellow line, but the inefficiency of this laser makes it almost useless for photocoagulation. Other sources are dye lasers (Fig. 22-1), one of which is the rhodamine 110 dye laser, which can be tuned from about 550 to 600 μm. It is pumped with relatively good efficiency by an argon gas laser. However, an impractically large argon laser would be required to provide rhodamine 110 laser output of about 1 W, a barely acceptable maximum.

Although the rhodamine 110 wavelengths are theoretically better than the two main wavelengths of argon, 488 and 513.5 μm, an examination of the three data curves, transmission through ocular media and absorption by melanin and hemoglobin, shows a relatively small advantage with the rhodamine 110 laser. The argon gas laser is stable and durable, two important factors in the ideal photocoagulator. However, if the technology of dye lasers improves sufficiently, the small theoretical advantages of the rhodamine 110 dye laser make it the ideal light source. The main advantage of the dye laser is its tunability, which provides the flexibility to either interact strongly with hemoglobin (by tuning to approximately 570 μm) or to avoid interaction with hemoglobin (by tuning to approximately 600 μm). This shift to 600 μm or longer could be used, for example, if

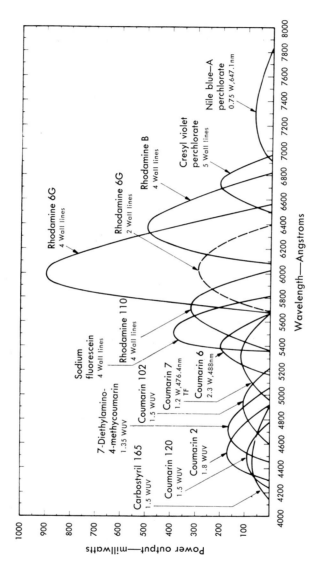

Fig. 22-1. Illustration of power output obtainable at various wavelengths, from commercially available dye laser (Coherent Radiation model 490). Most useful dye for maximum power output at 570 nm is rhodamine 110. (Courtesy Coherent Radiation, Inc., Palo Alto, California.)

there is blood in the vitreous, to avoid interaction with the vitreous while photocoagulating the retina.

DELIVERY SYSTEM

A binocular view of the retina or other ocular structures is better than a monocular view. Slit-lamp funduscopy through a three-mirror corneal diagnostic contact lens is the ideal method for viewing the retina for photocoagulation. The aiming beam should be an attenuated part of the treating beam, with a range in power from a few microwatts to a maximum no greater than 1 mW. It should be manipulated separately from the viewing optics.

The operator must be able to preselect length of exposure, power, and spot size. Power to 2 W should be available; spot size should be gradually variable from 50 to 1,000 μm in diameter; and time exposures of 0.05, 0.1, 0.2, 0.5, and 1 sec should be available. The power output should be continuously monitored. A foot pedal activator is better than a manual control, which frees the operator's hands to adjust the aiming and treating beam, lessening the chance of movement when the treating beam is fired.

A filter should cover the viewing optics during the treatment, to reduce reflection from the front surface of the contact lens into the operator's eye. Closure of the filter circuit should trigger the actual firing of the treating light.

Finally, several sensor systems should be built into the electrical systems to shut off the unit if a surge of electrical current or any other malfunction occurs.

The treating beam should be coaxial with the viewing optics; otherwise, treating in the far periphery is more difficult.

Since we introduced the system, it has been widely accepted. We developed such a system in 1966, and used it on animals in 1967 and 1968 and on patients since 1969.[2]

ARTICULATION OF LIGHT WITH DELIVERY SYSTEM

One last aspect of the ideal photocoagulator that needs discussion is the method by which the light is brought into the slit-lamp optics. Either a hollow arm with prisms or mirrors at the elbows, needed to give slit-lamp movement, or a fiber optics cable can be used. The former keeps coherence of the beam intact, but the arm can get out of alignment. The fiber optics cable destroys spatial coherence and makes refocusing of the beam more difficult than when it emerges from the hollow articulating arm, and the depth of field for the 50-μm spot size is much reduced. Therefore, a sturdy hollow articulating arm is preferable.

SUMMARY

Commercially available argon laser instruments have most characteristics of the ideal photocoagulator. The main possible improvement might be a continuous-wave light source in the yellow tunable laser from 570 to 600 μm.

REFERENCES

1. Krasnov, M. M.: Q-switched laser goniopuncture, Arch. Ophthalmol. **92:**37, 1974.
2. Little, H. L., Zweng, H. C., and Peabody, R. R.: Argon laser slit-lamp retinal photocoagulation, Trans. Am. Acad. Ophthalmol. Otolaryngol. **74:**85-97, 1970.

INDEX